2011
YEAR BOOK OF
SPORTS MEDICINE®

The 2011 Year Book Series

Year Book of Anesthesiology and Pain Management™: Drs Chestnut, Abram, Black, Gravlee, Lien, Mathru, and Roizen

Year Book of Cardiology®: Drs Gersh, Cheitlin, Elliott, Gold, Graham, and Thourani

Year Book of Critical Care Medicine®: Drs Dellinger, Parrillo, Balk, Dorman, Dries, and Zanotti-Cavazzoni

Year Book of Dermatology and Dermatologic Surgery™: Dr Del Rosso

Year Book of Diagnostic Radiology®: Drs Osborn, Abbara, Elster, Manaster, Oestreich, Offiah, Rosado de Christenson, Stephens, and Walker

Year Book of Emergency Medicine®: Drs Hamilton, Bruno, Handly, Mullin, Quintana, and Ramoska

Year Book of Endocrinology®: Drs Schott, Apovian, Clarke, Eugster, Ludlam, Meikle, Ovalle, Schinner, Schteingart, and Toth

Year Book of Gastroenterology™: Drs Talley, DeVault, Harnois, Pearson, Picco, Scolapio, Smith, and Vege

Year Book of Hand and Upper Limb Surgery®: Drs Yao and Steinmann

Year Book of Medicine®: Drs Barker, Garrick, Gersh, Khardori, LeRoith, Seo, Talley, and Thigpen

Year Book of Neonatal and Perinatal Medicine®: Drs Fanaroff, Benitz, Donn, Neu, Papile, Polin, and van Marter

Year Book of Neurology and Neurosurgery®: Drs Klimo and Rabinstein

Year Book of Obstetrics, Gynecology, and Women's Health®: Drs Dungan and Shulman

Year Book of Oncology®: Drs Arceci, Bauer, Gordon, Lawton, and Thigpen

Year Book of Ophthalmology®: Drs Rapuano, Cohen, Flanders, Hammersmith, Milman, Myers, Nelson, Penne, Pyfer, Sergott, Shields, and Vander

Year Book of Orthopedics®: Drs Morrey, Beauchamp, Huddleston, Swiontkowski, and Trigg

Year Book of Otolaryngology-Head and Neck Surgery®: Drs Sindwani, Balough, Franco, Gapany, and Mitchell

Year Book of Pathology and Laboratory Medicine®: Drs Raab, Parwani, Bejarano, and Bissell

Year Book of Pediatrics®: Dr Stockman

Year Book of Plastic and Aesthetic Surgery™: Drs Miller, Gosain, Gurtner, Gutowski, Ruberg, Salisbury, and Smith

Year Book of Psychiatry and Applied Mental Health®: Drs Talbott, Ballenger, Buckley, Frances, Krupnick, and Mack

Year Book of Pulmonary Disease®: Drs Barker, Jones, Maurer, Raza, Tanoue, and Willsie

Year Book of Sports Medicine®: Drs Shephard, Cantu, Feldman, Jankowski, Khan, Lebrun, Nieman, Pierrynowski, and Rowland

Year Book of Surgery®: Drs Copeland, Behrns, Daly, Eberlein, Fahey, Huber, Klodell, Mozingo, and Pruett

Year Book of Urology®: Drs Andriole and Coplen

Year Book of Vascular Surgery®: Drs Moneta, Gillespie, Starnes, and Watkins

2011

The Year Book of
SPORTS MEDICINE®

Editor-in-Chief
Roy J. Shephard, MD (Lond), PhD, DPE
Professor Emeritus of Applied Physiology, Faculty of Physical Education and Health, University of Toronto, Toronto, Ontario, Canada

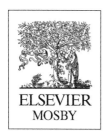

ELSEVIER
MOSBY

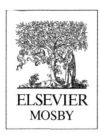

ELSEVIER
MOSBY

Vice President, Continuity Publishing: Kimberly Murphy
Editor: Jessica Demetriou
Production Supervisor, Electronic Year Books: Donna M. Skelton
Electronic Article Manager: Mike Sheets
Illustrations and Permissions Coordinator: Dawn Vohsen

Composition by TNQ Books and Journals Pvt Ltd, India

Printed and bound by CPI Group (UK) Ltd, Croydon, CR0 4YY

Transferred to Digital Print 2011

Editorial Office:
Elsevier, Inc.
Suite 1800
1600 John F. Kennedy Boulevard
Philadelphia, PA 19103-2899

International Standard Serial Number: 0162-0908
International Standard Book Number: 978-0-323-08426-0

Associate Editors

Robert C. Cantu, MA, MD, FACS, FAANS, FACSM

Clinical Professor of Neurosurgery, Boston University School of Medicine; Co-Director, Neurological Sports Injury Center at Brigham and Women's Hospital; Neurosurgery Consultant, Boston College Eagles and Boston Cannons Lacrosse Teams; Co-Director, Center for the Study of Traumatic Encephalopathy (CSTE), Boston University Medical Center, Boston, Massachusetts; Co-Founder and Chairman, Medical Advisory Board Sports Legacy Institute (SLI), Waltham, Massachusetts; Chairman, Department of Surgery, Chief, Neurosurgery Service, and Director, Service Sports Medicine, Emerson Hospital, Concord, Massachusetts; Adjunct Professor, Exercise and Sport Science, University of North Carolina; Medical Director, National Center for Catastrophic Sports Injury, Research, Chapel Hill, North Carolina; Senior Advisor, National Football League (NFL) Head, Neck and Spine Committee, New York, New York

Debbie Ehrmann Feldman, PT, PhD

Professor, Faculty of Medicine, School of Rehabilitation, Université de Montréal; and Physiotherapist, Montreal Children's Hospital, McGill University Health Centre, Montreal, Quebec, Canada

Catherine M. Jankowski, PhD

Assistant Research Professor, Division of Geriatric Medicine, University of Colorado Denver, Aurora, Colorado

Karim M. Khan, MD, PhD

Professor, Centre for Hip Health, Vancouver Coastal Health Research Institute, and the University of British Columbia; Department of Family Practice, University of British Columbia, Vancouver, British Columbia, Canada

Connie Lebrun, MD

Clinical Director, Glen Sather Sports Medicine Clinic; Associate Professor, Faculty of Physical Education and Recreation, University of Alberta, Edmonton, Alberta, Canada

David C. Nieman, DrPH

Professor, Appalachian State University, Boone, North Carolina; Director, The Human Performance Laboratory, North Carolina Research Campus, Kannapolis, North Carolina

Michael R. Pierrynowski, PhD

Associate Professor, School of Rehabilitation Science and the Department of Kinesiology, McMaster University, Hamilton, Ontario, Canada

Thomas Rowland, MD

Professor of Pediatrics, Tufts University School of Medicine, Boston; and Chief, Pediatric Cardiology, Baystate Medical Center, Springfield, Massachusetts

Table of Contents

Journals Represented

Journals represented in this YEAR BOOK are listed below.

Ageing Research Reviews
AJR American Journal of Roentgenology
American Journal of Cardiology
American Journal of Clinical Nutrition
American Journal of Emergency Medicine
American Journal of Epidemiology
American Journal of Preventive Medicine
American Journal of Public Health
American Journal of Sports Medicine
Annals of Internal Medicine
Annals of Surgery
Archives of Internal Medicine
Archives of Physical Medicine and Rehabilitation
Brain
Brain Research
British Journal of Cancer
British Journal of Sports Medicine
British Medical Journal
Canadian Medical Association Journal
Cancer Epidemiology, Biomarkers & Prevention
Circulation
Clinical Biomechanics
Clinical Endocrinology
Clinical Journal of Sport Medicine
Clinical Orthopaedics and Related Research
Critical Care Medicine
Current Opinion in Endocrinology, Diabetes and Obesity
Deutsche Zeitschrift fuer Sportmedizin
European Heart Journal
European Journal of Applied Physiology
European Urology
Exercise and Sport Sciences Reviews
Foot & Ankle International
Headache
Health Report
Heart
Human Reproduction
Hypertension
International Journal of Cardiology
International Journal of Obesity
International Journal of Sports Medicine
Journal of Aging and Physical Activity
Journal of Applied Physiology
Journal of Athletic Training
Journal of Bone and Joint Surgery
Journal of Bone and Mineral Metabolism
Journal of Clinical Endocrinology & Metabolism

Journal of Clinical Oncology
Journal of Clinical Pathology
Journal of Manipulative and Physiological Therapeutics
Journal of Neurology, Neurosurgery & Psychiatry
Journal of Orthopaedic & Sports Physical Therapy
Journal of Orthopaedic Research
Journal of Pain
Journal of Pediatric Orthopaedics
Journal of Pediatrics
Journal of Sports Medicine and Physical Fitness
Journal of the American College of Cardiology
Journal of the American College of Surgeons
Journal of the American Geriatrics Society
Journal of the American Medical Association
Journal of the European Academy of Dermatology and Venereology
Journal of Trauma
Maturitas
Medicine and Science in Sports and Exercise
Metabolism
Neurology
Neurourology and Urodynamics
New England Journal of Medicine
Pediatric Neurology
Pediatrics
PLoS Medicine
Proceedings of the National Academy of Sciences of the United States of America
Respiratory Medicine
Sports Medicine
Wilderness & Environmental Medicine
World Neurosurgery

STANDARD ABBREVIATIONS

The following terms are abbreviated in this edition: acquired immunodeficiency syndrome (AIDS), cardiopulmonary resuscitation (CPR), central nervous system (CNS), cerebrospinal fluid (CSF), computed tomography (CT), deoxyribonucleic acid (DNA), electrocardiography (ECG), health maintenance organization (HMO), human immunodeficiency virus (HIV), intensive care unit (ICU), intramuscular (IM), intravenous (IV), magnetic resonance (MR) imaging (MRI), ribonucleic acid (RNA), and ultrasound (US).

NOTE

The YEAR BOOK OF SPORTS MEDICINE is a literature survey service providing abstracts of articles published in the professional literature. Every effort is made to assure the accuracy of the information presented in these pages. Neither the editors nor the publisher of the YEAR BOOK OF SPORTS MEDICINE can be responsible for errors in the original materials. The editors' comments are their own opinions. Mention of specific products within this publication does not constitute endorsement.

To facilitate the use of the YEAR BOOK OF SPORTS MEDICINE as a reference tool, all illustrations and tables included in this publication are now identified as they appear in the original article. This change is meant to help the reader recognize that any illustration or table appearing in the YEAR BOOK OF SPORTS MEDICINE may be only one of many in the original article. For this reason, figure and table numbers will often appear to be out of sequence within the YEAR BOOK OF SPORTS MEDICINE.

Clinical Implications of Exercise Immunology for the Practicing Physician

David C. Nieman, DrPH, FACSM

Professor, Appalachian State University, Boone, North Carolina; Director, The Human Performance Laboratory, North Carolina Research Campus, Kannapolis, North Carolina

Introduction

Exercise immunology is a relatively new area of scientific endeavor, with the majority of papers published during the past 25 years.[1] Most studies have focused on the acute and chronic effects of various exercise workloads on the immune system and immunosurveillance against pathogens. For the practicing physician, 2 areas of investigation from exercise immunology have the greatest clinical and public health implications: (1) The chronic anti-inflammatory influence of exercise training; and (2) the reduction in risk of upper respiratory tract infections (URTI) from regular moderate exercise training.

The Chronic Anti-Inflammatory Influence of Exercise Training

Acute inflammation is a normal response of the immune system to infection and trauma. Intense and prolonged exercise similar to marathon race competition causes large but transient increases in total white blood cells (WBC) and a variety of cytokines including interleukin-6 (IL-6), IL-8, IL-10, IL-1 receptor antagonist (IL-1ra), granulocyte colony stimulating factor (GCSF), monocyte chemoattractant protein 1 (MCP-1). macrophage inflammatory protein 1 beta (MIP-1β), tumor necrosis factor-alpha (TNF-α), and macrophage migration inhibitory factor (MIF).[2,3] C-reactive protein (CRP) is also elevated after heavy exertion, but the increase is delayed in comparison to most cytokines. Despite regular increases in these inflammation biomarkers during each intense exercise bout, endurance athletes have lower levels when measured during rest in contrast to overweight and unfit adults. For example, mean CRP levels in long-distance runners (rested state) typically fall below 0.5 mg/L in comparison with 4.0 mg/L and higher in obese, postmenopausal women.[3,4]

The persistent increase in inflammation biomarkers is defined as chronic or systemic inflammation, and it is linked with multiple disorders and diseases including atherosclerosis and cardiovascular disease (CVD), the metabolic syndrome, diabetes mellitus, sarcopenia, arthritis, osteoporosis, chronic obstructive pulmonary disease, dementia, depression, and various types of cancers.[5-7] CRP is the most frequently measured inflammatory biomarker, and individuals with CRP values in the upper tertile of the adult population (>3.0 mg/L) have a 2-fold increase in CVD risk compared to those with a CRP concentration below 1.0 mg/L.[7] An elevated fasting IL-6 concentration is a significant component of the chronic low-grade inflammation that underlies the metabolic syndrome, CVD, diabetes, and various cancers.[8] Athletes typically have plasma IL-6 concentrations that fall below 1.0 pg/mL in contrast to values above 2.0 pg/mL in older and obese individuals.[3,8]

Physical Activity, Fitness, and Chronic Inflammation

Large population observational studies consistently show reduced WBC, CRP, IL-6, TNF-α, and other inflammatory biomarkers in adults with higher levels of physical activity and fitness, even after adjustment for potential confounders.[9-14] The inverse association between physical activity/fitness and inflammation is related in part to the effect of activity on fat mass.[11] In most studies, however, adjustment for body mass index (BMI) and adiposity attenuates but does not negate the strength of the relationship between inflammatory biomarkers and physical activity/fitness.[11,15] For example, in a study of 1002 community-dwelling adults (age range, 18-85 years), a general linear model (GLM) analysis adjusted CRP means for frequency of physical activity, BMI, and several other lifestyle and demographic factors.[15] BMI had the strongest effect on CRP followed by gender (higher in females), exercise frequency, age, and smoking status.

Randomized, controlled exercise-intervention studies provide equivocal support for the inverse relationship between increased physical activity and reduced systemic inflammation.[11,16-22] One explanation is that in comparison to the large variance evaluated in observational studies, the change in aerobic fitness and activity levels is typically of low magnitude in randomized exercise trials, the duration of training seldom extends beyond 6 months, and the number of subjects is relatively low.[17,18,20,21] Nonetheless, data from both study formats support that in order for reductions in chronic inflammation to be experienced, a large change in a combination of lifestyle factors is needed including weight loss, near daily moderate to vigorous physical activity of 30 to 60 minutes duration, avoidance of cigarette smoking, and increased intake of fruits and vegetables.[22,23] For example, if an obese older individual adds 3 weekly 30-minute walking sessions to the lifestyle, reductions in chronic inflammation are unlikely to be experienced unless the exercise workload is increased in combination with significant weight loss and improved diet quality.

Potential Mechanisms

When successful, exercise training may exert anti-inflammatory influences through a reduction in visceral fat mass and the induction of an acute anti-inflammatory environment with each bout of exercise that over time becomes chronic.[24,25] These effects may be mediated in part through muscle-derived peptides or myokines, but this proposed mechanism needs further testing.[25] Contracting skeletal muscles release myokines (eg, IL-6, IL-8, IL-15) that may exert both direct and chronic anti-inflammatory effects.

The first identified and most studied myokine is IL-6. During prolonged and intense exercise, IL-6 is produced by muscle fibers and stimulates the appearance in the circulation of other anti-inflammatory cytokines such as

IL-1ra and IL-10 (26). IL-6 also inhibits the production of the proinflammatory cytokine TNF-α and stimulates lipolysis and fat oxidation.[26] With weight loss from energy restriction and exercise, plasma levels of IL-6 fall, skeletal muscle TNF-α decreases, and insulin sensitivity improves.[27,28] Thus, IL-6 release from the exercising muscle may help mediate some of the health benefits of exercise including metabolic control of type 2 diabetes.[27,28]

Muscle IL-6 release, however, is very low during moderate physical activity. For example, during a 30-minute brisk walk on a treadmill, plasma IL-6 concentrations increased from 1.3 pg/mL to 2.0 pg/mL in female subjects.[29] The increase in IL-6 during brisk walking is probably insufficient to mediate anti-inflammatory and other beneficial health effects, and additional research is needed to determine the relative contribution of myokines compared to other exercise-induced factors. The acute exercise-induced increase in IL-6 after heavy exertion (eg, typically above 5 pg/mL, 10 pg/mL, and 50 pg/mL after 1-hour, 2-hour, and marathon-race running bouts, respectively) may indeed orchestrate anti-inflammatory influences, lipolysis, and improved insulin sensitivity, but this amount of physical activity is beyond levels achievable by most overweight/obese individuals.

A moderate exercise program of near-daily 30-minute walking bouts, without diet control, has small influences on visceral fat, even in long-term studies.[30] This is further evidence that the myokine hypothesis does not apply at the activity level attainable by most middle-aged and elderly individuals. Thus, moderate physical activity training must be increased to the highest levels acceptable to an individual (eg, 60 min/d) and combined with weight loss through tight control of energy intake and improved diet quality to achieve reductions in systemic inflammation.

URTI Risk Reduction from Regular Moderate Exercise Training

URTI is the most frequently occurring infectious disease in humans worldwide.[31-33] More than 200 different viruses cause the common cold, and rhinoviruses and coronaviruses are the culprits 25% to 60% of the time. The National Institute of Allergy and Infectious Diseases reports that people in the United States suffer 1 billion colds each year with an incidence of 2 to 4 for the average adult and 6 to 10 for children.[31] URTI imposes an estimated $40 billion burden in direct and indirect costs on the US economy.[32]

Low to high exercise workloads have a unique effect on URTI risk.[34] Regular physical activity improves immune function and lowers URTI risk while sustained and intense exertion has the opposite effect. Marathon race competitions and heavy exercise training regimens increase URTI risk, but relatively few individuals exercise at this level, limiting public health concerns. The second half of this article will review the benefits of regular moderate activity in improving immunosurveillance against pathogens and lowering URTI risk. This information has broad public health significance and appeal, and provides the clinician with an additional inducement to encourage increased physical activity among patients.

Moderate Physical Activity and URTI Risk

Several lines of evidence support the linkage between moderate physical activity and improved immunity and lowered infection rates: survey, animal, epidemiologic, and randomized training data. Survey data consistently support the common belief among fitness enthusiasts that regular exercise confers resistance against infection. In surveys, 80% to 90% of regular exercisers perceive themselves as less vulnerable to viral illnesses compared with sedentary peers.[35,36]

Animal studies are difficult to apply to the human condition, but in general, support the finding that moderate exercise lowers morbidity and mortality following pathogen inoculation, especially when compared with prolonged and intense exertion or physical inactivity. Mice infected with the herpes simplex virus, for example, and then exposed to 30 minutes of moderate exercise experience a lower mortality during a 21-day period compared with higher mortality rates after 2.5 hours of exhaustive exercise or rest.[37] Another study with mice showed that 3.5 months of moderate exercise training compared to no exercise prior to induced influenza infection decreased symptom severity and lung viral loads and inflammation.[38]

Retrospective and prospective epidemiologic studies have measured URTI incidence in large groups of moderately active and sedentary individuals. Collectively, the epidemiologic studies consistently show reduced URTI rates in physically active or fit individuals. A 1-year epidemiological study of 547 adults showed a 23% reduction in URTI risk in those engaging in regular versus irregular moderate to vigorous physical activity.[39] In a group of 145 elderly subjects, URTI symptomatology during a one-year period was reduced among those engaging in higher compared to lower amounts of moderate physical activity.[40] During a 1-year study of 142 males 33 to 90 years old, the odds of having at least 15 days with URTI was 64% lower among those with higher physical activity patterns.[41] A cohort of 1509 Swedish men and women 20 to 60 years old were studied for 15 weeks during the winter/spring.[42] Subjects in the upper tertile for physical activity experienced an 18% reduction in URTI risk, but this proportion improved to 42% among those with high perceived mental stress.

A group of 1002 adults (18-85 years old, 60% female, 40% male) were studied for 12 weeks (half during the winter, half during the fall) while monitoring URTI symptoms and severity using the Wisconsin Upper Respiratory Symptom Survey.[43,44] Subjects reported frequency of moderate to vigorous aerobic activity and rated their physical fitness level using a 10-point Likert scale. The number of days with URTI was 43% lower in subjects reporting an average of 5 or more days of aerobic exercise (20-minute bouts or longer) compared with those who were largely sedentary (≤1 d/wk). This relationship occurred after adjustment for important confounders including age, education level, marital status, gender, BMI, and perceived mental stress. The number of days with URTI was 46% lower when comparing subjects in the highest versus lowest tertile for perceived physical fitness, even after adjustment for confounders.

Regular physical activity may lower rates of infection for other types of diseases, but data are limited because of low disease prevalence. For example, women with a high frequency of walking experienced an 18% lower risk of pneumonia compared with women who walked the least.[45] In the same cohort, women who reported running or jogging more than 2 hours per week had a reduced pneumonia risk compared with women who spent no time running or jogging.[45]

Randomized experimental trials provide important data in support of the viewpoint that moderate physical activity reduces URTI symptomatology. In a randomized controlled study of 36 women (mean age, 35 years), subjects walked briskly for 45 minutes, 5 days a week, and experienced one-half the days with URTI symptoms (5.1 vs 10.8) during the 15-week period compared with that of the sedentary control group.[46]

The effect of exercise training (five 45 minute walking sessions per week at 60% to 75% maximum heart rate) and/or moderate energy restriction (1200-1300 kcal/d) on URTI was studied in obese women (N=91, body mass index 33.1 ± 0.6 kg/m^2) randomized to 1 of 4 groups: control, exercise, diet, exercise and diet.[47] Energy restriction had no significant effect on URTI incidence, and subjects from the 2 exercise groups were contrasted with subjects from the 2 nonexercise groups. The number of days with URTI for subjects in the exercise groups was reduced 40% relative to the nonexercise groups (5.6 vs 9.4), similar to the level of nonobese, physically active controls (N=30, 4.8 days with URTI).

In another study, 30 sedentary elderly women (mean age, 73 years) were assigned to walking or sedentary groups.[48,49] The exercise group walked 30 to 40 minutes, 5 days per week, for 12 weeks at 60% heart rate reserve. Incidence of URTI in the walking groups was 21% compared with 50% in the calisthenic control group during the study (September through November).

A 1-year randomized study of 115 overweight postmenopausal women showed that regular moderate exercise (166 minutes per week, approximately 4 days per week) lowered URTI risk compared to controls (who engaged in a stretching program).[50] In the final 3 months of the study, the risk of colds in the control group was more than 3-fold that of the exercisers.

Moderate Physical Activity and Enhanced Immunosurveillance

During moderate exercise several transient changes occur in the immune system.[29,51-53] Moderate exercise increases the recirculation of immunoglobulins, and neutrophils and natural killer cells, 2 cells that play a critical role in innate immune defenses. Animal data indicate that lung macrophages play an important role in mediating the beneficial effects of moderate exercise on lowered susceptibility to infection.[54] Stress hormones, which can suppress immunity, and proinflammatory and anti-inflammatory cytokines, indicative of intense metabolic activity, are not elevated during moderate exercise.[29]

Although the immune system returns to pre-exercise levels within a few hours after the exercise session is over, each session may represent an improvement in immune surveillance that reduces the risk of infection over the long term. Other exercise-immune related benefits include enhanced antibody-specific responses to vaccinations. For example, several studies indicate that both acute and chronic moderate exercise training improves the body's antibody response to the influenza vaccine.[55-58] In one study, a 45 minute moderate exercise bout just before influenza vaccination improved the antibody response.[55]

These data provide additional evidence that moderate exercise favorably influences overall immune surveillance against pathogens. Taken together, the data on the relationship between moderate exercise, enhanced immunity, and lowered URTI risk are consistent with guidelines urging the general public to engage in near-daily brisk walking.

Conclusions

Although methodology varies widely and evidence is still emerging,[59] epidemiologic and randomized exercise training studies consistently report a reduction in URTI incidence or risk of 18% to 67%. This is the most important finding for the practicing physician that has emerged from exercise immunology studies during the past 2 decades. Animal and human data indicate that during each exercise bout, transient immune changes take place that over time may improve immunosurveillance against pathogens, thereby reducing URTI risk. The magnitude of reduction in URTI risk with near-daily moderate physical activity exceeds levels reported for most medications and supplements, and it bolsters public health guidelines urging individuals to be physically active on a regular basis.

Regular physical activity should be combined with other lifestyle strategies to more effectively reduce URTI risk. These strategies include stress management, regular sleep, avoidance of malnutrition, and proper hygiene.[33,60-63] URTI is caused by multiple and diverse pathogens, making it unlikely that a unifying vaccine will be developed.[33] Thus, lifestyle strategies are receiving increased attention by investigators and public health officials, and a comprehensive lifestyle approach is more likely to lower the burden of URTI than a focus on physical activity alone.

The anti-inflammatory effect of near-daily physical activity may play a key role in many health benefits, including reduced cardiovascular disease, type 2 diabetes, various types of cancer, sarcopenia, and dementia.[9-18] This is an exciting area of scientific endeavor, and additional research is needed to determine how immune perturbations during each exercise bout accumulate over time to produce an anti-inflammatory influence. As with URTI, multiple lifestyle approaches to reducing chronic inflammation should be employed with a focus on weight loss, high volume of physical activity, avoidance of smoking, and improved diet quality.

References

1. Shephard RJ. Development of the discipline of exercise immunology. *Exerc Immunol Rev.* 2010;16:194-222.

2. Nieman DC, Henson DA, Smith LL, et al. Cytokine changes after a marathon race. *J Appl Physiol.* 2001;91:109-114.
3. Nieman DC, Dumke CL, Henson DA, McAnulty SR, Gross SJ, Lind RH. Muscle damage is linked to cytokine changes following a 160-km race. *Brain Behav Immun.* 2005;19:398-403.
4. Arsenault BJ, Earnest CP, Després JP, Blair SN, Church TS. Obesity, coffee consumption and CRP levels in postmenopausal overweight/obese women: importance of hormone replacement therapy use. *Eur J Clin Nutr.* 2009;63:1419-1424.
5. Khansari N, Shakiba Y, Mahmoudi M. Chronic inflammation and oxidative stress as a major cause of age-related diseases and cancer. *Recent Pat Inflamm Allergy Drug Discov.* 2009;3:73-80.
6. Devaraj S, Valleggi S, Siegel D, Jialal I. Role of C-reactive protein in contributing to increased cardiovascular risk in metabolic syndrome. *Curr Atheroscler Rep.* 2010;12:110-118.
7. Pearson TA, Mensah GA, Alexander RW, et al. Markers of inflammation and cardiovascular disease: application to clinical and public health practice: A statement for healthcare professionals from the Centers for Disease Control and Prevention and the American Heart Association. *Circulation.* 2003;107:499-511.
8. Dekker MJ, Lee S, Hudson R, et al. An exercise intervention without weight loss decreases circulating interleukin-6 in lean and obese men with and without type 2 diabetes mellitus. *Metabolism.* 2007;56:332-338.
9. Hsu FC, Kritchevsky SB, Liu Y, et al. Association between inflammatory components and physical function in the health, aging, and body composition study: a principal component analysis approach. *J Gerontol A Biol Sci Med Sci.* 2009; 64:581-589.
10. Lavoie ME, Rabasa-Lhoret R, Doucet E, et al. Association between physical activity energy expenditure and inflammatory markers in sedentary overweight and obese women. *Int J Obes (Lond).* 2010;34:1387-1395.
11. Beavers KM, Brinkley TE, Nicklas BJ. Effect of exercise training on chronic inflammation. *Clin Chim Acta.* 2010;411:785-793.
12. Ford ES. Does exercise reduce inflammation? Physical activity and C-reactive protein among U.S. adults. *Epidemiology.* 2002;13:561-568.
13. Borodulin K, Laatikainen T, Salomaa V, Jousilahti P. Associations of leisure time physical activity, self-rated physical fitness, and estimated aerobic fitness with serum C-reactive protein among 3,803 adults. *Atherosclerosis.* 2006;185:381-387.
14. Brooks GC, Blaha MJ, Blumenthal RS. Relation of C-reactive protein to abdominal adiposity. *Am J Cardiol.* 2010;106:56-61.
15. Shanely RA, Nieman DC, Henson DA, Jin F, Knab A, Sha W. Perceived fitness is predictive of decreased inflammation and oxidative stress. *Br J Sports Med.* In press.
16. Church TS, Earnest CP, Thompson AM, et al. Exercise without weight loss does not reduce C-reactive protein: the INFLAME study. *Med Sci Sports Exerc.* 2010; 42:708-716.
17. Arsenault BJ, Côté M, Cartier A, et al. Effect of exercise training on cardiometabolic risk markers among sedentary, but metabolically healthy overweight or obese post-menopausal women with elevated blood pressure. *Atherosclerosis.* 2009;207:530-533.
18. Kelley GA, Kelley KS. Effects of aerobic exercise on C-reactive protein, body composition, and maximum oxygen consumption in adults: a meta-analysis of randomized controlled trials. *Metabolism.* 2006;55:1500-1507.
19. Stewart LK, Earnest CP, Blair SN, Church TS. Effects of different doses of physical activity on C-reactive protein among women. *Med Sci Sports Exerc.* 2010; 42:701-707.
20. Thompson D, Markovitch D, Betts JA, Mazzatti D, Turner J, Tyrrell RM. Time course of changes in inflammatory markers during a 6-mo exercise intervention in sedentary middle-aged men: a randomized-controlled trial. *J Appl Physiol.* 2010;108:769-779.

21. Stewart LK, Flynn MG, Campbell WW, et al. The influence of exercise training on inflammatory cytokines and C-reactive protein. *Med Sci Sports Exerc.* 2007;39:1714-1719.

22. Christiansen T, Paulsen SK, Bruun JM, Pedersen SB, Richelsen B. Exercise training versus diet-induced weight-loss on metabolic risk factors and inflammatory markers in obese subjects: a 12-week randomized intervention study. *Am J Physiol Endocrinol Metab.* 2010;298:E824-E831.

23. Herder C, Peltonen M, Koenig W, et al. Anti-inflammatory effect of lifestyle changes in the Finnish Diabetes Prevention Study. *Diabetologia.* 2009;52: 433-442.

24. Brandt C, Pedersen BK. The role of exercise-induced myokines in muscle homeostasis and the defense against chronic diseases. *J Biomed Biotechnol.* 2010;2010: 520258. Epub 2010 Mar 9.

25. Pedersen BK. The diseasome of physical inactivity—and the role of myokines in muscle—fat cross talk. *J Physiol.* 2009;587:5559-5568.

26. Petersen AM, Pedersen BK. The anti-inflammatory effect of exercise. *J Appl Physiol.* 2005;98:1154-1162.

27. Ryan AS, Nicklas BJ. Reductions in plasma cytokine levels with weight loss improve insulin sensitivity in overweight and obese postmenopausal women. *Diabetes Care.* 2004;27:1699-1705.

28. Ferrier KE, Nestel P, Taylor A, Drew BC, Kingwell BA. Diet but not aerobic exercise training reduces skeletal muscle TNF-alpha in overweight humans. *Diabetologia.* 2004;47:630-637.

29. Nieman DC, Henson DA, Austin MD, Brown VA. Immune response to a 30-minute walk. *Med Sci Sports Exerc.* 2005;37:57-62.

30. Nicklas BJ, Wang X, You T, et al. Effect of exercise intensity on abdominal fat loss during calorie restriction in overweight and obese postmenopausal women: a randomized, controlled trial. *Am J Clin Nutr.* 2009;89:1043-1052.

31. National Institute of Allergy and Infectious Diseases. The common cold, http:// www.niaid.nih.gov/topics/commoncold. Accessed July 3, 2010.

32. Fendrick AM, Monto AS, Nightengale B, Sarnes M. The economic burden of non-influenza-related viral respiratory tract infection in the United States. *Arch Intern Med.* 2003;163:487-494.

33. Monto AS. Epidemiology of viral respiratory infections. *Am J Med.* 2002;112: 4S-12S.

34. Nieman DC. Is infection risk linked to exercise workload? *Med Sci Sports Exerc.* 2000;32:S406-S411.

35. Nieman DC. Immune function responses to ultramarathon race competition. *Med Sportiva.* 2009;13:189-196.

36. Shephard RJ, Kavanagh T, Mertens DJ, Qureshi S, Clark M. Personal health benefits of Masters athletics competition. *Br J Sports Med.* 1995;29:35-40.

37. Davis JM, Kohut ML, Colbert LH, Jackson DA, Ghaffar A, Mayer EP. Exercise, alveolar macrophage function, and susceptibility to respiratory infection. *J Appl Physiol.* 1997;83:1461-1466.

38. Sim YJ, Yu S, Yoon KJ, Loiacono CM, Kohut ML. Chronic exercise reduces illness severity, decreases viral load, and results in greater anti-inflammatory effects than acute exercise during influenza infection. *J Infect Dis.* 2009;200:1434-1442.

39. Matthews CE, Ockene IS, Freedson PS, Rosal MC, Merriam PA, Hebert JR. Moderate to vigorous physical activity and risk of upper-respiratory tract infection. *Med Sci Sports Exerc.* 2002;34:1242-1248.

40. Kostka T, Praczko K. Interrelationship between physical activity, symptomatology of upper respiratory tract infections, and depression in elderly people. *Gerontology.* 2007;53:187-193.

41. Kostka T, Drygas W, Jegier A, Praczko K. Physical activity and upper respiratory tract infections. *Int J Sports Med.* 2008;29:158-162.

42. Fondell E, Lagerros YT, Sundberg CJ, et al. Physical activity, stress, and self-reported upper respiratory tract infection. *Med Sci Sports Exerc.* 2011;43:272-279.

43. Nieman DC, Henson DA, Austin MD, Sha W. Upper respiratory tract infection is reduced in physically fit and active adults. *Br J Sports Med.* In press.
44. Barrett B, Brown R, Mundt M, et al. The Wisconsin Upper Respiratory Symptom Survey is responsive, reliable, and valid. *J Clin Epidemiol.* 2005;58:609-617.
45. Neuman MI, Willett WC, Curhan GC. Physical activity and the risk of community-acquired pneumonia in US women. *Am J Med.* 2010;123:281.e7-281.e11.
46. Nieman DC, Nehlsen-Cannarella SL, Markoff PA, et al. The effects of moderate exercise training on natural killer cells and acute upper respiratory tract infections. *Int J Sports Med.* 1990;11:467-473.
47. Nieman DC, Nehlsen-Cannarella SL, Henson DA, et al. Immune response to exercise training and/or energy restriction in obese women. *Med Sci Sports Exerc.* 1998;30:679-686.
48. Nieman DC, Henson DA, Gusewitch G, et al. Physical activity and immune function in elderly women. *Med Sci Sports Exerc.* 1993;25:823-831.
49. Nieman DC. Immune function. In: Gisolfi CV, Lamb DR, Nadel E, eds. *Perspectives in Exercise Science and Sports Medicine, Vol. 8: Exercise in Older Adults.* Carmel, IN: Cooper Publishing Group; 1995:435-461.
50. Chubak J, McTiernan A, Sorensen B, et al. Moderate-intensity exercise reduces the incidence of colds among postmenopausal women. *Am J Med.* 2006;119: 937-942.
51. Nehlsen-Cannarella SL, Nieman DC, Jessen J, et al. The effects of acute moderate exercise on lymphocyte function and serum immunoglobulin levels. *Int J Sports Med.* 1991;12:391-398.
52. Nieman DC. Exercise effects on systemic immunity. *Immunol Cell Biol.* 2000;78: 496-501.
53. Nieman DC, Nehlsen-Cannarella SL. The immune response to exercise. *Semin Hematol.* 1994;31:166-179.
54. Murphy DA, Davis JM, Brown AS, et al. Role of lung macrophages on susceptibility to respiratory infection following short-term moderate exercise training. *Am J Physiol Regul Integr Comp Physiol.* 2004;287:R1354-R1358.
55. Edwards DM, Burns VE, Reynolds T, Carroll D, Drayson M, Ring C. Acute stress exposure prior to influenza vaccination enhances antibody response in women. *Brain Behav Immun.* 2006;20:159-168.
56. Kohut ML, Arntson BA, Lee W, et al. Moderate exercise improves antibody response to influenza immunization in older adults. *Vaccine.* 2004;22:2298-2306.
57. Kohut ML, Lee W, Martin A, et al. The exercise-induced enhancement of influenza immunity is mediated in part by improvements in psychosocial factors in older adults. *Brain Behav Immun.* 2005;19:357-366.
58. Lowder T, Padgett DA, Woods JA. Moderate exercise early after influenza virus infection reduces the Th1 inflammatory response in lungs of mice. *Exerc Immunol Rev.* 2006;12:97-111.
59. Fondell E, Christensen SE, Bälter O, Bälter K. Adherence to the Nordic Nutrition Recommendations as a measure of a healthy diet and upper respiratory tract infection. *Public Health Nutr.* 2011;14:860-869.
60. Cohen S. Keynote Presentation at the Eight International Congress of Behavioral Medicine: the Pittsburgh common cold studies: psychosocial predictors of susceptibility to respiratory infectious illness. *Int J Behav Med.* 2005;12:123-131.
61. Spiegel K, Sheridan JF, Van Cauter E. Effect of sleep deprivation on response to immunization. *JAMA.* 2002;288:1471-1472.
62. Cohen S, Doyle WJ, Alper CM, Janicki-Deverts D, Turner RB. Sleep habits and susceptibility to the common cold. *Arch Intern Med.* 2009;169:62-67.
63. Keusch GT. The history of nutrition: malnutrition, infection and immunity. *J Nutr.* 2003;133:336S-340S.

1 Epidemiology, Prevention of Injuries, Lesions of Head and Neck

Quality and Content of Internet-Based Information for Ten Common Orthopaedic Sports Medicine Diagnoses
Starman JS, Gettys FK, Capo JA, et al (Carolinas Med Ctr, Charlotte, NC; et al)
J Bone Joint Surg Am 92:1612-1618, 2010

Background.—Although the use of the Internet to access health information has grown quickly, the emergence of quality controls for health information web sites has been considerably slower. The primary objective of this study was to assess the quality and content of Internet-based information for commonly encountered diagnoses within orthopaedic sports medicine.

Methods.—Ten common diagnoses within the scope of orthopaedic sports medicine were chosen. Custom grading templates were developed for each condition, and they included an assessment of web-site type, the accountability and transparency of the information (Health On the Net Foundation [HON] score), and the information content. Information content was divided into five subcategories: disease summary, pathogenesis, diagnostics, treatment and complications, and outcomes and prognosis. Two popular search engines were used, and the top ten sites from each were independently reviewed by three authors. Data were evaluated for interobserver variability, HON scores, information content scores, and subgroup score comparisons.

Results.—After eliminating duplicate sites, a total of 154 unique sites were reviewed. The most common web-site types were commercial (seventy-four sites) and academic (thirty-two sites). Average HON scores, on a 16-point scale, were 9.8, 9.5, and 8.5, for reviewers 1, 2, and 3, respectively. Average information content scores, on a 100-point scale, were 56.8, 56.0, and 54.8 for reviewers 1, 2, and 3, respectively. Average content scores in each subgroup ranged between 45% and 61% of the maximum possible score. The presence of the HONcode seal was associated with significantly higher HON (p = 0.0001) and content scores (p = 0.002).

Conclusions.—The quality and content of health information on the Internet is highly variable for common sports medicine topics. Patients should be encouraged to exercise caution and to utilize only well-known sites and those that display the HONcode seal of compliance with transparency and accountability practices.

▶ This is a fascinating study regarding the quality and content of Internet-based information that patients seek out for 10 common orthopedic sports medicine diagnoses. A total of 154 unique sites were reviewed, and these were found by searching Google and Yahoo!, which are the most common search engines used by patients. The Web sites were mainly commercial but also included academics, news articles, physician/group, personal, nonprofit, and other. Three independent reviewers looked at the content regarding disease summary, pathogenesis, diagnostics, treatment and complications, and outcomes and prognosis. Proper statistical methods were used to evaluate interobserver variability. A section of the grading sheet also evaluated each Web site for quality on the basis of the Health On the Net Foundation (HON) criteria. These were developed in 1996 by a Swiss-based nonprofit group to improve and monitor the transparency and purpose of Internet-based health information.[1] This can be thought of as a seal of approval for Internet sites displaying this logo.

Not surprisingly, nonprofit and education-based Web sites had the highest content and HON scores, while personal, news-related, and commercial sites had the lowest. The most reputable sites were WebMD and eMedicine. Unfortunately, only about a quarter of the Web sites reviewed displayed the HONcode compliance seal. Given that patients currently make extensive use of the Internet to look up health information related to their conditions, it behooves the practicing physician to be aware of this and, direct them accordingly to a reputable and accurate source. One family physician I know has actually made up a prescription pad for her patients, listing the most common informational Web sites for different medical problems. She will actually check off the most appropriate ones and hand the prescription to her patients. In this way, she is ensuring that they will benefit from the wealth of information that is readily available in electronic form while avoiding potential bias and lack of accountability on certain commercial sites. This article suggests that patients should be counseled to actually look for the HONcode seal of compliance on Web sites and, furthermore, that orthopedic residents and other health care professionals who use the Internet as a reference tool during their education would also benefit from this approach.

C. Lebrun, MD

Reference

1. Boyer C, Selby M, Scherrer JR, Appel RD. The Health On the Net Code of Conduct for medical and health Websites. *Comput Biol Med.* 1998;28:603-610.

The health and socioeconomic impacts of major multi-sport events: systematic review (1978-2008)

McCartney G, Thomas S, Thomson H, et al (Med Res Council Social and Public Health Sciences Unit, Glasgow; Sandside, Isle of Graemsay, Stromness, Orkney; et al)
BMJ 340:c2369, 2010

Objective.—To assess the effects of major multi-sport events on health and socioeconomic determinants of health in the population of the city hosting the event.

Design.—Systematic review.

Data Sources.—We searched the following sources without language restrictions for papers published between 1978 and 2008: Applied Social Science Index and Abstracts (ASSIA), British Humanities Index (BHI), Cochrane database of systematic reviews, Econlit database, Embase, Education Resources Information Center (ERIC) database, Health Management Information Consortium (HMIC) database, International Bibliography of the Social Sciences (IBSS), Medline, PreMedline, PsycINFO, Sociological Abstracts, Sportdiscus, Web of Knowledge, Worldwide Political Science Abstracts, and the grey literature.

Review Methods.—Studies of any design that assessed the health and socioeconomic impacts of major multi-sport events on the host population were included. We excluded studies that used exclusively estimated data rather than actual data, that investigated host population support for an event or media portrayals of host cities, or that described new physical infrastructure. Studies were selected and critically appraised by two independent reviewers.

Results.—Fifty four studies were included. Study quality was poor, with 69% of studies using a repeat cross-sectional design and 85% of quantitative studies assessed as being below 2+ on the Health Development Agency appraisal scale, often because of a lack of comparison group. Five studies, each with a high risk of bias, reported health related outcomes, which were suicide, paediatric health service demand, presentations for asthma in children (two studies), and problems related to illicit drug use. Overall, the data did not indicate clear negative or positive health impacts of major multi-sport events on host populations. The most frequently reported outcomes were economic outcomes (18 studies). The outcomes used were similar enough to allow us to perform a narrative synthesis, but the overall impact of major multisport events on economic growth and employment was unclear. Two thirds of the economic studies reported increased economic growth or employment immediately after the event, but all these studies used some estimated data in their models, failed to account for opportunity costs, or examined only short term effects. Outcomes for transport were also similar enough to allow synthesis of six of the eight studies, which showed that event related interventions— including restricted car use and public transport promotion—were

TABLE 1.—Impacts of Major Multi-Sport Events on Health and Determinants of Health

Study	Level of Evidence*	Event	Outcome	Impact†
Health				
Lee[17]	2+	2002 AG Busan, South Korea	Childhood asthma hospital admissions	↔
Friedman[18]	2−	1996 OG Atlanta, GA, USA	Childhood asthma acute care events	↓
Shin[16]	2+	1988 OG Seoul, South Korea	Suicide rates	↔
Indig[20]	2−	2000 OG Sydney, Australia	Hospital presentations related to illicit drugs	↑
Simon[19]	2−	1996 OG Atlanta	Paediatric health service demand	↑
Recreation				
Brown[23]	Qualitative	2002 CG Manchester, UK	Legacy programme implementation	N/A
MORI[21]	2−	2002 CG Manchester	Sports participation	↓
Truno[22]	2−	1992 OG Barcelona, Spain	Sports participation	↑
Newby[24]	2−	2002 CG Manchester	Satisfaction with green spaces	↑
Transport and the environment				
Lee[17]	2+	2002 AG Busan	Air pollution	↓
Potter[47]	2+	1996 OG Atlanta	Road traffic volume	↓
Fidell[52]	2−	1996 OG Atlanta	Airport noise episodes	↑
			Night time awakenings	↑
Friedman[18]	2−	1996 OG Atlanta	Air pollution	↓
			Road traffic volume	↓
Giuliano[49]	2−	1984 OG Los Angeles, CA, USA	Car commuting journey time	↓
Hallenbeck[50]	2−	1990 GWG Seattle, WA, USA	Road traffic volume	↔
Hensher[51]	2−	2000 OG Sydney	Commuting journey time	↓
Lee[48]	2−	2002 AG Busan	Air pollution	↑
			Road traffic volume	↓
Crime, housing, and demography				
Decker[56]	2+	1996 OG Atlanta	Demand for police services	↑
			Recorded crime	↓
Brunet[39]	2−	1992 OG Barcelona	House prices	↑
Halifax Plc[57]	2−	1992-2004 OG	House prices	↑
Hiller[58]	2−	1988 WO Calgary, AB, Canada	Population of immediate host area	↓
Hopkins[59]	2−	1996 OG Atlanta	"Urban camping law" introduction	N/A
Greater London Authority[31]	2−	1992-2004 OG	House prices	↑
Newby[24]	2−	2002 CG Manchester	Perceived supermarket access	↑
			Satisfaction with local area	↑
			Satisfaction with house and its condition	↑
			Reported vandalism to own property	↓
Lybbert[32]	2−	1980 and 1988 WO; 1984 and 1996 OG	Migration to Olympic regions	↑
Volunteers				
Downward[54]	2−	2002 CG Manchester	Volunteers' participation in sport	↔
			Likelihood of event volunteers volunteering after event	↔
Kemp[55]	2−	1994 WO Lillehammer, Norway, and 2000 OG Sydney	Perceived skills development	↑

(*Continued*)

TABLE 1. *(continued)*

Study	Level of Evidence*	Event	Outcome	Impact[†]
Lumsdon[53]	Qualitative	2002 CG Manchester	Experience of event volunteers	↑↓
			Volunteers' participation in sport	↔
			Volunteers' participation in further voluntary work	↔
Culture				
Hargreaves[63]	2−	1992 OG Barcelona	Catalan identity	↓
Kolstad[62]	2−	1994 WO Lillehammer	Adoption of Olympic values	↔
Waitt[61]	2−	2000 OG Sydney	Community spirit	↑
			Pride	↑
Owen[60]	Qualitative	2000 OG Sydney	Local democracy	↓

See web table F for full critical appraisal and results for all included studies.

Abbreviations: AG, Asian Games; CG, Commonwealth Games; GWG, Goodwill Games; OG, Olympic Games; WO, Winter Olympic Games.

Editor's Note: Please refer to original journal article for full references.

*Level of evidence as per web table E.

[†] ↑=increase; ↓=decrease; ↔=no change; ↑↓=mixed impacts for this outcome; N/A=not applicable (that is, the outcome cannot be described as a simple increase or decrease).

associated with significant short term reductions in traffic volume, congestion, or pollution in four out of five cities.

Conclusions.—The available evidence is not sufficient to confirm or refute expectations about the health or socioeconomic benefits for the host population of previous major multi-sport events. Future events such as the 2012 Olympic Games and Paralympic Games, or the 2014 Commonwealth Games, cannot be expected to automatically provide benefits. Until decision makers include robust, long term evaluations as part of their design and implementation of events, it is unclear how the costs of major multi-sport events can be justified in terms of benefits to the host population (Table 1).

▶ I was personally interested to read this article as I live in a small town midway between Vancouver and Whistler, sites of the 2010 Winter Olympic Games, and have had first-hand experience of the community impact of a major sporting event. Those promoting the Games predicted vast economic benefits for our area. The day that the final decision to host the Games was announced, there was indeed a 50% rise in the price of property in this region, and this was followed by a frantic speculative construction boom. But 4 months following the games, much of the new housing has been abandoned, half constructed, with the contractors unpaid; a new golf course has declared bankruptcy; and 2 new hotels are avoiding creditors. Local shopkeepers found that the time involved in reaching the sites of competition and passing security were such that visitors had little time or energy to visit their stores or eat in local restaurants. The main new athletic facility, a vast skating oval in the city of Richmond, had to be dismantled and converted to a gymnasium immediately after the Games because of political arguments concerning supposed competition with another rink previously built for the Calgary Olympic Winter Games. Two positive consequences of the event were the construction of a rail link from Vancouver airport to the city and major upgrades to the Vancouver-Whistler highway, although arguably population pressures would have forced such construction even if the Games had not been hosted. So, I would agree with this review that the case has not yet been made for tangible economic benefits resulting from hosting a major athletic event. However, the experience in Vancouver does support the conclusion of some short-term increase in the use of public transportation consequent upon Draconian restrictions of car use during the Games (Table 1). Many of the volunteers involved in the Games also found this to have been a very worthwhile experience.

R. J. Shephard, MD (Lond), PhD, DPE

Sports injuries and illnesses during the Winter Olympic Games 2010
Engebretsen L, Steffen K, Alonso JM, et al (IOC Med Commission, Lausanne, Switzerland; Oslo Sports Trauma Res Ctr, Norway; International Association of Athletics Federations (IAAF), Monte-Carlo, Spain; et al)
Br J Sports Med 44:772-780, 2010

Background.—Identification of high-risk sports, including their most common and severe injuries and illnesses, will facilitate the identification of sports and athletes at risk at an early stage.

Aim.—To analyse the frequencies and characteristics of injuries and illnesses during the XXI Winter Olympic Games in Vancouver 2010.

Methods.—All National Olympic Committees' (NOC) head physicians were asked to report daily the occurrence (or non-occurrence) of newly sustained injuries and illnesses on a standardised reporting form. In addition, the medical centres at the Vancouver and Whistler Olympic clinics reported daily on all athletes treated for injuries and illnesses.

Results.—Physicians covering 2567 athletes (1045 females, 1522 males) from 82 NOCs participated in the study. The reported 287 injuries and 185 illnesses resulted in an incidence of 111.8 injuries and 72.1 illnesses per 1000 registered athletes. In relation to the number of registered athletes, the risk of sustaining an injury was highest for bobsleigh, ice hockey, short track, alpine freestyle and snowboard cross (15−35% of registered athletes were affected in each sport). The injury risk was lowest for the Nordic skiing events (biathlon, cross country skiing, ski jumping, Nordic combined), luge, curling, speed skating and freestyle moguls (less than 5% of registered athletes). Head/cervical spine and knee were the most common injury locations. Injuries were evenly distributed between training (54.0%) and competition (46.0%; p=0.18), and 22.6% of the injuries resulted in an absence from training or competition. In skeleton, figure and speed skating, curling, snowboard cross and biathlon, every 10th athlete suffered from at least one illness. In 113 illnesses (62.8%), the respiratory system was affected.

Conclusion.—At least 11% of the athletes incurred an injury during the games, and 7% of the athletes an illness. The incidence of injuries and illnesses varied substantially between sports. Analyses of injury mechanisms in high-risk Olympic winter sports are essential to better direct injury-prevention strategies.

▶ This is the first report of surveillance of injuries and illnesses during a Winter Olympic Games. This study was conducted by a group of experts selected by the International Olympic Committee (IOC). The same research group carried out a similar study during the Beijing 2008 Summer Olympics, but only injuries were included in that survey.[1] They used a standard reporting form that was relatively simple to encourage compliance from the National Olympic Committee (NOC) reporting doctors and physiotherapists. By crosschecking the results with reported injuries and illnesses from the medical centers at the Vancouver and Whistler Olympic Polyclinics, and also the reports from the technical delegates of each sport, the investigators managed to capture a significant number of the injuries and illnesses incurred during training and competition. At least 11% of the athletes incurred an injury during the games, and 7% of the athletes an illness. This study also identified significant differences in reported injuries and illnesses in the different sports.

Injury surveillance and epidemiology is the first step in injury prevention, following the 4-stage model of Willem van Mechelan.[2] The goal is to identify athletes at high risk of injury early, and to provide them with the tools for injury prevention. The IOC is currently developing and promoting a periodic health assessment system for athletes participating in Olympic and Paralympic sports, as well as for the young elite athletes. This should help the NOCs to identify health problems in advance in their athletes and maximize the health protection of their elite athletes.

C. Lebrun, MD

References

1. Junge A, Engebretsen L, Mountjoy ML, et al. Sports injuries during the Summer Olympic Games 2008. *Am J Sports Med.* 2009;37:2165-2172.
2. van Mechelen W, Hlobil H, Kemper HC. Incidence, severity, aetiology and prevention of sports injuries. A review of concepts. *Sports Med.* 1992;14:82-99.

Injury Incidence and Predictors on a Multiday Recreational Bicycle Tour: The Register's Annual Great Bike Ride Across Iowa, 2004 to 2008
Boeke PS, House HR, Graber MA (Univ of Iowa Hosps and Clinics)
Wilderness Environ Med 21:202-207, 2010

Objective.—The "Register's Annual Great Bike Ride Across Iowa" (RAGBRAI) is a 7-day recreational bicycle ride with more than 10,000 participants covering 500 miles. The heat and humidity of late July in Iowa, the prevalence of amateur riders, and the consumption of alcohol can combine creating the potential for a significant number of injuries.

The purpose of this study is to determine the type, quantity, and severity of injuries on RAGBRAI and gather data on the factors related to these incidents.

Methods.—This retrospective chart review examined ambulance "run sheets" for patients requiring transport to the hospital from the bike route between 2004 and 2008. These run sheets included name, age, chief complaint, anatomic location of injuries, medications administered, procedures performed, and a full narrative describing the initial scene, patient's account of the incident, services provided, and ongoing condition of the patient while en route to the hospital. Chi-square tests, Pearson's correlation tests, and t tests were applied to determine significant statistical outcomes.

Results.—From 2004 to 2008, Care Ambulance Inc provided on-route medical services for 419 RAGBRAI participants. Of these participants, 190 (45.3%) required transport to a local hospital by Care Ambulance Inc. Females were more likely to require transport, as they comprised 46.3% of transported patients while only representing 35% of all RAGBRAI participants ($P = .001$). For men, increasing age was a significant predictor of transport, particularly males between the ages of 60 and 69 years old ($P = .01$). Of the 148 run sheets where mechanism of incident was documented, 114 incidents were caused by rider factors (77.0%), 29 by road factors (19.6%), and 5 by bicycle factors (3.4%). Higher heat indexes were correlated with an increased number of dehydration cases ($r = 0.979$, $P = .02$). Of participants who reported with minor injuries to a mobile first aid station and did not require transport, 90.1% had not imbibed any alcohol. Bony injuries were more common above the waistline as 39/45 (86.7%) fractures occurred to the clavicle, shoulder/proximal humerus, hand, or head. The most common bony injury each year of RAGBRAI was a clavicle fracture, which represented 44.4% of all recorded fractures from 2004 to 2008. Lacerations and abrasions were also more common above the waist, as 63.5% (127/200) of soft tissue injuries requiring treatment were either to the head or upper extremities. No specific event day showed any correlation with increased injury ($P > .05$).

Conclusions.—This study suggests that females and older males are more likely to require transport for injuries sustained on RAGBRAI, the majority of injuries occur around the head and upper extremities, dehydration case load is correlated with heat index, and that incidents are usually caused by rider factors. This research could be used by multiday recreational bicycle tour organizers to continue educating riders on riding carelessness and etiquette and prepare medical services for certain quantities and types of injuries.

▶ Multiday recreational bike tours take place every year in 44 states. The Register's Annual Great Bicycle Ride Across Iowa (RAGBRAI) is the grandfather of these events. The longevity and large attendance of RAGBRAI provided the opportunity to evaluate the incidence and mechanisms of injury in recreational cyclists. The authors compiled injury reports from the ambulance service and mobile first aid stations that attended to riders over 5 years of RAGBRAI (2004-2008). This time frame included approximately 50 000 riders of whom 65% were men and approximately half were aged 40 to 59 years. The main message of this survey is that about 77% of injuries requiring transport to a medical facility are caused by rider factors such as falls/loss of balance and entanglement with other riders. Road factors were associated with 19% of injuries and bicycle factors only 3%. In confirmation of previous studies, dehydration requiring medical attention was significantly correlated with heat index. The incidence of medical transport was greater in women than men and men older than 60 years compared with other age groups. The medical issues of older men were likely related to deconditioning including symptoms such as dyspnea, tachycardia, or chest pain. The reasons for greater incidence of medical transport in women riders are not clear but could be because of the greater willingness of women than men to seek medical attention. The day of the event (day 1-7) was not significantly related to injury incidence. Rider education regarding bicycle handling and proper hydration may reduce injuries during these recreational events.

C. M. Jankowski, PhD

Behaviour, the Key Factor for Sports Injury Prevention
Verhagen EALM, van Stralen MM, van Mechelen W (VU Univ Med Ctr, Amsterdam, the Netherlands)
Sports Med 40:899-906, 2010

Safety in sports and physical activity is an important prerequisite for continuing participation in sports, as well as for maintenance of a healthy physically active lifestyle. For this reason, prevention, reduction and control of sports injuries are important goals for society as a whole. Recent advances in sports medicine discuss the need for research on real-life injury prevention. Such views call for a more behavioural approach when it comes to actual sports injury prevention. Nevertheless, the role of behaviour in sports injury prevention remains under-researched. In order to push the field of sports injury prevention forward, this article provides an overview of the relationship between behaviour and sports injury risk.

Different types of behaviour relate to injury risk factors and injury mechanisms. Behaviour that influences risk factors and injury mechanisms is not confined only to the athlete. Various types of behaviour by, for example, the coach, referee, physical therapist or sports associations, also influence risk factors and injury mechanisms. In addition, multiple behaviours often act together. Some types of behaviour may directly affect injury risk and are by definition a risk factor. Other behaviours may only affect risk factors and injury mechanisms, and influence injury risk indirectly.

Recent ideas on injury prevention that call for studies on real-life injury prevention still rely heavily on preventive measures that are established through efficacy research. A serious limitation in such an approach is that one expects that proven preventive measures will be adopted if the determinants and influences of sports safety behaviours are understood. Therefore, if one truly wants to prevent sports injuries in a real-life situation, a broader research focus is needed. In trying to do so, we need to look at lessons learned from other fields of injury prevention research.

▶ Prevention of illness and injury in sport is of paramount importance, and it is also the latest focus of research in sport medicine. Early models by van Mechelen[1] and Meeuwisse[2] established the sequence of prevention, beginning with identification of the problem (ie, injury surveillance and epidemiology). The next steps include determination of risk factors and injury mechanisms, institution of some type of intervention, and then repeat surveillance to determine the impact of the intervention. Meeuwisse further described the complex interplay between internal and external risk factors and included the concept of a predisposed athlete and an inciting event. Bahr and Krosshaug[3] elaborated on this theory and presented a more comprehensive model for injury causation.

More recently, however, sport scientists have begun to look toward examples in the behavioral and/or social science fields to assess the effects of behavior on injury prevention and injury risk factors. This article eloquently outlines the different influences that may enter into play—starting with the behavior of the athlete, coach, referee, rehabilitation specialist, or sports association (Fig 1 in the original article). The authors suggest that effective implementation of injury prevention strategies must also take into account the potential for individual or group behavior to mitigate their effectiveness. As also pointed out in this article, the role of behavior in injury prevention has been underresearched to date, so this is an essential area for future attention. Although not specifically discussed here, another key issue is knowledge translation—taking the findings of well-designed studies with valid findings from bench, or theory, to bedside, field of play, or real-life injury prevention, through effective dissemination of the new information. Here again, behavior will be a necessary component and will include other important features such as teaching strategies, modes of learning, retention of new knowledge, and changes in established habits. The field of injury prevention in sport is indeed exciting and challenging!

C. Lebrun, MD

References

1. van Mechelen W, Hlobil H, Kemper HC. Incidence, severity, aetiology and prevention of sports injuries. A review of concepts. *Sports Med*. 1992;14:82-99.
2. Meeuwisse W. Assessing causation in sport injury: a multifactorial approach. *Clin J Sport Med*. 1994;4:166-170.
3. Bahr R, Krosshaug T. Understanding injury mechanisms: a key component of preventing injuries in sport. *Br J Sports Med*. 2005;39:324-329.

Investigation of Baseline Self-Report Concussion Symptom Scores

Piland SG, Ferrara MS, Macciocchi SN, et al (Univ of Southern Mississippi, Hattiesburg; Univ of Georgia, Athens; Shepherd Spinal Inst, Atlanta, GA; et al)

J Athl Train 45:273-278, 2010

Context.—Self-reported symptoms (SRS) scales comprise one aspect of a multifaceted assessment of sport-related concussion. Obtaining SRS assessments before a concussion occurs assists in determining when the injury is resolved. However, athletes may present with concussion-related symptoms at baseline. Thus, it is important to evaluate such reports to determine if the variables that are common to many athletic environments are influencing them.

Objective.—To evaluate the influence of a history of concussion, sex, acute fatigue, physical illness, and orthopaedic injury on baseline responses to 2 summative symptom scales; to investigate the psychometric properties of all responses; and to assess the factorial validity of responses to both scales in the absence of influential variables.

Design.—Cross-sectional study.

Setting.—Athletic training facilities of 6 National Collegiate Athletic Association institutions.

Patients or Other Participants.—The sample of 1065 was predominately male (n = 805) collegiate athletes with a mean age of 19.81 ± 1.53 years.

Main Outcome Measure(s).—Participants completed baseline measures for duration and severity of concussion-related SRS and a brief health questionnaire.

Results.—At baseline, respondents reporting a previous concussion had higher composite scores on both scales ($P \leq .01$), but no sex differences were found for concussion-related symptoms. Acute fatigue, physical illness, and orthopaedic injury increased composite SRS scores on both duration and severity measures ($P \leq .01$). Responses to both scales were stable and internally consistent. Confirmatory factor analysis provided strong evidence for the factorial validity of the responses of participants reporting no fatigue, physical illness, or orthopaedic injury on each instrument.

Conclusions.—A history of concussion, acute fatigue, physical illness, and orthopaedic injury increased baseline SRS scores. These conditions need to be thoroughly investigated and controlled by clinicians before baseline SRS measures are collected.

▶ This well-done study underscores the importance of obtaining a baseline self-report symptom score before a concussion occurs, as many athletes will have a number of concussion symptoms being experienced at baseline. Following a concussion, it can only be expected to come back to baseline number of symptoms rather than being truly asymptomatic. These authors found that variables that included a history of a previous concussion, current fatigue, other physical illness, and/or orthopedic injury all altered the normal baseline self-reported symptom scores. They recommend therefore that if an athlete is experiencing fatigue, physical illness, or orthopedic injury, baseline testing should be postponed until the athlete recovers. An athlete with a history of concussion or elevated self-reported symptom score should be thoroughly evaluated. I might take this 1 step further that in the assessment of an athlete, he/she should be screened for such conditions as depression, anxiety disorder, panic attack, or migraine. Virtually all of these conditions will have a positive self-report symptom score at baseline that is unrelated to the concussion. Such an athlete after a concussion will have an elevated symptom report score, but when he/she is back to his/her true baseline he/she will still be symptomatic but at a baseline reduced level. This has significant obvious implications in terms of making return-to-play criteria. If an individual had baseline elevated symptom score that is unrelated to previous concussion, they would need to only return to that level before being safely able to return to play.

The authors further stress the value of using symptom report scales but typically use the Likert-type scaling rather than a simple yes/no answer in terms of whether symptoms are experienced. It is also stressed that capturing information beyond simply the presence of symptoms, namely their duration, severity, and intensity, is important as well.

R. C. Cantu, MD, MA

Concussion or Mild Traumatic Brain Injury: Parents Appreciate the Nuances of Nosology

Gordon KE, Dooley JM, Fitzpatrick EA, et al (Dalhousie Univ, Halifax, Nova Scotia, Canada; IWK Health Centre, Halifax, Nova Scotia, Canada)
Pediatr Neurol 43:253-257, 2010

We explored whether parents of our pediatric patients valued the diagnostic terms "concussion," "minor traumatic brain injury," and "mild traumatic brain injury" as equivalent or nonequivalent. 1734 of 2304 parents attending a regional pediatric emergency department completed a brief questionnaire assessing the equivalence or nonequivalence of the diagnostic terms "concussion," "minor traumatic brain injury," and "mild traumatic brain injury" in a pairwise fashion. Many parents viewed these diagnostic terms as equivalent, when assessed side by side. For those who considered these diagnostic terms nonequivalent, concussion was regarded as considerably "better" (or less "worse") than minor traumatic brain injury ($P < 0.001$, χ^2 test) or mild traumatic brain injury ($P < 0.001$, χ^2 test). A moderate degree of variability was evident in parent/guardian responses. As a group, parents reported that concussion or mild/minor traumatic brain injuries are valued equivalently. However, many parents considered them different, with concussion reflecting a "better" (or less "worse") outcome.

▶ Many of us who manage patients with concussion, especially those with postconcussion syndrome, do not like to equate the term concussion with a minor or mild traumatic brain injury because a brain injury that can cause life-changing alterations in cognitive or emotional function certainly is arguably not mild or minor. Thus, this author prefers the term concussion as a traumatic brain injury without the adjective. This article takes a look at what are parental attitudes toward concussion in terms of whether it is a minor or mild brain injury or is perceived as being a lesser injury. While most parents did consider the terms concussion and a mild or minor brain injury equivalent, many other parents considered concussion as reflecting an even less severe injury. This article poignantly points out the need for education to correct this misconception. The opportunity for such education currently exists in 9 states, where concussion education is mandated for not only coaches and athletes but also their parents. As hopefully other states adopt similar education, the opportunity for correcting misconceptions about the severity of concussion will be afforded.

R. C. Cantu, MD, MA

Assessment of metabolic brain damage and recovery following mild traumatic brain injury: a multicentre, proton magnetic resonance spectroscopic study in concussed patients

Vagnozzi R, Signoretti S, Cristofori L, et al (Univ of Rome 'Tor Vergata', Rome, Italy; S. Camillo Hosp, Rome, Italy; Ospedale Maggiore di Verona 'Borgo Trento', Italy; et al)
Brain 133:3232-3242, 2010

Concussive head injury opens a temporary window of brain vulnerability due to the impairment of cellular energetic metabolism. As experimentally demonstrated, a second mild injury occurring during this period can lead to severe brain damage, a condition clinically described as the second impact syndrome. To corroborate the validity of proton magnetic resonance spectroscopy in monitoring cerebral metabolic changes following mild traumatic brain injury, apart from the magnetic field strength (1.5 or 3.0 T) and mode of acquisition, we undertook a multicentre prospective study in which a cohort of 40 athletes suffering from concussion and a group of 30 control healthy subjects were admitted. Athletes (aged 16–35 years) were recruited and examined at three different institutions between September 2007 and June 2009. They underwent assessment of brain metabolism at 3, 15, 22 and 30 days post-injury through proton magnetic resonance spectroscopy for the determination of N-acetylaspartate, creatine and choline-containing compounds. Values of these representative brain metabolites were compared with those observed in the group of non-injured controls. Comparison of spectroscopic data, obtained in controls using different field strength and/or mode of acquisition, did not show any difference in the brain metabolite ratios. Athletes with concussion exhibited the most significant alteration of metabolite ratios at Day 3 post-injury (N-acetylaspartate/creatine: -17.6, N-acetylaspartate/choline: -21.4; $P < 0.001$ with respect to controls). On average, metabolic disturbance gradually recovered, initially in a slow fashion and, following Day 15, more rapidly. At 30 days post-injury, all athletes showed complete recovery, having metabolite ratios returned to values detected in controls. Athletes self-declared symptom clearance between 3 and 15 days after concussion. Results indicate that N-acetylaspartate determination by proton magnetic resonance spectroscopy represents a non-invasive tool to accurately measure changes in cerebral energy metabolism occurring in mild traumatic brain injury. In particular, this metabolic evaluation may significantly improve, along with other clinical assessments, the management of athletes suffering from concussion. Further studies to verify the effects of a second concussive event occurring at different time points of the recovery curve of brain metabolism are needed.

▶ The recognition and management of sport-related concussion continues to rely on clinical judgment. It had long been recognized that a biologic marker of concussion occurrence and subsequent resolution would greatly enhance the diagnosis and management of this condition. At the time of the Zurich Third International Concussion Consensus Conference in November 2008, preliminary work from Italy suggested that magnetic resonance spectroscopy and, in particular, the ratios of N-acetylaspartate/creatine-containing compounds (NAA/Cr) and N-acetylaspartate/choline-containing compounds (NAA/Cho) had promise for being biologic markers of concussion. This now fairly robust study using this technology to compare a cohort of 40 athletic concussions with 30 control subjects over a 3-year period in a multicenter study suggests that this technology may indeed be specific and sensitive enough to diagnose when a concussion has occurred and when metabolic equilibrium has been established and therefore safe return to sports could occur. Because the findings were similar at each of the 3 centers involved in the study, it suggests that as long as there are standardized volumes of interest allowed, the acquisition of reproducible data is possible so that differences in magnetic resonance scanners should not be considered as a source of confounding variability. What was found in each of the 3 centers was a significant reduction in NAA/Cr and NAA/Cho ratios peaking at day 3, normalizing more by day 15, and having reached baseline levels by day 30. Many of these athletes were asymptomatic, far short of the 30 days that it took for these metabolic studies to normalize. While this study needs to be confirmed by others at independent centers, it nonetheless suggests that a noninvasive brain marker of at least the metabolic effects of a concussive brain injury has been found. Whether the 30-day window suggested in this study is necessary for optimal management of sport-related concussion will require further study.

R. C. Cantu, MD, MA

Clinical Report—Sport-Related Concussion in Children and Adolescents
Halstead ME, the Council on Sports Medicine and Fitness
Pediatrics 126:597-615, 2010

Sport-related concussion is a "hot topic" in the media and in medicine. It is a common injury that is likely underreported by pediatric and adolescent athletes. Football has the highest incidence of concussion, but girls have higher concussion rates than boys do in similar sports. A clear understanding of the definition, signs, and symptoms of concussion is necessary to recognize it and rule out more severe intracranial injury. Concussion can cause symptoms that interfere with school, social and family relationships, and participation in sports. Recognition and education are paramount, because although proper equipment, sport technique, and adherence to rules of the sport may decrease the incidence or severity of concussions, nothing has been shown to prevent them. Appropriate management is essential for reducing the risk of long-term symptoms and complications. Cognitive and physical rest is the mainstay of management after diagnosis, and neuropsychological testing is a helpful tool in the management of concussion. Return to sport should be accomplished by using a progressive exercise program while evaluating for any return of signs or symptoms. This report serves as a basis for understanding the diagnosis and management of concussion in children and adolescent athletes.

▶ This document is essentially a position statement by the American Academy of Pediatrics on sport-related concussion in children and adolescents. It is authored by Mark E Halstead, MD and Kevin Walter. It is a thoughtful, comprehensive, and accurate portrayal of the state of our knowledge regarding concussion diagnosis, management, and treatment in the eyes of this coauthor of the 3 international concussion consensus statements, the National Athletic Trainers' Association and the American College of Sports Medicine concussion documents. While the information provided is not new and there is no unique information contained, it is a comprehensive thoughtful treatment of this subject that is useful not only to pediatricians but also to all individuals diagnosing and managing concussion, not only at the pediatric/adolescent level but at older ages as well.

R. C. Cantu, MD, MA

Measurement of Head Impacts in Youth Ice Hockey Players
Reed N, Taha T, Keightley M, et al (Univ of Toronto, Ontario, Canada; et al)
Int J Sports Med 31:826-833, 2010

Despite growing interest in the biomechanical mechanisms of sports-related concussion, ice hockey and the youth sport population has not been studied extensively. The purpose of this pilot study was: 1) to describe the biomechanical measures of head impacts in youth minor ice hockey players; and, 2) to investigate the influence of player and game characteristics on the number and magnitude of head impacts. Data was collected from 13 players from a single competitive Bantam boy's (ages 13–14 years) AAA ice hockey team using telemetric accelerometers implanted within the players' helmets at 27 ice hockey games. The average linear acceleration, rotational acceleration, Gadd Severity Index and Head Injury Criterion of head impacts were recorded. A significantly higher number of head impacts per player per game were found for wingers when compared to centre and defense player positions (df = 355, t = 3.087, p = 0.00218) and for tournament games when compared to regular season and playoff games (df = 355, t = 2.641, p = 0.086). A significant difference in rotational acceleration according to player position ($F_{2,1812}$ = 4.9551, p = 0.0071) was found. This study is an initial step towards a greater understanding of head impacts in youth ice hockey.

▶ Most of the work to date using the Head Impact Telemetry System to record head impact location and linear and rotational accelerations has been carried out in college football and ice hockey players. More recently, some data have been collected on high school football players, and plans are under way to record these data in National Football League athletes during the 2011 season. While there is debate among biomechanists of the accuracy of the linear accelerations recorded and rotational accelerations computed by this system, especially for off-center tangential impacts, there is no question about recording the number and location of impacts. For this reason alone, especially as long-term effects of repeated head impacts seem more related to the number of impacts rather than just observed concussions, collecting these data is to be encouraged.

To date, very little data have been collected in youth sports, and these authors are to be commended for studying the number and biomechanical characteristics of head impacts sustained by youth (13- to 14-year-old) ice hockey players. That wingers, probably because they more often chase pucks into the corners along the boards, sustain more impacts to the head per contest were sustained in tournament play than regular season games most likely reflects the intensity of play.

Though this is a small pilot study in 13 male youth players, its significant findings support a larger youth study being carried out.

R. C. Cantu, MD, MA

Collision Type and Player Anticipation Affect Head Impact Severity Among Youth Ice Hockey Players

Mihalik JP, Blackburn JT, Greenwald RM, et al (Univ of North Carolina at Chapel Hill; Simbex, Lebanon, NH; et al)
Pediatrics 125:e1394-e1401, 2010

Objective.—The objective was to determine how body collision type and player anticipation affected the severity of head impacts sustained by young athletes. For anticipated collisions, we sought to evaluate different body position descriptors during delivery and receipt of body collisions and their effects on head impact severity. We hypothesized that head impact biomechanical features would be more severe in unanticipated collisions and open-ice collisions, compared with anticipated collisions and collisions along the playing boards, respectively.

Methods.—Sixteen ice hockey players (age: 14.0 ± 0.5 years) wore instrumented helmets from which biomechanical measures (ie, linear acceleration, rotational acceleration, and severity profile) associated with head impacts were computed. Body collisions observed in video footage captured over a 54-game season were evaluated for collision type (open ice versus along the playing boards), level of anticipation (anticipated versus unanticipated), and relative body positioning by using a new tool developed for this purpose.

Results.—Open-ice collisions resulted in greater head linear ($P = .036$) and rotational ($P = .003$) accelerations, compared with collisions along the playing boards. Anticipated collisions tended to result in less-severe head impacts than unanticipated collisions, especially for medium-intensity impacts (50th to 75th percentiles of severity scores).

Conclusion.—Our data underscore the need to provide players with the necessary technical skills to heighten their awareness of imminent collisions and to mitigate the severity of head impacts in this sport.

▶ This is a thoughtful, well-conducted study with positive suggestions as to how concussions may be prevented at the youth level and in older populations as well. By clearly documenting in this study of youth ice hockey players that the biomechanical forces imparted were greater when the player did not anticipate the impact, it clearly underscored the need to afford players proper instruction to develop the technical skills to heighten their awareness of imminent collisions and thus attenuate the severity of head impacts. While much attention has been focused in the past years as to the importance of helmets and their role in attenuating forces in athletic head collisions, this study clearly shows that forces sustained by the head with open-ice collisions can be attenuated when the individual senses that the collision is imminent and properly braces his/her neck. This awareness of impending open-ice collisions will likely afford a reduction in concussion occurrence.

R. C. Cantu, MD, MA

Emergency Department Visits for Concussion in Young Child Athletes

Bakhos LL, Lockhart GR, Myers R, et al (Brown Univ, Providence, RI)
Pediatrics 126:e550-e556, 2010

Objectives.—The objective of this study was to characterize emergency department (ED) visits for pediatric sport-related concussion (SRC) in pre— high school— versus high school—aged athletes.

Methods.—A stratified probability sample of US hospitals that provide emergency services in the National Electronic Injury Surveillance System (1997—2007) and All Injury Program (2001—2005) was used. Concussion-related ED visits were analyzed for 8- to 13- and 14- to 19-year-old patients. Population data were obtained from the US Census Bureau; sport participation data were obtained from National Sporting Goods Association.

Results.—From 2001 to 2005, US children who were aged 8 to 19 years had an estimated 502 000 ED visits for concussion. The 8- to 13-year-old group accounted for ~35% of these visits. Approximately half of all ED visits for concussion were SRC. The 8- to 13-year-old group sustained 40% of these, which represents 58% of all concussions in this group. Approximately 25% of all SRC visits in the 8- to 13-year-old group occurred during organized team sport (OTS). During the study period, ~4 in 1000 children aged 8 to 13 years and 6 in 1000 children aged 14 to 19 years had an ED visit for SRC, and 1 in 1000 children aged 8 to 13 years and 3 in 1000 children aged 14 to 19 years had an ED visit for concussion sustained during OTS. From 1997 to 2007, although participation had declined, ED visits for concussions in OTS in 8- to 13-year-old children had doubled and had increased by >200% in the 14- to 19-year-old group.

Conclusions.—The number of SRCs in young athletes is noteworthy. Additional research is required.

▶ While the limitations of this study, which looked at emergency department diagnoses of concussion for the prehigh school 8- to 13-year-old age group as compared with the high school 14-to-19-year-old age group, are significant in that many, if not most, athletic concussions do not make their way to emergency departments, it is nonetheless striking that the number of sport-related concussions in the prehigh school age group was as high as 40% compared with 58% in the high school age group. What was particularly striking was the fact that in the prehigh school age group, there had been a 200% increase in sport-related concussions during the period of this study, while there has been a dramatic reduction in overall sport participation. While this is most probably because of the increased awareness and diagnosis of concussion and more appropriate management, it points out the need for more emphasis in this age group. Presently, there are no evidence-based guidelines for concussion management, including return-to-play guidelines that are based exclusively on the youth age group. While prospective studies of this age group certainly need to be done, because of the limitations of this study, I do not believe it should serve as anything other than stimulus for more studies on concussion incidence in our prehigh school athletes.

R. C. Cantu, MD, MA

High School Concussions in the 2008-2009 Academic Year: Mechanism, Symptoms, and Management
Meehan WP III, d'Hemecourt P, Dawn Comstock R (Children's Hosp Boston, MA; et al)
Am J Sports Med 38:2405-2409, 2010

Background.—An estimated 136 000 concussions occur per academic year in high schools alone. The effects of repetitive concussions and the potential for catastrophic injury have made concussion an injury of significant concern for young athletes.

Purpose.—The objective of this study was to describe the mechanism of injury, symptoms, and management of sport-related concussions using the High School Reporting Information Online (HS RIO) surveillance system.

Study Design.—Descriptive epidemiology study.

Methods.—All concussions recorded by HS RIO during the 2008-2009 academic year were included. Analyses were performed using SPSS software. Chi-square analysis was performed for all categorical variables. Statistical significance was considered for $P < .05$.

Results.—A total of 544 concussions were recorded. The most common mechanism (76.2%) was contact with another player, usually a head-to-head collision (52.7%). Headache was experienced in 93.4%; 4.6% lost consciousness. Most (83.4%) had resolution of their symptoms within 1 week. Symptoms lasted longer than 1 month in 1.5%. Computerized neuropsychological testing was used in 25.7% of concussions. When neuropsychological testing was used, athletes were less likely to return to play within 1 week than those for whom it was not used (13.6% vs 32.9%; $P < .01$). Athletes who had neuropsychological testing appeared less likely to return to play on the same day (0.8% vs 4.2%; $P = .056$). A greater proportion of injured, nonfootball athletes had computerized neuropsychological testing than injured football players (23% vs 32%; $P = .02$).

Conclusion.—When computerized neuropsychological testing is used, high school athletes are less likely to be returned to play within 1 week of their injury. Concussed football players are less likely to have computerized neuropsychological testing than those participating in other sports. Loss of consciousness is relatively uncommon among high school athletes who sustain a sport-related concussion. The most common mechanism is contact with another player. Some athletes (1.5%) report symptoms lasting longer than 1 month.

▶ These authors used Dawn Comstock's high school reporting information online surveillance system. Their findings were primarily similar to a number of previous publications, namely the most common mechanism of concussion was head-to-head collision with another player, headache was the most common concussion symptom, and loss of consciousness was seen in a small percentage of total concussions. Most of their players had symptoms clear within 1 week, and symptoms lasted greater than a month in less than 2% of athletes.

What was new with regard to this publication though was the fact that in a quarter of concussions, computerized, neuropsychological testing was used. When neuropsychological testing was used, the athletes were less likely to return to play within 1 week than when it was not used. They also found that athletes who underwent neuropsychological testing were much less likely to return to play on the same day. Because these data were collected, there has been a recommendation by the Zurich International Concussion Conference and the Lystedt Law legislation, which is now passed in 9 states, that suggests that anyone suspected or diagnosed with a concussion be held out of competition and not be allowed to return the same day. This has also been the recommendation largely adopted at the collegiate level and National Football League level as well in 2010.

The limitations of this study are well discussed by the authors, namely that all data entered into the online reporting are by athletic trainers who themselves have their own individual criteria for diagnosis, management, and return-to-play protocols for their athletes. Therefore, the definition of concussion, determination of recovery, and approach to assessment and management is not standardized in this study.

R. C. Cantu, MD, MA

Frequency and Location of Head Impact Exposures in Individual Collegiate Football Players

Crisco JJ, Fiore R, Beckwith JG, et al (The Warren Alpert Med School of Brown Univ and Rhode Island Hosp, Providence; Brown Univ, Providence, RI; Simbex, Lebanon, NH; et al)
J Athl Train 45:549-559, 2010

Context.—Measuring head impact exposure is a critical step toward understanding the mechanism and prevention of sport-related mild traumatic brain (concussion) injury, as well as the possible effects of repeated subconcussive impacts.

Objective.—To quantify the frequency and location of head impacts that individual players received in 1 season among 3 collegiate teams, between practice and game sessions, and among player positions.

Design.—Cohort study.

Setting.—Collegiate football field.

Patients or Other Participants.—One hundred eighty-eight players from 3 National Collegiate Athletic Association football teams.

Intervention(s).—Participants wore football helmets instrumented with an accelerometer-based system during the 2007 fall season.

Main Outcome Measure(s).—The number of head impacts greater than 10 *g* and location of the impacts on the player's helmet were recorded and analyzed for trends and interactions among teams (A, B, or C), session types, and player positions using Kaplan-Meier survival curves.

Results.—The total number of impacts players received was nonnormally distributed and varied by team, session type, and player position. The maximum number of head impacts for a single player on each team was 1022 (team A), 1412 (team B), and 1444 (team C). The median number of head impacts on each team was 4.8 (team A), 7.5 (team B), and 6.6 (team C) impacts per practice and 12.1 (team A), 14.6 (team B), and 16.3 (team C) impacts per game. Linemen and linebackers had the largest number of impacts per practice and per game. Offensive linemen had a higher percentage of impacts to the front than to the back of the helmet, whereas quarterbacks had a higher percentage to the back than to the front of the helmet.

Conclusions.—The frequency of head impacts and the location on the helmet where the impacts occur are functions of player position and session type. These data provide a basis for quantifying specific head impact exposure for studies related to understanding the biomechanics and clinical aspects of concussion injury, as well as the possible effects of repeated subconcussive impacts in football.

▶ Using the Head Impact Telemetry's (HIT's) system for recording head impact location and frequency in collegiate football players, these authors, I believe, have carried out an extremely important study. Whereas the HIT's system has its critics with regard to the accuracy of the actual linear accelerations and calculated rotational accelerations, such criticism of the location and occurrence of such accelerations does not exist. With colleagues at the Boston University Center for the Study of Traumatic Encephalopathy, we have published articles that suggest that the incidence of chronic traumatic encephalopathy is most related to total brain trauma, not just recorded concussions. Thus this article, which records total impacts of greater than 10 g, is most meaningful in allowing the medical profession and researchers to understand the total number of impacts sustained at the college football level. These authors found that as many as nearly 1500 impacts may be sustained in a season and that while the incidence of impacts per game is nearly 3 times greater than that for practice, since most of the time is spent practicing, most impacts were sustained during practice. The implications of this finding become extremely important at the National Football League (NFL) level where there is discussion of increasing the season from 16 to 18 games. The only way this could be done without significantly increasing the head impact exposure to these players would be to reduce the amount of head impacts that they receive during preseason, during the season practice, and at off-season mini camps. Understanding that it is doable to keep the total amount of head impacts the same if practice patterns were dramatically altered, namely that the amount of hitting and full contact in practice was dramatically reduced, takes on key importance.

These authors also found that linemen and linebackers have the highest numbers of head impacts and that most of them were to the front of the head for all positions, except the quarterback for whom this highest number of recorded impacts were to the back of the head. This likely reflects the blindside hit on quarterbacks and quarterbacks being hit from the front but driven backwards, striking the back of their heads on the turf.

These authors are to be complimented on a well-done article whose importance has significant ramifications for athletes at all levels, including the NFL.

R. C. Cantu, MD, MA

Investigating baseline neurocognitive performance between male and female athletes with a history of multiple concussion
Covassin T, Elbin R, Kontos A, et al (Michigan State Univ, East Lansing; Humboldt State Univ, Arcata, CA)
J Neurol Neurosurg Psychiatry 81:597-601, 2010

Objective.—The purpose of this study was to examine, using a dose–response model, sex differences in computerised neurocognitive performance among athletes with a history of multiple concussions.

Design.—Retrospective with randomly selected concussion cases from four levels/numbers of previous concussion.

Setting.—Multicentre analysis of NCAA student-athletes.

Participants.—Subjects included a total of 100 male and 88 female NCAA athletes.

Intervention.—Sex and four mutually exclusive groups of self-reported concussion history: (1) no history of concussion, (2) one previous concussion, (3) two previous concussions, (4) three or more previous concussions.

Main Outcome Measurements.—Neurocognitive performance as measured by a computerised neurocognitive test battery (Immediate Post-concussion Assessment Cognitive Testing (ImPACT)).

Results.—A dose–response gradient was found for two or more previous concussions and decreased neurocognitive performance. Females with a history of two and three or more concussions performed better than males with a history of two (p=0.001) and three or more concussions (p=0.012) on verbal memory. Females performed better than males with a history of three or more concussions (p=0.021) on visual memory. Finally, there was a significant difference for sex on both motor processing speed and reaction-time composite scores. Specifically, males performed worse than females on both processing speed (p=0.029) and reaction time (p=0.04).

Conclusion.—The current study provided partial support for a dose–response model of concussion and neurocognitive performance decrements beginning at two or more previous concussions. Sex differences should be considered when examining the effects of concussion history on computerised neurocognitive performance.

▶ The lead author has previously used Immediate Postconcussion Assessment Cognitive Testing (ImPACT) looking at scores in females compared with males after a concussion. She has reported that females generally took longer to recover back to baseline. They also found that females performed significantly higher than males on verbal memory in athletes without a concussion. Here, the authors compare sex differences and computerized neurocognitive test performance among athletes with a history of multiple concussions with those with no concussions. They purport to show that the athletes who have had more than 2 concussions perform slightly worse than those who have had no concussions, and that males with a history of 3 or more concussions perform worse than females with 3 or more concussions on verbal memory. The serious limitation of this study is that the males in this study were largely taken from collision sports, such as football and ice hockey. These are sports with a known 6 to 8 times incidence of unreported concussion as compared with the recognized incidence of concussion by the sideline medical team. Therefore, it is very probable that the males in this study had many more concussions than the 2 or 3 that were reported, and this could have had a profound impact on the scores recorded.

Another serious limitation is that we do not know the scores of the athletes before sustaining their third concussion. Because it was not possible to compare what one's initial ImPACT score may have been with what was recorded after a third recognized concussion, it is possible that this group may have, as a group, scored lower even without a concussion.

Finally, another major limiting feature of this study is that concussion severity was not quantified. Assuming that all concussions are equal, which is essentially what this dose-related response does, it is not without serious limitations.

A final limitation of the study is that it does involve questionnaire self-report and all the limitations attendant with that.

R. C. Cantu, MD, MA

Psychological approaches to treatment of postconcussion syndrome: a systematic review
Al Sayegh A, Sandford D, Carson AJ (Royal Edinburgh Hosp, Morningside Terrace, UK; Lancashire NHS Foundation Trust, Chorley, UK; Univ of Edinburgh, UK)
J Neurol Neurosurg Psychiatry 81:1128-1134, 2010

Background and Aim.—Postconcussion syndrome (PCS) is a term used to describe the complex, and controversial, constellation of physical, cognitive and emotional symptoms associated with mild brain injury. At the current time, there is a lack of clear, evidence-based treatment strategies. In this systematic review, the authors aimed to evaluate the potential efficacy of cognitive behavioural therapy (CBT) and other psychological treatments in postconcussion symptoms.

Methods.—Four electronic databases were searched up to November 2008 for studies of psychological approaches to treatment or prevention of postconcussion syndrome or symptoms.

Results.—The search identified 7763 citations, and 42 studies were included. This paper reports the results of 17 randomised controlled trials for psychological interventions which fell into four categories: CBT for PCS or specific PCS symptoms; information, reassurance and education; rehabilitation with a psychotherapeutic element and mindfulness/relaxation. Due to heterogeneity of methodology and outcome measures, a meta-analysis was not possible. The largest limitation to our findings was the lack of high-quality studies.

Conclusion.—There was evidence that CBT may be effective in the treatment of PCS. Information, education and reassurance alone may not be as beneficial as previously thought. There was limited evidence that multifaceted rehabilitation programmes that include a psychotherapeutic element or mindfulness/relaxation benefit those with persisting symptoms. Further, more rigorous trials of CBT for postconcussion symptoms are required.

▶ Postconcussion syndrome is a controversial diagnosis that involves a constellation of physical, cognitive, and emotional symptoms associated with a mild brain injury. These authors essentially studied the world's literature in treating this condition, lumping treatments into 4 categories: (1) cognitive brain therapy; (2) information, reassurance, and education; (3) rehabilitation programs with a psychotherapeutic element; and (4) mindfulness-based interventions using a stress/relaxation component. The authors concluded that while category 2 involving information and education had a role, its benefit was not nearly as strong as might be expected. Psychotherapeutic rehabilitation programs were not uniformly shown to be beneficial, nor were mindfulness-based interventions, except stress reduction, which was generally associated with fewer symptoms. Of all the categories, cognitive-based therapies seem to hold the most promise, but virtually all the studies were limited in their numbers and duration of follow-up.

Therefore, it was concluded by these authors and supported by this reviewer that ideal management and therapy of postconcussion syndrome remains a work in progress. What is needed is not further small studies; we need a large, comprehensive, multicentered study with rigorous randomized controlled trials that might study all the modalities discussed, but especially that of cognitive-based therapy for postconcussion syndrome.

R. C. Cantu, MD, MA

World Cup Soccer; a Major League Soccer Superstar's Career-Ending Injury, Concussion; and WORLD NEUROSURGERY: A Common Thread
Cantu RC (Boston Univ School of Medicine, MA)
World Neurosurg 74:224-225, 2010

Background.—Concussion is a traumatic injury to the brain caused by an impulsive force transmitted to the head after a direct or indirect impact involving the head, face, neck, or other area. Among its clinical signs and symptoms are physical findings, behavioral changes, impaired or altered cognition, sleep disturbances, somatic symptoms, and/or emotional symptoms. Often the onset of signs and symptoms is sudden and their resolution is spontaneous, so athletes, coaches, and trainers may not even suspect the problem and do not report it.

Soccer and Concussion.—Head collisions in the act of heading the ball are the most common cause of concussion in both male and female soccer players. The position of goalie is associated with the highest risk for concussion. The reported concussion incidence is higher for women than men. High school athletes have a slower rate of recovery than college athletes. It may be possible to alter concussion risk by changing the rules to limit heading of the ball, the specific mechanism identified to cause most concussions in soccer. Headgear may also protect against concussions, but current studies have not looked specifically at headgear's relationship to concussion rates or severity. In addition, the pathophysiology and biomechanical forces that produce concussion and its possible consequences, such as postconcussion syndrome and chronic traumatic encephalopathy, remain poorly understood.

> *Case Report.*—Taylor Twellman was a superstar Major League Soccer player in the United States a couple of years ago. He is the youngest and fastest player to reach 100 goals. However, after nine concussions and perhaps a premature return to play after the ninth one, he developed persistent postconcussion syndrome and had his career cut short at age 28 years. He is now a television broadcaster for soccer and attended the Fédération Internationale de Football Association (FIFA) World Cup in South Africa in that capacity.

Connections.—The International Concussion Conferences that FIFA, the International Ice Hockey Federation, the International Olympic Committee, and the International Rugby Union have sponsored have produced consensus statements that dramatically advanced concussion awareness, understanding, and management. Just as Twellman has recently begun a new career, the journal *World Neurosurgery* is in its infancy. It now faces the challenge of conveying the implications of neurosurgical knowledge, including such topics as concussion, to a worldwide audience.

▶ In the last several years, there have been a number of high-profile National Football League (NFL) players who have had their careers ended with a postconcussion syndrome. There also have been now over 20 NFL deceased players whose brains have been studied and shown to have chronic traumatic encephalopathy. This report of a Major League Soccer superstar Taylor Twellman, who was the youngest and fastest player in league history to reach the 100-goal plateau, chronicles his postconcussion syndrome that derailed and terminated his career at the height of his talents. This report thus points out that in soccer and other sports at risk for head trauma, persistent postconcussion syndrome can be a career-ending injury. This report also suggests that female soccer players are at greater risk of concussion than male players, with a higher incidence of reported concussion and a recovery rate that appears to be slower.

R. C. Cantu, MD, MA

Second Impact Syndrome: Concussion and Second Injury Brain Complications
Wetjen NM, Pichelmann MA, Atkinson JLD (Mayo Clinic, Rochester, MN)
J Am Coll Surg 211:553-557, 2010

Second impact syndrome was first described in 1973 by Richard Schneider in 2 young athletes who experienced initial concussive syndromes and subsequently died after a relatively minor second head injury. Saunders and Harbaugh coined the term *second impact syndrome* in their 1984 description of a 19-year-old college football player who suffered a head injury with brief loss of consciousness, returned to play, reported a headache, and on the 4th day collapsed, became unresponsive, and died. Postmortem examination revealed no space-occupying hematoma and extensive cerebral edema. It is the second collision impact, absence of space-occupying hematoma, and subsequent rapid and profound brain swelling that identify and mark the second impact syndrome. The severe brain swelling and absence of impact hematoma are identical to first head injury findings duplicated in head injury laboratory investigations and identified in clinical series of severe head injury patients.

Statistics as to the occurrence of second impact syndrome do not exist and the actual prevalence and incidence remain unknown. Second impact syndrome has always had proponents and detractors. Multiple head injury experts have discussed this phenomenon as a worrisome corollary in virtually every article or chapter on sport-related head injury. However, others have been suspicious that the pure form is rare, and some have called into question its existence, commenting ". . . it is fear of this entity that underpins concussion guidelines regarding return to sport." The latter statement prompted a strong rebuttal from a long-term and fully fledged head injury investigator who noted that, although the syndrome might be uncommon, its existence is a reality and is identifiable at some level virtually every year. In addition, it would be naïve to suggest return to play guidelines are solely in place as a consequence of possible second impact syndrome, when there are multiple reasons to protect a concussed athlete from re-exposure to play too early. Second impact syndrome is only a small determinant for return to play guidelines, and other factors, such as reported concussions are endemic in contact play and sport and are probably under-reported in high school football players; laboratory evidence and clinical series of concussed athletes reveal an increased susceptibility to additional concussions; repetitive concussions have prolonged neuropsychiatric effects; and recurrent concussions are related to substantial late-life cognitive impairment. Return to play guidelines after sport-related traumatic brain injury are beyond the scope of this article, but are founded and invested in athletic safety by assuring that the celerity of thought and clarity of mentation have returned to normal so that athletic mental and physical reflexes are not still impaired, which would make the athlete more susceptible to any subsequent injury; and recognizing that concussed athletes are more susceptible to a second concussion and that permanent sequelae might result. The reader is referred to return to play guidelines and their continued evolution, for which there are multiple sources.

Head injury research during the last century has clinically and experimentally produced clear evidence that severe first impact head injury—induced cerebral autoregulatory failure, with simultaneous catecholamine-induced marked blood pressure elevation, leads to rapid and often fatal malignant brain swelling. It is highly probable that the same events occur in the second impact syndrome as well, only in tandem sequence with lesser energies and generally in young people and children, but with the same devastating results.

▶ This is a thoughtful article that discusses the pathophysiology of head injury in general and the lack of autoregulation as well as the stress-induced catecholamine surge that occurs with traumatic brain injury. There are more than 20 cases of the second impact syndrome in the world's literature and undoubtedly countless cases that have not been reported. That it is because of a lack of autoregulation that allows for rapid vascular engorgement and brain herniation is well recognized. What is not well understood is why it is as rare as it appears to be.

These authors present the theory that it is the initial mild concussive brain injury that produces the cerebral autoregulatory failure, which can last hours or days, and that it is the subsequent stress-inducing second impact that produces the catecholamine release, which leads to rapid blood pressure elevation and massive vascular engorgement in a brain with failed autoregulation. As for why it's as rare as it is, the authors suggest that a concussive level brain injury uncommonly produces autoregulatory failure. In addition, the stress-induced secondary injury is also of a relatively mild nature and produces a modest catecholamine release and resultant blood pressure elevation. Therefore, it is not common that this entity is observed on athletic fields. This explanation could explain why an injury early in a football game could lead to loss of autoregulation, and a second injury later in the game could lead to the catecholamine surge in the presence of loss of autoregulation, which results in the vascular engorgement. Because the loss of autoregulation can last days, it would also explain why an athlete a week or more after an initial concussion could still be susceptible to this entity. While the catecholamine release can occur from a second head injury, this theory suggests that the second injury could be any injury to the body that provokes the catecholamine release.

This is a new way of looking at the second impact syndrome and one that undoubtedly will stimulate further research and reflection.

R. C. Cantu, MD, MA

Early Predictors of Postconcussive Syndrome in a Population of Trauma Patients With Mild Traumatic Brain Injury

Dischinger PC, Ryb GE, Kufera JA, et al (The Univ of Maryland School of Medicine, Baltimore)
J Trauma 66:289-297, 2009

Purpose.—The purpose of this analysis was to determine which of the initial symptoms after mild traumatic brain injury (MTBI) can best predict the development of persistent postconcussive syndrome (PCS).

Methods.—One hundred eighty MTBI patients admitted to a level I trauma center were enrolled in a prospective study and 110 followed for 3 months. MTBI was defined as a Glasgow Coma Score of 13 to 15 with a transient loss of consciousness or report of being dazed or confused. PCS was defined as the persistence of four or more symptoms long term. Patients were screened at admission and at 3 days to 10 days and 3 months. Symptom checklists were administered to ascertain the presence of symptoms (cognitive, emotional, and physical) after concussion. For a subset of patients that were physically able, balance tests were also conducted. Stepwise logistic regression was used to identify which symptoms best predicted PCS.

Results.—The mean age of the subjects was 35 years, and 65% were men. Physical symptoms were the most prevalent in the 3 days to 10 days postinjury with most declining thereafter to baseline levels. Emotional and cognitive symptoms were less prevalent but more likely to remain elevated at 3 months; 41.8% of subjects reported PCS at 3 months. The strongest individual symptoms that predicted long-term PCS included anxiety, noise sensitivity (NS), and trouble thinking; reported by 49%, 27%, and 31% of the subjects at 3 days to 10 days, respectively. In multivariate regressions including age, gender, and early symptoms, only anxiety, NS and gender remained significant in the prediction of PCS. Interactions revealed that the effect of anxiety was seen primarily among women. NS had an odds ratio of 3.1 for PCS at 3 months.

Conclusions.—After MTBI, anxiety among women and NS are important predictors of PCS. Other physical symptoms, while more prevalent are poor predictors of PCS.

▶ This is a very useful article that looks at whether there are initial symptoms reported after a concussion that allow one to predict the likelihood of a postconcussion syndrome occurring. The authors found that while physical symptoms such as headache, dizziness, blurred vision, fatigue, and sensitivity to light and noise occurred with greater frequency initially after a concussion, they were not significant predictors of a postconcussion syndrome and in fact had returned to baseline levels by 3 months. On the other hand, cognitive and emotional symptoms, while having declined from the initial levels immediately after a concussion, still had not returned to baseline levels at 3 months. The authors found that in women, anxiety was the symptom that best predicted a postconcussion syndrome. Female subjects were 50 times more likely to have a postconcussion syndrome if they initially reported anxiety, whereas other symptoms that predicted a postconcussion syndrome included difficulty thinking and noise sensitivity. Besides allowing the clinician the opportunity to recognize based on symptoms those at greater risk for postconcussion syndrome, if anxiety is identified, especially in women, it suggests that early intervention may well be useful and that early referral for psychiatric or neuropsychological help may be of benefit.

One serious limitation of this study is that it was carried out in a trauma center, and most individuals suffered other injuries in addition to a cerebral concussion. This greatly limited their ability to carry out balance testing as part of the assessment initially. It also means that the especially emotional responses may be influenced by the nonbrain injuries that the individual sustained. Nonetheless, this is a study that is well done within its limitations and certainly warrants being seen if it can be replicated by others.

R. C. Cantu, MD, MA

Headaches After Concussion in US Soldiers Returning From Iraq or Afghanistan
Theeler BJ, Flynn FG, Erickson JC (William Beaumont Army Med Ctr, Fort Bliss, TX; Madigan Traumatic Brain Injury Program, Fort Lewis, WA; Madigan Army Med Ctr, Fort Lewis, WA)
Headache 50:1262-1272, 2010

Objectives.—To determine the prevalence, characteristics, impact, and treatment patterns of headaches after concussion in US Army soldiers returning from a deployment to Iraq or Afghanistan.

Methods.—A cross-sectional study was conducted with a cohort of soldiers undergoing postdeployment evaluation during a 5-month period at the Madigan Traumatic Brain Injury Program at Ft. Lewis, WA. All soldiers screening positive for a deployment-related concussion were given a 13-item headache questionnaire.

Results.—A total of 1033 (19.6%) of 5270 returning soldiers met criteria for a deployment-related concussion. Among those with a concussion, 957 (97.8%) reported having headaches during the final 3 months of deployment. Posttraumatic headaches, defined as headaches beginning within 1 week after a concussion, were present in 361 (37%) soldiers. In total, 58% of posttraumatic headaches were classified as migraine. Posttraumatic headaches had a higher attack frequency than nontraumatic headaches, averaging 10 days per month. Chronic daily headache was present in 27% of soldiers with posttraumatic headache compared with 14% of soldiers with nontraumatic headache. Posttraumatic headaches interfered with duty performance in 37% of cases and caused more sick call visits compared with nontraumatic headache. In total, 78% of soldiers with posttraumatic headache used abortive medications, predominantly over-the-counter analgesics, and most perceived medication as effective.

Conclusions.—More than 1 in 3 returning military troops who have sustained a deployment-related concussion have headaches that meet criteria for posttraumatic headache. Migraine is the predominant headache phenotype precipitated by a concussion during military deployment. Compared with headaches not directly attributable to head trauma, posttraumatic headaches are associated with a higher frequency of headache attacks and an increased prevalence of chronic daily headache.

▶ Headache is the most common symptom documented following a concussion. Its occurrence though does not seem to predict whether one is going to have long-term symptoms or a postconcussion syndrome. Other than the onset of the headaches occurring immediately after the head trauma and not having been experienced prior to the head trauma, there are no defining clinical features of posttraumatic headaches that separate them from other primary headache disorders. This study of returning soldiers from Iraq and Afghanistan looked at the incidence of posttraumatic headaches, which were defined as occurring within 1 week of a concussion. Slightly more than a third of returning soldiers with a concussion had posttraumatic headaches using this definition. It is of interest to this commentator that a 1-week definition was used, and in my experience, posttraumatic headaches following a concussion are almost experienced the same day or within 24 hours. Slightly more than half of these posttraumatic concussion headaches met migraine criteria of being exacerbated by physical activity, being unilateral in nature, and associated with nausea, vomiting, or photophonosensitivity.

An unexpected finding was that 60% of returning soldiers had a history of deployment-related concussion but headaches that did not meet the posttraumatic headache definition of occurring within 1 week of the head trauma. This unusually high incidence of headache following a concussion makes me wonder whether some of those headaches that occurred days after but less than 7 days after a concussion shared features with this larger group. Because of this unusually high occurrence of chronic headaches in this population, it makes it possible that emotional and/or stress-related factors are present in this population.

A limitation of this study is that there was not a predeployment screening for either prior head trauma or pre-existing headaches, which could have significantly contributed to this unusually high incidence of chronic headaches following concussion in these soldiers. Another limitation of this study is that it did not examine the mechanism of concussion, for example, primary blast injury versus blunt trauma, number of concussions, or severity of concussion. It also did not address other potential contributing factors such as psychiatric conditions, including posttraumatic stress disorder.

R. C. Cantu, MD, MA

Postconcussion Syndrome After Mild Traumatic Brain Injury in Western Greece

Spinos P, Sakellaropoulos G, Georgiopoulos M, et al (Patras Med School, Greece)
J Trauma 69:789-794, 2010

Background.—The prevalence of postconcussion syndrome (PCS) in the first weeks after mild traumatic brain injury varies from 40% to 80%. However, as many as 50% of patients report symptoms for up to 3 months and 10% to 15% for more than a year. The objective of this study is to analyze the characteristics and estimate the prevalence of PCS in an adult Greek population.

Methods.—This prospective study was performed in the University Hospital of Patras in Western Greece. Patients with mild traumatic brain injury (n = 539) were randomly recruited on admission between May 2006 and May 2008. Overall, 223 patients (223 of 539, 41.5%) met the Colorado Medical Society guidelines for concussion; 141 men (63%) and 82 women (37%) with a median age of 30 years (range, 18.5–57.5 years) were included in the study. Patient follow-up consisted of telephone interviews at 1 month, 3 months, and 6 months postinjury, when they were asked about experiencing common postconcussion symptoms (International Classification of Diseases—10th revision criteria).

Results.—The rate of PCS at 1 month, 3 months, and 6 months postinjury was estimated to be 10.3%, 6%, and 0.9%, respectively. The syndrome was more frequent among women (17%) and individuals with bleeding diathesis (26%) compared with men (6.4%) and patients without clotting disorders (8.5%), respectively. In addition, higher rates of PCS affected patients who sustained assaults compared with other types of accidents.

Conclusion.—The prevalence of PCS was remarkably higher in previous studies. Cultural differences regarding symptom expectation and the lack of compensation might explain the low rate of chronic symptoms in Greeks.

▶ Postconcussion syndrome incidence varies widely in different published reports. Most of the reports have come from American studies. Most individuals writing about postconcussion syndrome recognize that the origin of symptoms include not only pathophysiologic brain injury but also psychological or emotional reactions to the symptoms that individuals may be experiencing as well as other factors such as litigation. Therefore, this study, which looked at the incidence of postconcussion syndrome as defined by postconcussion symptoms that met the *International Classification of Diseases, Tenth Revision*, criteria in a moderately large study of Western Greece individuals, allows one to see what the incidence might be without some of the Western influences playing a role. Indeed, it was of interest that the incidence of postconcussion syndrome postinjury was only 10% at 1 month, 6% at 3 months, and 0.9% at 6 months. As was found in other studies, women were twice as likely to have postconcussion syndrome as men. These very low incidences probably are related to cultural differences among the Greeks and the fact there is no litigation compensation playing a role.

R. C. Cantu, MD, MA

Postconcussive Symptoms and Neurocognitive Function After Mild Traumatic Brain Injury in Children

Sroufe NS, Fuller DS, West BT, et al (Univ of Michigan, Ann Arbor; et al)
Pediatrics 125:e1331-e1339, 2010

Objectives.—We describe children's postconcussive symptoms (PCSs), neurocognitive function, and recovery during 4 to 5 weeks after mild traumatic brain injury (MTBI) and compare performance and recovery with those of injured control group participants without MTBIs.

Methods.—A prospective, longitudinal, observational study was performed with a convenience sample from a tertiary care, pediatric emergency department. Participants were children 10 to 17 years of age who were treated in the emergency department and discharged. The MTBI group included patients with blunt head trauma, Glasgow Coma Scale scores of 13 to 15, loss of consciousness for ≤30 minutes, posttraumatic amnesia of ≤24 hours, altered mental status, or focal neurologic deficits, and no intracranial abnormalities. The control group included patients with injuries excluding the head. The Post-Concussion Symptom Questionnaire and domain-specific neurocognitive tests were completed at baseline and at 1 and 4 to 5 weeks after injury.

Results.—Twenty-eight MTBI group participants and 45 control group participants were compared. There were no significant differences in demographic features. Control group participants reported some PCSs; however, MTBI group participants reported significantly more PCSs at all times. Among MTBI group participants, PCSs persisted for 5 weeks after injury, decreasing significantly between 1 and 4 to 5 weeks. Patterns of recovery on the Trail-Making Test Part B differed significantly between groups; performance on other neurocognitive measures did not differ.

Conclusions.—In children 10 to 17 years of age, self-reported PCSs were not exclusive to patients with MTBIs. However, PCSs and recovery patterns for the Trail-Making Test Part B differed significantly between the groups.

▶ This was an interesting study that compared postconcussion symptoms and neurocognitive performance in a group of individuals who sustained a mild traumatic brain injury by Glasgow Coma Scale of 13 to 15 as compared with a second group that had largely orthopedic injuries and other injuries that did not involve the head. Both groups had postconcussion symptoms, but the brain-injured group had a much greater number of postconcussion symptoms and the rate at which those symptoms cleared over a 5-week period was much more rapid than the non—brain-injured group. The performance on neurocognitive testing also was different between the 2 groups. This is yet another example of pointing out that postconcussion symptoms are not unique to brain injured individuals, but the rate at which they recover and the profiles of performance on neurocognitive studies are different from individuals who have suffered largely orthopedic injuries. It was of interest that both groups did show improvement in the neurocognitive studies over time reinforcing the importance of understanding the learning effect of repeating such testing.

R. C. Cantu, MD, MA

Epidemiology of Postconcussion Syndrome in Pediatric Mild Traumatic Brain Injury

Barlow KM, Crawford S, Stevenson A, et al (Univ of Calgary, Alberta, Canada; Alberta Children's Hosp Res Inst for Children and Maternal Health, Calgary, Canada)
Pediatrics 126:e374-e381, 2010

Background.—Much disagreement exists as to whether postconcussion syndrome (PCS) is attributable to brain injury or to other factors such as trauma alone, preexisting psychosocial problems, or medicolegal issues. We investigated the epidemiology and natural history of PCS symptoms in a large cohort of children with a mild traumatic brain injury (mTBI) and compared them with children with an extracranial injury (ECI).

Methods.—This investigation was a prospective, consecutive controlled-cohort study of 670 children who presented to a tertiary referral emergency department with mTBI and 197 children who presented with ECI. For all participants, data were collected by use of a telephone interview of a parent 7 to 10 days after injury. If a change from preinjury symptoms was reported by a parent, follow-up continued monthly until symptom resolution. Outcomes were measured by using the Post Concussion Symptom Inventory, Rivermead Postconcussion Symptom Questionnaire, Brief Symptom Inventory, and Family Assessment Device.

Results.—There was a significant difference between the mTBI and ECI groups in their survival curves for time to symptom resolution (log rank

[Mantel-Cox] 11.15, $P < .001$). Three months after injury, 11% of the children in the mTBI group were symptomatic (13.7% of children older than 6 years) compared with 0.5% of the children in the ECI group. The prevalence of persistent symptoms at 1 year was 2.3% in the mTBI group and 0.01% in the ECI group. Family functioning and maternal adjustment did not differ between groups.

Conclusions.—Among school-aged children with mTBI, 13.7% were symptomatic 3 months after injury. This finding could not be explained by trauma, family dysfunction, or maternal psychological adjustment. The results of this study provide clear support for the validity of the diagnosis of PCS in children.

▶ This is a very useful prospective study of a large number, 670 children who presented to a tertiary emergency department with a mild traumatic brain injury and 197 children who presented to the same emergency department with primarily orthopedic injuries. The intent of the study was to contrast these 2 populations and to see if among the school-age children with mild traumatic brain injury there was a significantly greater incidence of postconcussion syndrome at 3 months and 1 year time as compared with the group of individuals with primarily orthopedic nonbrain injuries.

There was a clear-cut, highly statistically significant difference between the incidence of postconcussion syndrome in the head-injured group as compared with the orthopedic-injured group at 3 months and at 1 year. This lends direct support to the fact that the occurrence of postconcussion syndrome in head-injured individuals in most instances is due to the head injury itself and not due to psychological factors. Also of significance in this study is that while there was a 2.3% incidence of postconcussion symptoms in the head-injured group at 1 year, this is a relatively small fraction of the 14% that was present at 3 months. Therefore, this study lends reassurance that in most pediatric aged children, postconcussion symptoms will clear in 1 year's time. The role of proper education and reassurance soon after injury has been shown to reduce postconcussion symptoms in adults, yet there is no such evidence in children. Clearly, further research in this area is warranted.

R. C. Cantu, MD, MA

Longitudinal Changes in the Health-Related Quality of Life During the First Year After Traumatic Brain Injury
Lin M-R, Chiu W-T, Chen Y-J, et al (Taipei Med Univ, Taiwan; Cathay General Hosp, Taipei, Taiwan; et al)
Arch Phys Med Rehabil 91:474-480, 2010

Objective.—To track the health-related quality of life (HRQL) at discharge and at 6 and 12 months after a traumatic brain injury (TBI) and examine factors associated with changes in each HRQL domain.

Design.—Longitudinal cohort study.

Setting.—Using codes of the *International Classification of Diseases*, eligible participants who had a newly diagnosed TBI were identified from discharge records of 4 hospitals in northern Taiwan. Information on the HRQL and injury-related characteristics at the initial and 2 follow-up assessments was collected by extracting medical records and conducting telephone interviews.

Participants.—Subjects (N = 158) participated in the initial assessment, and 147 and 146, respectively, completed the follow-up assessments at 6 and 12 months after injury.

Interventions.—Not applicable.

Main Outcome Measure.—The brief version of the World Health Organization Quality of Life (WHOQOL-BREF) with 4 domains of physical capacity, psychologic well being, social relationships, and environment.

Results.—Scores on all WHOQOL-BREF domains except social relationships greatly improved over the first 6 months and showed continued improvement at 12 months after injury. The domain scores of the WHOQOL-BREF at discharge were significantly associated with the pre-injury HRQL level, marital status, alcohol consumption at the time of injury, Glasgow Outcome Scale (GOS) level, cognition, activities of daily living, social support, and depressive status. However, after adjusting for these baseline differences, only the GOS level and depressive status significantly influenced longitudinal changes in the psychologic and social domains over the 12-month period. Changes in the physical and environmental domains were not significantly associated with any characteristics of the study.

Conclusions.—During the first year after a TBI, the magnitude of HRQL recovery differed across different HRQL domains. Many factors may have significant associations with the initial domain scores of HRQL after TBI; however, only a few factors can significantly influence longitudinal changes in the HRQL.

▶ This study describes health-related quality of life over the span of 1 year postinjury for 158 persons with a traumatic brain injury. There was improvement in health-related quality of life in all 4 domains of the brief version of the World Health Organization Quality of Life questionnaire: physical capacity, psychological well-being, social relationships, and environment; however, after adjustment for preinjury scores and other covariates, there was no significant change in the social relationship domain. Severity and depressive status were associated with changes in psychologic and social domains. These results highlight the need for development of improved interventions at the social level. Limitations of the study were that preinjury assessment of health-related quality of life was done retrospectively, that is, collected at the hospital discharge interview, and the sample had a lower representation of those with severe traumatic brain injury. There may also be problems with validity of telephone interviews and recall among persons with traumatic brain injury. A possible solution would have been the use of proxy respondents for some of the persons with cognitive impairments.

D. E. Feldman, PT, PhD

Pediatric Concussions in United States Emergency Departments in the Years 2002 to 2006
Meehan WP III, Mannix R (Children's Hosp Boston, MA)
J Pediatr 157:889-893, 2010

Objectives.—To estimate the incidence and demographics of concussions in children coming to emergency departments (EDs) in the United States and describe the rates of neuroimaging and follow-up instructions in these patients.

Study Design.—This is a cross-sectional study of children 0 to 19 years old diagnosed with concussion from the National Hospital Ambulatory Medical Care Survey. National Hospital Ambulatory Medical Care Survey collects data on approximately 25 000 visits annually to 600 randomly selected hospital emergency and outpatient departments. We examined visits to United States emergency departments between 2002 and 2006. Simple descriptive statistics were used.

Results.—Of the 50 835 pediatric visits in the 5-year sample, 230 observations, representing 144 000 visits annually, were for concussions. Sixty-nine percent of concussion visits were by males. Thirty percent were sports-related. Sixty-nine percent of patients diagnosed with a concussion had head imaging. Twenty-eight percent of patients were discharged without specific instructions to follow-up with an outpatient provider for further treatment.

Conclusions.—Approximately 144 000 pediatric patients present to emergency departments each year with a concussion. Most of these patients undergo computed tomography of the head, and nearly one-third are discharged without specific instructions to follow-up with an outpatient provider for further treatment.

▶ This was a study of children who presented in emergency departments in the United States over a 5-year period. Perhaps the most striking finding was that the most common mechanism of concussion was a sports-related injury. With this in mind, it was particularly discouraging that nearly a similar percentage of children were not given instructions in terms of following up with an outpatient provider. Only by proper follow-up and assessment could it be determined when one has recovered from concussion and when one could safely return to the sports-related activity that caused the concussion in the first place.

The authors correctly pointed out that the severity of a concussion could not be determined nor should it be at the time of the initial assessment in the emergency department, as delayed symptoms could not be predicted with accuracy and the duration that symptoms might last could not be predicted with accuracy. Since the severity of a concussion is most related to the number, duration, and severity of symptoms, this is something that should never be totally concluded until one has made a complete recovery from a concussion.

It was also of interest that nearly 70% of concussions were assessed with a computerized axial tomography scan to rule out a structural lesion. This certainly does raise the concern for the amount of radiation that is given in a situation where the likelihood of a structural lesion might be quite low if symptoms are minimal and improving at the time the individual is seen in the emergency department.

This is a useful article that points out how the care delivered for concussion could be improved in our emergency departments, which I suspect has been improved in the years since this study was done.

R. C. Cantu, MD, MA

Biomechanical Properties of Concussions in High School Football
Broglio SP, Schnebel B, Sosnoff JJ, et al (Univ of Illinois at Urbana-Champaign, IL; Univ of Oklahoma, Norman; et al)
Med Sci Sports Exerc 42:2064-2071, 2010

Introduction.—Sport concussion represents the majority of brain injuries occurring in the United States with 1.6—3.8 million cases annually. Understanding the biomechanical properties of this injury will support the development of better diagnostics and preventative techniques.

Methods.—We monitored all football related head impacts in 78 high school athletes (mean age = 16.7 yr) from 2005 to 2008 to better understand the biomechanical characteristics of concussive impacts.

Results.—Using the Head Impact Telemetry System, a total of 54,247 impacts were recorded, and 13 concussive episodes were captured for analysis. A classification and regression tree analysis of impacts indicated that rotational acceleration (>5582.3 rad·s^{-2}), linear acceleration (>96.1 g), and impact location (front, top, and back) yielded the highest predictive value of concussion.

Conclusions.—These threshold values are nearly identical with those reported at the collegiate and professional level. If the Head Impact Telemetry System were implemented for medical use, sideline personnel can expect to diagnose one of every five athletes with a concussion when the impact exceeds these tolerance levels. Why all athletes did not sustain a concussion when the impacts generated variables in excess of our threshold criteria is not entirely clear, although individual differences between participants may play a role. A similar threshold to concussion in adolescent athletes compared with their collegiate and professional counterparts suggests an equal concussion risk at all levels of play.

▶ Using the Head Impact Telemetry System (HIT), these authors recorded a total of 54 247 impacts in which 13 concussive episodes were documented in a 4-year study of high school football players. The authors concluded that when there were rotational accelerations greater than 5582.3 radians per second squared and linear accelerations greater than 96.1g and the impact was to the front, top, or back of the helmet, the highest predictive value of concussion was attained. Using these 3 criteria, the authors had a positive predictive value of 13.4%. Like other studies, this study used HIT's data on collegiate athletes and theoretically calculated data on professional football players. Also similar to other studies, this study tried to explain why the positive predictive value is not higher. Perhaps a more basic question is whether the HIT's system itself accurately reflects the head impact accelerations that are received by football players on the field. Whereas the system probably does function and has been validated with regard to hits through the center of gravity of the head, we know that many hits to the helmet, if not most, are tangential in nature, and it is probable that the recordings for these hits may be falsely low. It is also known that the helmet deforms when it is hit and also slides on the scalp. The role of fit, hair gel, and do-rags worn by many players today on the accuracy of these recordings is not currently known. Thus, it may be that the reason why we are not able to use these biomechanical data to better predict concussion is that the data themselves are far less reliable than suggested by validation studies that are carried out in the laboratory and involve hits to hybrid 3 mounted head forms that are truly through the center of gravity.

R. C. Cantu, MD, MA

Ski Helmets Could Attenuate the Sounds of Danger
Tudor A, Ruzic L, Bencic I, et al (Univ of Rijeka, Croatia; Univ of Zagreb, Croatia)
Clin J Sport Med 20:173-178, 2010

Objective.—To determine whether a ski helmet reduces skiers' hearing particularly sounds that can warn skiers of potentially dangerous situations.

Design.—Randomized repeated measures (first part), environmental field measurements (second part).

Setting.—Audiology Centre of Rijeka Medical School, ski slopes at Platak resort.

Participants.—Thirty healthy subjects not used to wearing a helmet each served as their own control.

Intervention.—Ski cap, ski helmet, and no intervention in randomized order.

Main Outcome Measurements.—Laboratory open-field audiometric testing: bareheaded, ski cap, and ski helmet (0.125-8 kHz protocol), and environmental A-weighted sound measurements on the slope for potentially dangerous situations like snowboarder breaking or skier passing by. In both parts of the study, the sound pressure levels (dB) and sound spectrum frequencies were analyzed.

Results.—First part—No differences were found between bare head and wearing only a ski cap. Significant sound attenuation characteristics of the helmet were determined for frequencies 2, 4, and 8 kHz ($P < 0.001$).

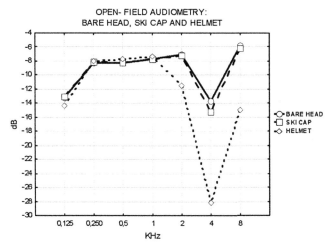

FIGURE 2.—Mean thresholds were calculated for all 3 situations. The dotted line shows sound attenuation that is most apparent between 1 and 8 kHz. (Reprinted from Tudor A, Ruzic L, Bencic I, et al. Ski helmets could attenuate the sounds of danger. *Clin J Sport Med.* 2010;20:173-178, with permission from Lippincott Williams & Wilkins.)

Second part—High sound pressure levels were found for all the danger sounds measured on the slope, especially at frequencies that were most affected by helmet sound attenuation (2-8 kHz) in previously conducted laboratory tests.

Conclusions.—Helmets could influence the level of the hearing threshold in frequencies between 2 and 8 KHz. The spectrum of danger sounds on the slope has high pressure levels at frequencies that were most affected by helmet sound attenuation characteristics (2-8 kHz), so the helmet wearers might misinterpret the sounds of potentially dangerous situations because the sound might be distorted (Fig 2).

▶ I learned about the potential of safety equipment to cause a drastic loss of sensory input during my years of research at the UK Chemical Defence Research Establishment. The respirators designed at that establishment were excellent in terms of protecting personnel against chemical warfare agents, but they imposed many severe ergonomic penalties, not the least of which were a restriction of the visual field and difficulties in speaking and in hearing.[1] However, relatively little attention has been given to the sensory limitations imposed by the protective equipment used in sports. One report noted that 21% of those wearing ski helmets felt their hearing was impaired,[2] and a second survey found that 35% of ski patrollers cited potential hearing loss as a reason for not wearing helmets.[3] This study by Tudor and associates is based on careful audiometry. The subjects were not normally involved in skiing to avoid bias from previous opinions. Observations demonstrated a substantial loss of hearing in the frequency band judged as most critical to safety (2-8 kHz, Fig 2). Helmet wearers were able to hear warning sounds at an intensity of over 20 to 30 dB, meaning noises louder than quiet conversation, but often the information was distorted, so that there seems to be a need for the re-education of skiers regarding the characteristics of dangerous noises when wearing a protective helmet. There may also be scope for a study identifying the number of accidents caused by misinterpretations of sound when wearing a helmet.

R. J. Shephard, MD (Lond), PhD, DPE

References

1. Shephard RJ. The design and use of respirators. In: Davies CN, ed. *Ergonomics of the Respirator.* London: Pergamon Press; 1961.
2. Ruzic L, Tudor A. Injury risk ski behavior in helmet wearers and non-wearers. In: Senner V, Fatenbauer V, Bohm H, eds. *Abstracts of the XVII Congress of the International Society for Skiing Safety.* Munchen: Tecnhische Universitaet; 2009:15-16.
3. Evans B, Gervais JT, Heard K, et al. Ski patrollers: reluctant role models for helmet use. *Int J Inj Contr Saf Promot.* 2009;16:9-14.

The effectiveness of helmet wear in skiers and snowboarders: a systematic review
Cusimano MD, Kwok J (St Michael's Hosp, Toronto, Ontario, Canada; Injury Prevention Res Office, Toronto, Ontario, Canada)
Br J Sports Med 44:781-786, 2010

Objective.—To summarise the best available evidence to determine the impact of helmet use on head injuries, neck injuries and cervical spine injuries in skiers and snowboarders.

Data Sources.—Relevant publications were identified through electronic searches of MEDLINE, PubMed, EMBASE, CINAHL and the Cochrane Library databases (1966—2009) in addition to manual reference checks of all included articles.

Review Methods.—45 articles were identified through our systematic literature search. Of these, 10 studies met the inclusion criteria after two levels of screening. Two independent reviewers critically appraised the studies. Data were extracted on the primary outcomes of interest: Head injury, neck injury and cervical spine injury. Studies were assessed for quality by the criteria of Downs and Black.

Results.—Studies reviewed indicate that helmet wear reduces the risk of head injuries in skiing and snowboarding. Four case-control studies reported a reduction in the risk of head injury with helmet use ranging from 15% to 60%. Another cohort study found a significantly lower incidence of head injuries involving loss of consciousness in helmet users (p<0.05). The five remaining studies suggested a major protective effect of helmets by indicating that none or few of the head-injured and deceased participants wore a helmet.

Conclusions.—There is strong evidence to support the protective value of helmets in reducing the risk of head injuries in skiing and snowboarding.

There is no good evidence to support the claim that the use of helmets leads to an increase risk of cervical spine injuries or neck injuries.

▶ Injuries to the head, neck, and cervical spine in skiers and snowboarders are common because of falls or collisions with other skiers or snowboarders and collisions with fixed inanimate objects, such as trees. It has been presumed that the use of helmets during these sports would help to prevent concussions, but some have questioned whether the use of helmets will actually increase cervical spine injuries, particularly in children who have a greater head-to-body ratio. However, there are no large-scale trials (certainly no double-blind randomized control trials [RCTs], for obvious reasons), and evidence to support the latter concept has been somewhat limited.

This systematic review was only able to identify 10 studies that met the inclusion criteria after 2 levels of screening by independent reviewers. There were 4 case-control series (the next strongest level of evidence after RCTs), 3 case series, 2 retrospective cohort studies, and 1 cross-sectional study. By critically analyzing the results of these studies and calculating odds ratios, the authors of this review were able to conclude that helmet use does significantly reduce the risk of concussions (up to 15%-60%) without increasing the risk of neck or cervical spine injuries. This will be important information for policymakers, ski resort owners, parents, and participants in these fast high-impact winter sports. There was no indication of the types of helmets used in these studies. Therefore, the next critical area to research relates to the manufacturing, testing, and standardized approval of such helmets.

C. Lebrun, MD

Cheerleading-Related Injuries in the United States: A Prospective Surveillance Study

Shields BJ, Smith GA (The Res Inst at Nationwide Children's Hosp, Columbus, OH; Ohio State Univ College of Medicine, Columbus)
J Athl Train 44:567-577, 2009

Context.—Cheerleading injuries are on the rise and are a significant source of injury to females. No published studies have described the epidemiology of cheerleading injuries by type of cheerleading team and event.

Objective.—To describe the epidemiology of cheerleading injuries and to calculate injury rates by type of cheerleading team and event.

Design.—Prospective injury surveillance study.

Setting.—Participant exposure and injury data were collected from US cheerleading teams via the Cheerleading RIO (Reporting Information Online) online surveillance tool.

Patients or Other Participants.—Athletes from enrolled cheerleading teams who participated in official, organized cheerleading practices, pep rallies, athletic events, or cheerleading competitions.

Main Outcome Measure(s).—The numbers and rates of cheerleading injuries during a 1-year period (2006–2007) are reported by team type and event type.

Results.—A cohort of 9022 cheerleaders on 412 US cheerleading teams participated in the study. During the 1-year period, 567 cheerleading injuries were reported; 83% (467/565) occurred during practice, 52% (296/565) occurred while the cheerleader was attempting a stunt, and 24% (132/563) occurred while the cheerleader was basing or spotting 1 or more cheerleaders. Lower extremity injuries (30%, 168/565) and strains and sprains (53%, 302/565) were most common. Collegiate cheerleaders were more likely to sustain a concussion ($P = .01$, rate ratio [RR] = 2.98, 95% confidence interval [CI] = 1.34, 6.59), and All Star cheerleaders were more likely to sustain a fracture or dislocation ($P = .01$, RR = 1.76, 95% CI = 1.16, 2.66) than were cheerleaders on other types of teams. Overall injury rates for practices, pep rallies, athletic events, and cheerleading competitions were 1.0, 0.6, 0.6, and 1.4 injuries per 1000 athlete-exposures, respectively.

Conclusions.—We are the first to report cheerleading injury rates based on actual exposure data by type of team and event. These injury rates are lower than those reported for other high school and collegiate sports; however, many cheerleading injuries are preventable.

▶ This assessment of cheerleading injuries reminds us that prevention of injuries during exercise activities should not be limited to just competitive athletes. Anyone who has watched a good cheerleading squad cannot help being impressed with the athleticism that goes into this activity. Therefore, that significant injuries can occur in the course of cheerleading comes as no surprise. It would seem important that cheerleaders view themselves like the competitors they cheer on. They need to be physically ready for their strenuous activities and that includes proper training, stretching, and diet—all the components that we know go into successful athletic play. One can expect that a fit cheerleader will be less prone to the injuries outlined in this article.

T. Rowland, MD

Skeletal Scintigraphy in Pediatric Sports Medicine

Zukotynski K, Grant FD, Curtis C, et al (Dana-Farber Cancer Inst and Harvard Med School, Boston, MA; Children's Hosp Boston and Harvard Med School, MA)
AJR Am J Roentgenol 195:1212-1219, 2010

Objective.—Athletes can have pain derived from fractures or alternate pathology. Skeletal scintigraphy may detect abnormalities before anatomic imaging and provides a practical tool for whole-body imaging. However, study interpretation in children can be challenging. This pictorial essay describes a technique for pediatric skeletal scintigraphy and reviews findings commonly encountered in athletes.

Conclusion.—Skeletal scintigraphy complements anatomic findings in pediatric athletes. Familiarity with imaging technique and study interpretation can improve diagnosis.

▶ New methods for early diagnosis of serious sports injuries are always welcome. This article introduces the imaging technique of skeletal scintigraphy for detecting pathology in young athletes. As the authors point out, interpretation of abnormal findings, particularly in youth, can be challenging. What we now need to see is whether a learning curve in the use of this methodology will confirm its clinical use or whether the challenges of interpretation will serve as a difficult obstacle. Issues of cost and availability will also need to be considered as the use of this technique evolves.

T. Rowland, MD

2 Other Musculoskeletal Injuries

Standardization of Adverse Event Terminology and Reporting in Orthopaedic Physical Therapy: Application to the Cervical Spine
Carlesso LC, Macdermid JC, Santaguida LP (McMaster Univ, Hamilton, Ontario, Canada; St Joseph's Health Centre, London, Ontario, Canada)
J Orthop Sports Phys Ther 40:455-463, 2010

Synopsis.—Orthopaedic physical therapy is considered safe, based on a lack of reported harms. Most of the research until now has focused on benefits. Consideration of benefits and harm involves informed consent, clinical decision making, and cost-benefit analyses. Benefits and harms are treatment and dosage specific. There is currently an insufficient number of dosage trials in orthopaedic physical therapy to identify optimal dosage for common interventions, including exercise and manual therapy. Published cases of severe adverse events following chiropractic manipulation illustrate the need for physical therapy to have high-quality data documenting the safety of orthopaedic physical therapy, including cervical manipulation. A recent systematic review identified poor reporting standards of harms within clinical research in this area. Lack of standardization of terminology has contributed to this problem. Pharmacovigilence provides a framework for terms that orthopaedic physical therapy can adapt and thereafter adopt into clinical practice and research. Adverse events are unexpected events that occur following an intervention without evidence of causality. Where temporality of an event is highly suggestive of causality, the term "adverse reaction" may be more appropriate. Future studies in orthopaedic physical therapy should adopt the CONSORT statement extension on the reporting of harms, published in 2004, to ensure better reporting. Consistent reporting of harms in both research and clinical practice requires professional consensus on terminology pertaining to harms, as well as defining what constitutes an adverse event or an adverse reaction. Widespread consultation and consensus should support optimal definitions and processes and facilitate their implementation into practice. This paper is focused on theoretical considerations and evidence in terms of harm reporting within physical therapy using cervical manual therapy as an example.

▶ This article highlights an important and often neglected issue: the reporting (or lack thereof) of adverse events or harms. The example of cervical spine manual physical therapy is used to illustrate the need for standardization of terminology and inclusion of the patient perspective. In their systematic review, the authors show the differences in reporting of harms in cervical spine manual therapy trials. They conclude with 5 recommendations regarding reporting of harms: (1) using defined and clear terms to describe harms in physical therapy; (2) the adoption of consistent clinical documentation in reporting of harms in physical therapy practice; (3) the establishment of reporting harms as an important component of physical therapy clinical research; (4) using the extended Consolidated Standards of Reporting Trials criteria for reporting harms in randomized clinical trials in physical therapy research; and (5) development of clear evidence-based tools to assist patients in making informed decisions regarding orthopedic physical therapy and transfer of these tools for use in clinical settings.

D. E. Feldman, PT, PhD

A Comparison of Neck Movement In the Soft Cervical Collar and Rigid Cervical Brace in Healthy Subjects

Whitcroft KL, Massouh L, Amirfeyz R, et al (Univ of Bristol, UK; Bristol Royal Infirmary, UK; et al)
J Manipulative Physiol Ther 34:119-122, 2011

Objective.—The soft cervical collar has been prescribed for whiplash injury but has been shown to be clinically ineffective. As some authors report superior results for managing whiplash injury with a cervical brace, we were interested in comparing the mechanical effectiveness of the soft collar with a rigid cervical brace. Therefore, the purpose of this study was to measure ranges of motion in subjects without neck pain using a soft cervical collar and a rigid brace compared with no orthosis.

Methods.—Fifty healthy subjects (no neck or shoulder pain) aged 22 to 67 years were recruited for this study. Neck movement was measured using a cervical range of motion goniometer. Active flexion, extension, right and left lateral flexion, and right and left rotation were assessed in each subject under 3 conditions: no collar, a soft collar, and a rigid cervical brace.

Results.—The soft collar and rigid brace reduced neck movement compared with no brace or collar, but the cervical brace was more effective at reducing motion. The soft collar reduced movement on average by 17.4%; and the cervical brace, by 62.9%. The effect of the orthoses was not affected by age, although older subjects had stiffer necks.

Conclusion.—Based on the data of the 50 subjects presented in this study, the soft cervical collar did not adequately immobilize the cervical spine.

▶ Whiplash injuries are common. Conservative treatment of whiplash-associated disorders often includes various interventions to relieve pain and stiffness and promote mobility and function. Although immobilization appears to be contraindicated, short-term use of collars are still used at times to relieve pain, especially in the acute phase. This study compares the use of soft cervical collars and rigid cervical braces in healthy subjects to determine just how much movement is limited by these devices. Not surprisingly, the results indicate that the soft collar does not limit much of the cervical range of motion. The authors conclude that the soft cervical collar does not adequately immobilize the cervical spine. While this may be true, the effect of the soft cervical collar to decrease pain in the acute phase following a whiplash injury needs to be evaluated. However, based on current evidence, long-term immobilization by any device after injury is not recommended.

D. E. Feldman, PT, PhD

A Comparison of Thoracolumbosacral Orthoses and SpineCor Treatment of Adolescent Idiopathic Scoliosis Patients Using the Scoliosis Research Society Standardized Criteria

Gammon SR, Mehlman CT, Chan W, et al (Univ of Cincinnati, OH; et al)
J Pediatr Orthop 30:531-538, 2010

Background.—SpineCor is a relatively new bracing system that uses dynamic bracing concepts in the treatment of adolescent idiopathic scoliosis (AIS). Limited data are available regarding its effectiveness. This study compared treatment outcomes of 2 groups of AIS patients treated via either a conventional rigid thoracolumbosacral orthoses (TLSO) or a SpineCor nonrigid orthosis.

Methods.—We identified 2 scoliosis patient cohorts: 35 patients treated with a TLSO and 32 patients treated with a SpineCor orthosis. All patients included in these groups conformed with the Scoliosis Research Society (SRS) standardized criteria for AIS bracing: (1) Risser ≤2, (2) curve magnitude 25 to 40 degrees, (3) age ≥10 years. Outcomes were SRS standardized with failure being defined as curve progression ≥6 degrees, or ever exceeding 45 degrees, or having surgery recommended before skeletal maturity. All patients were followed through the completion of brace treatment or attainment of other treatment end points. The Yates corrected χ^2 test and unpaired *t* test were used for data analysis.

Results.—The 35 patients (32 girls, 3 boys) in the TLSO group had an average age of 13 years (range: 11.1-16.8) and an average primary curve magnitude of 33 degrees (range: 25-40 degrees). Follow-up averaged 2 years (range: 8-61 m) from the beginning of brace treatment. The 32 patients (28 girls, 4 boys) in the SpineCor group had an average age of 13 years (range: 11-15.2) and an average primary curve magnitude of 31 degrees (range: 25-40 degrees). Follow-up for this group averaged 2 years and 6 months (range: 13-73 mo) from the beginning of brace treatment. No significant difference ($P = 0.75$) was found using the more strict outcome measure (≤ 5-degree curve progression) as the success rates were 60% (21/35) for TLSO and 53% (17/32) for SpineCor. Similarly, no significant difference ($P = 0.62$) was found using the more liberal outcome measure (never reached 45 degrees) as the success rates were 80% (28/35) for TLSO and 72% (23/32) for SpineCor.

Conclusions.—We were unable to identify any significant differences in brace treatment outcomes when comparing TLSO and SpineCor treated patients.

▶ The treatment of adolescent idiopathic scoliosis (AIS) is largely conservative. There are a number of braces on the market, but the most commonly used are the traditional thoracolumbosacral rigid orthosis (TLSO) and more recently, the SpineCor nonrigid orthosis. The significance of this article is that it is the largest study to date using the Scoliosis Research Society (SRS) standardized criteria for AIS bracing. Although this was a retrospective cohort study, a reasonable number of patients using each brace were evaluated using either a strict outcome measure ($\leq 5°$ curve progression) or a more liberal outcome measure (never reach 45°). The success rates of bracing and outcomes when comparing the TLSO- and SpineCor-treated patients were not significantly different. Similarly, the percentage of patients requiring surgery or having surgery prior to skeletal maturation was not different between groups. Further prospective studies using larger number of patients are needed to further validate these findings. It will also be very interesting to evaluate both the compliance and quality of life in patients using these 2 orthoses. The more dynamic SpineCor brace fits under the clothing and is not as evident as the more rigid TLSO brace. As both appear to be similarly effective, these characteristics may determine patient preference and physician prescribing practices.

C. Lebrun, MD

A two-year sonographic follow-up after intratendinous injection therapy in patients with tennis elbow
Zeisig E, Fahlström M, Öhberg L, et al (Univ of Umeå, Sweden)
Br J Sports Med 44:584-587, 2010

Background.—Tennis elbow is a tendinopathy affecting the upper extremity. Recent studies have shown high sensitivity for ultrasound (US) examination and high specificity for colour Doppler (CD) examination. There are no mid- or long-term follow-up investigations of the tendon structure and blood flow using these techniques.

Objective.—To use US and CD to study structure and blood flow in the extensor origin in patients with tennis elbow treated with intratendinous injections.

Design.—Follow-up study.

Setting.—Sports Medicine Unit, Umeå University.

Patients.—25 patients (28 elbows), mean age 46 years (range 27–66), treated with intratendinous injections due to chronic pain from tennis elbow.

Method.—US and CD examination of the extensor origin was carried out at inclusion and at follow-up two years after intratendinous injection treatment with polidocanol and/or a local anaesthetic.

Main Outcome Measurements.—US (structure) and CD (blood flow) findings.

Results.—All patients had structural tendon changes and high blood flow at inclusion when given the injection treatment. At the two-year follow-up, structural tendon changes were seen in 20/28 elbows and high blood flow was seen in 4/28 elbows. The majority of patients with a good clinical result after treatment had no visible blood flow (17/20), but the structural changes showed no relation to a good result (13/20 remaining changes).

Conclusions.—Doppler findings, but not structure, might be related to the clinical result after intratendinous injection treatment of tennis elbow (Fig 1).

▶ This study is important because of 2 separate findings, the first being an improvement in symptoms of tendinopathy in the 25 patients (28 elbows) with tennis elbow who were treated with ultrasound (US)-guided intratendinous injections of polidocanol and/or a local anesthetic. The second is because of the use of high-sensitivity US examination using color Doppler (CD) examination in an attempt to visualize the pathology. This useful tool is being increasingly used in clinical settings both in Europe and North America to diagnose and treat various musculoskeletal pathologies. Many of the US Primary Care Sports Medicine Fellowship programs are now teaching the use of diagnostic US, and curricula are being developed. While it is true that a trained radiologist with a special interest in diagnostic US will be more skilled in conducting and interpreting these studies, nevertheless, primary care physicians can benefit from using diagnostic US to diagnose many common sport medicine soft tissue conditions and to guide various interventions such as injections.

As noted in most of the previous studies, there was essentially no change in the gray-scale US appearance of the lateral elbows on scanning in those patients with an improvement in their symptoms. There is only 1 previous investigation that has reported resolution of the sonographic findings.[1] However, there was a diminution in the areas of high blood flow, as visualized with CD (Fig 1a-e). This study is strengthened by the fact that a single experienced radiologist with 25 years of experience performed and interpreted all the scans both at baseline and at the 2-year follow-up time (and at the time of the second examination, he was blinded to whether or not that elbow had been treated).

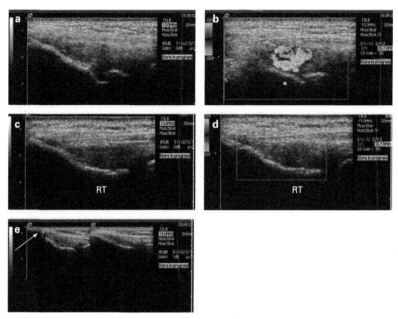

FIGURE 1.—Patients clinically diagnosed to have tennis elbow. The extensor origin is shown in a longitudinal view. (a) Grey-scale ultrasonography (US) shows irregular structure and hypoechogenity in the extensor origin. (b) Colour Doppler (CD) shows blood-flow inside the area with structural changes in the extensor origin. (c) US of the same patient two years later. (d) CD shows no blood-flow inside the area with structural changes in the extensor origin after two years. (e) US of the extensor origin on both sides after two years, the affected (left) and unaffected (right). Note the bone spur (arrow). (Reprinted from Zeisig E, Fahlström M, Öhberg L, et al and reproduced with permission from the BMJ Publishing Group. A two-year sonographic follow-up after intratendinous injection therapy in patients with tennis elbow. *Br J Sports Med.* 2010;44:584-587.)

It remains to be seen what the most effective intratendinous injection is for these chronic tendinopathies: corticosteroids, local anesthetic, polidocanol, platelet-rich plasma, or autologous blood. Perhaps it is simply the act of needling or disrupting the tissue in the abnormal areas of tendinopathy that is responsible for stimulating healing. Further studies using larger groups of subjects and different modes of imaging are needed to help answer these questions.

C. Lebrun, MD

Reference

1. Lind B, Ohberg L, Alfredson H. Sclerosing polidocanol injections in mid-portion Achilles tendinosis: remaining good clinical results and decreased tendon thickness at 2-year follow-up. *Knee Surg Sports Traumatol Arthrosc.* 2006;14:1327-1332.

The Value of Using Radiographic Criteria for the Treatment of Persistent Symptomatic Olecranon Physis in Adolescent Throwing Athletes

Matsuura T, Kashiwaguchi S, Iwase T, et al (The Univ of Tokushima Graduate School, Japan; Tokyo Kosei-nenkin Hosp, Japan; Tokushima Natl Hosp, Japan)
Am J Sports Med 38:141-145, 2010

Background.—Previously published reports present a variety of nonoperative and operative treatments for a persistent olecranon physis. However, the radiographic indication for the operative treatment is not clear.

Hypothesis.—Our radiographic classification of persistent olecranon physis is helpful in formulating treatment decisions.

Study Design.—Cohort study; Level of evidence, 3.

Methods.—Sixteen male baseball players with persistent olecranon physis were retrospectively evaluated. The mean age at first presentation was 14.7 years (range, 12-17 years). The lesion was classified into 2 stages based on radiographic appearance. Stage I demonstrated widening of the olecranon epiphyseal plate when compared with the contralateral elbow on the lateral view. Sclerotic change indicated stage II. All patients underwent nonoperative treatment for at least 3 months. Follow-up radiographs were taken at 1-month intervals. Operative treatment was provided to the patients whose condition had failed to improve after nonoperative treatment.

Results.—Of the 16 patients, 12 had stage I lesions and 4 had stage II lesions. Nonoperative management produced healing in 91.7% of patients with stage I lesions and none of the patients with stage II lesions.

Conclusion.—Our radiographic classification of persistent olecranon physis is useful for treatment decision making. In addition, our results demonstrated that sclerotic change is a high predictive indicator of the need for operative treatment.

▶ This is an interesting case series on 16 male baseball players with symptomatic olecranon physis injury. The authors put forth a radiologic classification that may be useful to indicate treatment plans. However, this is an extremely small sample with only 4 patients in their stage II category. Furthermore, it appears that bone age may work to classify patients to appropriate treatment as well because 4 of 5 who did not heal with conservative treatment had closed physes. Thus, having a closed physis with this condition may be an indication for surgical intervention. Nevertheless, it does appear that the radiologic classification is helpful, but confirmation in a larger sample should be done.

D. E. Feldman, PT, PhD

A Meta-analysis Examining Clinical Test Utility for Assessing Superior Labral Anterior Posterior Lesions

Meserve BB, Cleland JA, Boucher TR (Dartmouth Hitchcock Med Ctr, Lebanon, NH; Franklin Pierce College, Concord, NH; Plymouth State Univ, NH)
Am J Sports Med 37:2252-2258, 2009

Background.—The reported accuracy of clinical tests for superior labral anterior posterior lesions is extremely variable. Pooling results from multiple studies of higher quality is necessary to establish the best clinical tests to use.

Hypothesis.—Certain clinical tests are superior to others for diagnosing the presence or absence of a superior labral anterior posterior lesion.

Study Design.—Meta-analysis.

Methods.—A literature search of MEDLINE (1966-2007), CINAHL (1982-2007), and BIOSIS (1995-2007) was performed for (labrum OR labral OR SLAP OR Bankart) AND (shoulder OR shoulder joint OR glenoid) AND (specificity OR sensitivity AND specificity). Identified articles were reviewed for inclusion criteria. Sensitivity and specificity values were recorded from each study and used for meta-analysis.

Results.—Six of 198 identified studies satisfied the eligibility criteria. Active compression, anterior slide, crank, and Speed tests were analyzed using receiver operating characteristic curves. The accuracy of the anterior slide test was significantly inferior to that of the active compression, crank, and Speed tests. There was no significant difference in test accuracy found among active compression, crank, and Speed tests. Between studies, methodological scores did not significantly affect sensitivity and specificity values.

Conclusion.—The anterior slide test is a poor test for detecting the presence of a labral lesion in the shoulder. Active compression, crank, and

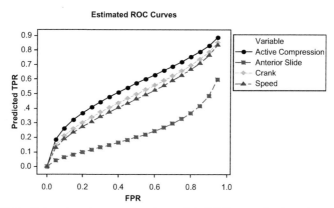

FIGURE 2.—Estimated receiver operating characteristic (ROC) curves for the active compression, anterior slide, crank, and Speed tests. (Reprinted from Meserve BB, Cleland JA, Boucher TR. A meta-analysis examining clinical test utility for assessing superior labral anterior posterior lesions. *Am J Sports Med.* 2009;37:2252-2258, with permission from The Author(s).)

Speed tests are more optimal choices. Clinicians should choose the active compression test first, crank second, and Speed test third when a labral lesion is suspected (Fig 2).

▶ The need for simple, practical, and evidence-based clinical tests cannot be emphasized enough. This article is a step toward fulfilling this need. It is important to note that conducting a systematic review and pooling the data for a meta-analysis of diagnostic studies have challenges. This study systematically investigated the diagnostic accuracy of 3 commonly used tests for labral injuries. A strength of this meta-analysis was that the authors used the rigorous Cochrane criteria. The practical conclusion was that clinicians can use the active compression test as a screening tool (high sensitivity) followed by the crank test and the Speed test in that order as confirmatory tests (higher specificity) (Fig 2). To increase certainty, clinicians are advised to combine the findings of the 3 tests. Given that these tests can all be done quickly, I recommend that clinicians use the combination. This study suggests that the anterior slide test adds very little; it may now disappear from favor.

K. Khan, MD

Pain Relief, Motion, and Function after Rotator Cuff Repair or Reconstruction May Not Persist after 16 Years

Borgmästars N, Paavola M, Remes V, et al (ORTON Orthopaedic Hosp, Tenholantie, Helsinki, Finland; Helsinki Univ Hosp, Finland)
Clin Orthop Relat Res 468:2678-2689, 2010

Background.—Short- to medium-term rotator cuff repair reportedly relieves pain in 82% to 97% of patients and provides normal or almost normal shoulder function in 82% to 92%. However, it is unknown whether pain relief and function persist long term.

Questions/Purposes.—We asked whether, after rotator cuff repair or reconstruction, pain relief, ROM, shoulder strength, and function remained over the long term.

Patients and Methods.—We retrospectively reviewed 75 patients who underwent rotator cuff repair between 1980 and 1989. There were 55 men and 20 women. Their mean age at surgery was 52 years. The minimum followup was 16 years (mean, 20 years; range 16—25 years).

Results.—Twenty-eight of the 75 patients (37%) had persistent relief of pain lasting for 20 years. In the remaining 47 patients, alleviation of pain lasted, on average, 14 years (range, 0—24 years). Mean flexion and abduction strength increased postoperatively but during long-term followup decreased to less than preoperative levels. External rotation also decreased. At the last followup, the Constant-Murley score averaged 66 (range, 10—98) in men and 60 (range, 29—89) in women. In the Simple Shoulder Test questionnaire, the mean number of yes answers was eight of 12. Of the 75 patients, 32 (43%) reported impairment in activities of daily living owing to an index shoulder complaint. Severe degenerative changes of the glenohumeral joint were evident in 14 patients (19%).

Conclusions.—The early high functional scores after primary rotator cuff repair or reconstruction of the types we performed in the 1980s did not persist. The function achieved postoperatively was lost, as ROM and strength decreased to less than preoperative values. However, alleviation of pain was long-standing in most patients. Based on our data, we should warn patients to expect less than permanent relief with those repairs. We cannot say whether the same will apply to currently performed types of repairs.

Level of Evidence.—Level IV, therapeutic study. See Guidelines for Authors for a complete description of levels of evidence.

▶ The very long-term consequence of rotator cuff repair surgeries is largely unknown. This knowledge gap prompted the Borgmastars research team to report pain relief, shoulder range of motion, and shoulder function for a group of 75 patients 16 to 25 years post surgery. Their major findings suggest that the patient's shoulder pain was lessened but shoulder function, range of motion, and force all diminished when they compared the follow-up scores with the preoperative and postoperative values. The authors report several limitations of their study that include that acromial osteotomy is rarely used today, calling into question the usefulness of their findings, and that patient selection and recruitment biases significantly limit generalizability. Although the authors discuss that decreases in shoulder function, range of motion, and force are expected consequences of aging, this article would have benefited from a statistical analysis that adjusted for age. Because of the limitations of this article, its clinical relevance is minor. However, it does advocate the need for very long-term follow-up of patients who receive rotator cuff surgical repairs using standardized outcome measures.

M. R. Pierrynowski, PhD

Healing of a painful intervertebral disc should not be confused with reversing disc degeneration: Implications for physical therapies for discogenic back pain
Adams MA, Stefanakis M, Dolan P (Univ of Bristol, UK)
Clin Biomech 25:961-971, 2010

Background.—Much is known about intervertebral disc degeneration, but little effort has been made to relate this information to the clinical problem of discogenic back pain, and how it might be treated.

Methods.—We re-interpret the scientific literature in order to provide a rationale for physical therapy treatments for discogenic back pain.

Interpretation.—Intervertebral discs deteriorate over many years, from the nucleus outwards, to an extent that is influenced by genetic inheritance and metabolite transport. Age-related deterioration can be accelerated by physical disruption, which leads to disc "degeneration" or prolapse. Degeneration most often affects the lower lumbar discs, which are loaded most severely, and it is often painful because nerves in the peripheral anulus or vertebral endplate can be sensitised by inflammatory-like changes arising from contact with blood or displaced nucleus pulposus. Surgically-removed human discs show an active inflammatory process proceeding from the outside-in, and animal studies confirm that effective healing occurs only in the outer anulus and endplate, where cell density and metabolite transport are greatest. Healing of the disc periphery has the potential to relieve discogenic pain, by re-establishing a physical barrier between nucleus pulposus and nerves, and reducing inflammation.

Conclusion.—Physical therapies should aim to promote healing in the disc periphery, by stimulating cells, boosting metabolite transport, and preventing adhesions and re-injury. Such an approach has the potential to accelerate pain relief in the disc periphery, even if it fails to reverse age-related degenerative changes in the nucleus.

▶ The authors of this review article do an excellent job of synthesizing the evidence regarding the properties of the painful intervertebral disk and indicating that physical therapy may be an effective way to promote healing. They present evidence that human disk degeneration can be initiated by mechanical loading and that genetics also exert influences on disk aging and degeneration. Disk degeneration is strongly associated with back pain particularly structural defects, such as disk extrusions, complete radial fissures, end plate defects, and loss of annulus height. Furthermore, severe back pain is associated with end plate damage, increased sensory innervations of that end plate, and inflammatory changes in the adjacent vertebrae. Pain sensitization (mechanical allodynia) is important in the outer annulus, and there is evidence that an intact outer annulus is effective against progression of inflammation. Based on this synthesis of the evidence, the authors suggest that treatment for discogenic pain should aim at reducing inflammation and re-establishing a physical barrier between nucleus pulposus and nerve cells in the outer annulus, vertebral end plate, and nerve roots (ie, directing the disk periphery). The suggestions are to avoid reinjury during the acute inflammatory phase by suggesting that a patient should rest initially. The authors make an important point: physical causes of back pain should not be neglected and avoidance of early morning flexion when disks are swollen can reduce recurrent attacks. During the reparative phase and remodeling phase, physical therapy is important. Graduated exercises and mobilization should be done. However, further research is needed to quantify the optimal levels of loading and movement for disk healing. Finally, the authors suggest that correct identification of the pain source would be helpful to target the physical therapy intervention. They suggest ways for this identification and propose rehabilitation protocols to reflect the different pain sources.

D. E. Feldman, PT, PhD

Preference, Expectation, and Satisfaction in a Clinical Trial of Behavioral Interventions for Acute and Sub-Acute Low Back Pain

George SZ, Robinson ME (Univ of Florida, Gainesville)
J Pain 11:1074-1082, 2010

The equivalency of behavioral interventions has led to the consideration of whether patient-related factors influence clinical trial outcomes. The primary purpose of this secondary analysis was to determine if treatment preference and patient expectation were predictors of trial outcomes and if selected patient-satisfaction items were appropriate as outcome measures. Perceived effectiveness, treatment preference, and patient expectation were assessed before random assignment, and patient satisfaction was assessed 6 months later. Patient preference was associated with perceived effectiveness for those with no treatment preference and those preferring graded exposure. Higher patient expectation was associated with higher perceived effectiveness ratings for all treatments in the clinical trial. Patients with no strong treatment preferences had larger 6-month improvements in pain intensity and disability, while patients with higher expectations had lower disability at baseline, 4 weeks, and 6 months. Patient satisfaction rates did not differ based on treatment received. Patient satisfaction was highest with treatment delivery and much lower

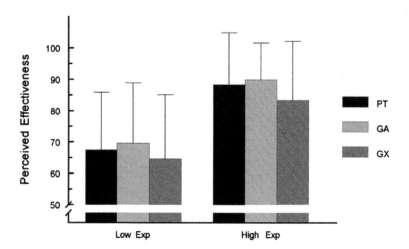

Figure Key

Y-axis indicates perceived effectiveness rating of treatment (0 – 100)

Low Exp = low expectation of symptom relief, High Exp = high expectation of symptom relief, PT = physical therapy, GA = physical therapy with graded activity, GX = physical therapy with graded exposure, and NP = no strong treatment preference

Error bars = 1 standard deviation

FIGURE 2.—Perceived effectiveness ratings based on patient expectation. (Reprinted from George SZ, Robinson ME. Preference, expectation, and satisfaction in a clinical trial of behavioral interventions for acute and sub-acute low back pain. *J Pain*. 2010;11:1074-1082, with permission from the American Pain Society.)

with treatment effect. Patient satisfaction was uniformly associated with expectations being met, but only satisfaction with treatment effect was associated with lower pain and disability scores. These data support assessment of treatment preference and patient expectation as predictors and patient satisfaction as an outcome measure in low back pain (LBP) clinical trials.

Perspective.—These data indicate treatment preference potentially impacts rate of improvement for patients with low back pain. Patient expectation did not impact rate of improvement, but those with higher expectations had lower pain and disability scores throughout the trial. Optimal assessment of patient satisfaction should include items that separately consider treatment delivery and effect (Fig 2).

▶ The main point of this study was to assess whether patient preferences and patient expectations have an effect on outcome for patients with low back pain who were involved in a clinical trial. In terms of patient preferences (for type of treatment), the researchers actually found that having no strong treatment preference was associated with the largest improvements in pain intensity and disability. Thus, the authors suggest that perhaps those persons without preset notions may do better than those who had treatment preferences. With respect to expectations, the findings do support a difference in terms of higher perceived effectiveness for those with higher expectations (Fig 2) as well as lower disability scores at baseline, 4 weeks, and 6 months for those with higher treatment expectations. Although there are limitations, notably the crude nature of measuring patient expectations, the study does indicate that it may be important to assess patient expectations when conducting a clinical trial of behavioral interventions.

D. E. Feldman, PT, PhD

Motivational Enhancement Therapy in Addition to Physical Therapy Improves Motivational Factors and Treatment Outcomes in People With Low Back Pain: A Randomized Controlled Trial
Vong SK, Cheing GL, Chan F, et al (The Hong Kong Polytechnic Univ, Hung Hom, Kowloon, China; Univ of Wisconsin, Madison; et al)
Arch Phys Med Rehabil 92:176-183, 2011

Objectives.—To examine whether the addition of motivational enhancement treatment (MET) to conventional physical therapy (PT) produces better outcomes than PT alone in people with chronic low back pain (LBP).

Design.—A double-blinded, prospective, randomized, controlled trial.

Setting.—PT outpatient department.

Participants.—Participants (N=76) with chronic LBP were randomly assigned to receive 10 sessions of either MET plus PT or PT alone.

Intervention.—MET included motivational interviewing strategies and motivation-enhancing factors. The PT program consisted of interferential therapy and back exercises.

Main Outcome Measures.—Motivational-enhancing factors, pain intensity, physical functions, and exercise compliance.

Results.—The MET-plus-PT group produced significantly greater improvements than the PT group in 3 motivation-enhancing factors; proxy efficacy (P<.001), working alliance (P<.001), and treatment expectancy (P=.011). Furthermore, they performed significantly better in lifting capacity (P=.015), 36-Item Short Form Health Survey General Health subscale (P=.015), and exercise compliance (P=.002) than the PT group. A trend of a greater decrease in visual analog scale and Roland-Morris Disability Questionnaire scores also was found in the MET-plus-PT group than the PT group.

Conclusion.—The addition of MET to PT treatment can effectively enhance motivation and exercise compliance and show better improvement in physical function in patients with chronic LBP compared with PT alone.

▶ There are many studies on the subject of physical therapy for low back pain; evidence shows that exercise and multidisciplinary interventions are effective. Improving motivation in patients is an important strategy for physical therapists, so that patients commit to achieving behavioral changes and ultimately have better health outcomes. This randomized controlled trial sets out to evaluate the benefits of adding a specific intervention to enhance motivation (motivational enhancement therapy [MET]) to physical therapy programs for patients with low back pain. The results support the use of MET to enhance motivation outcomes, such as proxy efficacy (patients' confidence in their therapists' ability to function effectively on their behalf), working alliance, and treatment expectance, as well as health outcomes, such as improved lifting capacity and general health. There was also better compliance to the home exercise program. The study underscores the importance of using motivational strategies when dealing with patients with chronic low back pain.

D. E. Feldman, PT, PhD

Causes of Radiculopathy in Young Athletes With Spondylolysis
Sairyo K, Sakai T, Amari R, et al (The Univ of Tokushima, Japan)
Am J Sports Med 38:357-362, 2010

Background.—The main clinical symptom of lumbar spondylolysis is lower back pain. Radiculopathy rarely occurs without vertebral slippage.

Hypothesis.—Spondylolysis in young athletes can cause lumbar radiculopathy.

Study Design.—Case series; Level of evidence, 4.

Methods.—Ten patients (7 males and 3 females) were included in this study. The age of the patients ranged from 12 to 27 years. We employed plain radiography, computed tomography, magnetic resonance imaging, and selective radiculography if needed.

Results.—The pathomechanism was classified into nonspondylolytic radiculopathy (3 cases) and spondylolytic radiculopathy (7 cases). In the nonspondylolytic group, 1 patient had a juxta-facet cyst at L4-5 and 2 patients had a herniated nucleus pulposus. In the other group, spondylolytic-related factors caused radiculopathy, and spondylolysis was in the early or progressive stage in all 7 patients. Radiologic findings indicated that radiculopathy was caused by extraosseous hematoma or edema in the vicinity of the fracture site. The radiculopathy disappeared within a month of nonoperative management, and radiologic abnormalities disappeared 3 to 6 months later.

Conclusion.—Radiculopathy can occur together with lumbar spondylolysis without slippage in young athletes. We propose extraosseous hematoma or edema at the site of spondylolysis as the unique pathomechanism causing radiculopathy in young athletes. Radiculopathy is rare in athletes with spondylolysis. Magnetic resonance imaging is a useful tool to clarify the pathologic changes that induce the radiculopathy for both spondylolytic and nonspondylolytic factors.

▶ This case series consists of a small sample of 10 young athletes who complained of leg pain and back pain. The authors proceed to use radiographs, computed tomography (CT), and magnetic resonance imaging (MRI) on these athletes to better understand the cause of radiculopathy. They divide their group into 2 categories: those with nonspondylolytic radiculopathy (who happened to be in the terminal stage of lysis on CT scan) and those with spondylolytic radiculopathy (who happened to be in the early or progressive stage of lysis). It appears that all the patients who had early- or progressive-stage spondylolysis appear to get better with conservative treatment (ie, stop sports temporarily and wear a brace). MRI findings of those in the spondylolytic radiculopathy group revealed extraosseous hematoma and edema at the site of the fracture, which may irritate the adjacent nerve root. Perhaps only those persons with later-stage spondylolysis should undergo further investigation using MRI because treatment in these cases may require surgery or other interventions.

D. E. Feldman, PT, PhD

The Effects of Exercise for the Prevention of Overuse Anterior Knee Pain: A Randomized Controlled Trial
Coppack RJ, Etherington J, Wills AK (The Centre for Human Performance, Headley Court, Surrey, UK)
Am J Sports Med 2011 [Epub ahead of print]

Background.—Anterior knee pain (AKP) is the most common activity-related injury of the knee. The authors investigated the effect of an exercise intervention on the incidence of AKP in UK army recruits undergoing a 14-week physically arduous training program.

Hypothesis.—Modifying military training to include targeted preventative exercises may reduce the incidence of AKP in a young recruit population.

Study Design.—Randomized controlled trial; Level of evidence, 1.

Methods.—A single-blind cluster randomized controlled trial was performed in 39 male and 11 female training groups (median age: 19.7 years; interquartile range, 17-25) undergoing phase 1 of army recruit training. Each group was randomly assigned to either an intervention (n = 759) or control (n = 743) protocol. The intervention consisted of 4 strengthening and 4 stretching exercises completed during supervised physical training lessons (7 per week). The control group followed the existing training syllabus warm-up exercises. The primary outcome was a diagnosis of AKP during the 14-week training program.

Results.—Forty-six participants (3.1%; 95% confidence interval [CI], 2.3-4.1) were diagnosed with AKP. There were 36 (4.8%; 95% CI, 3.5-6.7) new cases of AKP in the control group and 10 (1.3%; 0.7-2.4) in the intervention group. There was a 75% reduction in AKP risk in the intervention group (unadjusted hazard ratio = 0.25; 95% CI, 0.13-0.52; $P < .001$). Three participants (0.4%) from the intervention group were discharged from the military for medical reasons compared to 25 (3.4%) in the control group.

Conclusion.—A simple set of lower limb stretching and strengthening exercises resulted in a substantial and safe reduction in the incidence of AKP in a young military population undertaking a physical conditioning program. Such exercises could also be beneficial for preventing this common injury among nonmilitary participants in recreational physical activity (Table 1).

▶ This is the first randomized controlled trial to demonstrate prevention of overuse anterior knee pain (AKP) using a targeted exercise intervention. Preventing AKP is important because it is the most common knee disorder, accounting for 25% to 40% of all knee problems presenting to sports medicine clinics. The intervention included multiple sets of progressive strengthening and stretching exercises (Table 1) performed daily for 14 weeks by young military recruits. The risk of AKP was reduced by 75% in the intervention group compared with the control group. There were no adverse events. It is not clear what component of the exercise intervention is most closely related to the prevention of AKP. The closed chain kinetic exercises have been shown to increase quadriceps activation patterns and improve patellofemoral joint alignment. The emphasis on eccentric exercise may have increased the muscular capacity to absorb high patellofemoral forces during the early stages of basic military training. Stretching of soft tissue has been shown to reduce pain and increase flexibility in patients with AKP, but there is scientific evidence to support the protective effects of stretching. This was a highly controlled study because of the military population, standardization of other physical activity during basic training, the supervision of the exercises, the reporting of AKP in real time as opposed to retrospectively, and the diagnostic criteria of AKP. It is unclear if the intervention would be beneficial for

TABLE 1.—Anterior Knee Pain Prevention Training Program (PTP)[a]

Exercise	Weeks of Program				
	1-3	4-6	7-9	10-12	13-14
Isometric hip abduction against a wall in standing, sec[b]	10	10	15	15	20
Forward lunges—knee over the forward foot, repetitions[b]	10	12	12	14	14
Single-legged step downs from a 20-cm step, repetitions[b]	10	10	12	12	14
Single-legged squats to 45° of knee flexion with isometric gluteal muscle contraction, repetitions[b]	10	10	12	12	14
Quadriceps (hip and knee) stretches, sec[c]	20	20	20	20	20
Iliotibial band (lateral thigh) stretches, sec[c]	20	20	20	20	20
Hamstring stretches, sec[c]	20	20	20	20	20
Calf (gastrocnemius) stretches, sec[c]	20	20	20	20	20

[a]All stretches measured in seconds.
[b]Exercises performed during formal physical training session warm-up. All repetitions completed in sets of 3.
[c]Stretching exercises performed during formal physical training session warm-down.

long-term prevention of AKP and whether there is a dose-response and effectiveness in older or less active populations.

C. M. Jankowski, PhD

ACL Research Retreat V: An Update on ACL Injury Risk and Prevention, March 25–27, 2010, Greensboro, NC
Shultz SJ, Schmitz RJ, Nguyen A-D, et al (Univ of North Carolina at Greensboro; College of Charleston, SC; et al)
J Athl Train 45:499-508, 2010

Background.—Many factors, individually or in concert, probably contribute to noncontact anterior cruciate ligament (ACL) injury. An update on the risk and prevention of ACL injury was issued after the fifth ACL Research Retreat in March 2010. The updated and refined consensus statement addresses hormonal and anatomical risk factors, neuromechanical factors in ACL injury, and risk factor screening and prevention.

Neuromuscular and Biomechanical Factors.—Research shows that during dynamic sports postures considered high risk, the ACL is loaded by several sagittal and nonsagittal mechanisms. In vivo, ACL strain is related to maximal load and timing of ground reaction forces. Motivation and fatigue alter biomechanical and neuromuscular factors. Fatigue may increase risk of ACL injury through altered lower limb biomechanical and neuromuscular factors. Lower limb factors vary with trunk, core, and upper body mechanics. Hip position and stiffness affect lower limb biomechanics. A certain profile or profiles may cause noncontact ACL rupture. How trunk and hip biomechanical factors for in vivo ACL strain during highly dynamic activity cause injury is unclear. Variable neuromuscular and biomechanical factors may alter the risk of indirect or noncontact ACL injury. Athletes with ACL injuries have slower reaction times, slower processing speed, and visual-spatial disorientation, but whether these lead to injury is unknown. It is unclear how many episodes are needed to cause gross ACL failure and whether one or many high-risk neuromuscular and biomechanical profiles contribute to ACL injury.

Anatomical and Structural Factors.—Female ACLs are shorter, smaller cross-sectionally, and have less volume than male ACLs even after body anthropometry adjustments. The femoral notch height is larger and the femoral notch angle smaller in female than male subjects. Femoral notch width predicts ACL size in males but not females; femoral notch angle predicts ACL size in females but not males. Female ACLs are less stiff and fail at a lower load than male ACLs. The percentage of area occupied by collagen fiber is less in females than males. Injured individuals have smaller ACLs, higher posterior slopes of the lateral tibia, similar medial tibial slopes, and a reduced condylar depth on the medial tibial plateau. They also demonstrate an anterior medial ridge on the intercondylar notch. Laxity differs between genders. Compared to male subjects, females have greater genu recurvatum, anterior knee laxity, and general joint laxity, 25% to 30% greater frontal-plane and transverse-plane laxity and less torsional stiffness. With greater joint laxity, subjects have altered knee-joint neuromechanics during weight bearing and increased risk of injury. Women have greater anterior pelvic tilt, hip anterversion, tibiofemoral angle, and quadriceps angle than men. Maturity alters lower extremity alignment, with changes occurring at different rates between men and women. Research does not indicate whether and how physical activity influences these anatomical and structural factors. Meniscal geometry's effects on ACL strain and failure during activity are unknown. The influence of anatomical and structural factors on knee-joint neuromechanics and body composition on lower extremity neuromechanical strategies and ACL injury rate remain to be determined.

Hormonal Factors.—Menstrual cycle phase alters the likelihood of suffering an ACL injury. Such injury is more likely during the preovulatory phase. Sex hormone receptors are located on the human ACL and in skeletal muscle. Hormone profiles are somewhat consistent within an individual woman from month to month but differ greatly from woman to woman. Variability is reduced by taking multiple samples over repeated days. Laxity also varies substantially through the menstrual cycle but is fairly predictable within the same individual from month to month. A single measurement in a single phase is not sufficient to represent the same hormone profile or time point in a particular menstrual phase in all women. Mechanical and molecular ACL properties are altered by estrogen and the interaction of several sex hormones, secondary messengers, remodeling proteins, and mechanical stresses. ACL tissue characteristics change in a time-dependent manner as a result of sex hormones and other remodeling agents. Animal models show interactions among mechanical stress, hormones, and altered ACL structure and metabolism. The mechanisms by which hormones affect ACL injury are yet to be determined. Dynamic motion control may or may not be influenced by sex hormones' effects on skeletal muscle structure and function. The relationship between soft tissue changes and hormone fluctuations must be explored. Physically active female subjects need to be assessed for interactions among mechanical stress on the ACL, hormone profiles, and altered ACL structure and metabolism.

Risk Factor Screening and Prevention.—Training programs can alter the biomechanical and neuromuscular variables that may contribute to ACL injury. These programs should incorporate balance training, plyometric training, education, strengthening, and feedback. However, their protective effects tend to be transient. Field assessment and screening tools help identify persons at higher risk for ACL injury. ACL injuries can have long-term effects, including osteoarthritis. A previous personal or family history of ACL injury may be a risk factor for repeat ACL injury. Which programs offer the most protective effects remains to be determined. How long a training stimulus is needed to be protective and how long the protective effect lasts has yet to be determined. The age at which protective interventions are most effective is unknown. Whether preventive programs should be targeted to sports, ages, or individual athletes' needs is not yet clear, nor is their effect on athletic performance known. How to manage familial or personal ACL injury history has not been determined. Whether the risk factors and mechanisms of ACL injury are the same for children and adults is unknown. The ability to prevent ACL injury through organized programs may differ and barriers to such programs or facilitating factors remain to be identified.

Conclusions.—The advances in knowledge concerning ACL injury risk and prevention have influenced medicine's current understanding, reshaped what is unknown, and identified future directions that need to be taken. Further research is needed in the identified areas.

▶ This is the fifth in a series of anterior cruciate ligament (ACL) retreats designed to (1) present and discuss the most recent research on ACL injury risk and prevention and (2) identify new research directives aimed at understanding the epidemiology, risk factors, and prevention of noncontact ACL injury. This ACL Research Retreat V was hosted by the Department of Kinesiology at the University of North Carolina at Greensboro. This year, 75 clinicians and researchers representing 6 countries participated in a number of keynote presentations and 40 podium and poster presentations. The participants revisited and updated the consensus statement from the 2008 ACL Research Retreat IV. Three separate interest groups discussed neuromuscular and biomechanical factors, anatomical and structural factors, hormonal factors, and risk factor screening and prevention. In each of these specific areas, What We Know, What We Don't Know, and Where We Go From Here, are concisely outlined, with the appropriate references. Therefore, this article serves as a single-source up-to-date summary, for clinicians and researchers alike, of the latest knowledge regarding the multifactorial etiology of ACL injuries, as well as risk factors and injury-prevention strategies. This group of scientists is to be commended for their ongoing investigations and interest in this significant knee ligament injury that so often leads to an increased disease burden of osteoarthritis in later life.

C. Lebrun, MD

Two- to 4-Year Follow-up to a Comparison of Home Versus Physical Therapy-Supervised Rehabilitation Programs After Anterior Cruciate Ligament Reconstruction

Grant JA, Mohtadi NGH (Univ of Calgary Sport Medicine Ctr, Alberta, Canada)
Am J Sports Med 38:1389-1394, 2010

Background.—There have been no long-term follow-up studies comparing a predominantly home-based rehabilitation program with a standard physical therapy program after anterior cruciate ligament (ACL) reconstruction. Demonstrating the long-term success of such a cost-effective program would be beneficial to guide future rehabilitation practice.

Purpose.—To determine whether there were any differences in long-term outcome between recreational athletes who performed a physical therapy-supervised rehabilitation program and those who performed a primarily home-based rehabilitation program in the first 3 months after ACL reconstruction.

Study Design.—Randomized clinical trial; Level of evidence, 1.

Methods.—Patients were randomized before ACL reconstruction surgery to either the physical therapy-supervised (17 physical therapy sessions) or home-based (4 physical therapy sessions) program. Eighty-eight of the original 129 patients returned 2 to 4 years after surgery to assess their long-term clinical outcomes. Primary outcome was the ACL quality of life questionnaire (ACL QOL). Secondary outcomes were bilateral difference in knee extension and flexion range of motion, sagittal plane knee laxity, relative quadriceps and hamstring strength, and objective International Knee Documentation Committee score. Unpaired t tests and a chi-square test were used for the comparisons.

Results.—The home-based group had a significantly higher mean ACL QOL score (80.0 ± 16.2) than the physical therapy-supervised group (69.9 ± 22.0) a mean of 38 months after surgery ($P = .02$, 95% confidence interval [CI]: 1.7, 18.4). The mean change in ACL QOL score from before surgery to follow-up was not significantly different between the groups (physical therapy = 40.0, home = 45.8, $P = .26$, 95% CI: −15.8, 4.4). There were no significant differences in the secondary outcome measures.

Conclusion.—This long-term study upholds the short-term findings of the original randomized clinical trial by demonstrating that patients who participate in a predominantly home-based rehabilitation program in the first 3 months after ACL reconstruction have similar 2- to 4-year outcomes compared with those patients who participate in a more clinically supervised program.

▶ Rehabilitation is extremely important post anterior cruciate ligament reconstruction surgery. The process typically lasts several months. This study aimed to assess long-term outcomes for persons who underwent 17 physical therapy—supervised sessions versus those who did their therapy at home (albeit having 4 sessions with a physical therapist to instruct and guide their home therapy). The authors followed up on patients 2 to 4 years following their enrollment in a randomized clinical trial. Although they conclude that those in the home therapy group had a higher quality of life score, there was no significant difference in change in quality of life score. Because there were losses to follow-up (ie, only 88 of the original 129 patients participated in this follow-up study), this study cannot be considered as a randomized trial (there could have been selection bias because of losses to follow-up). Thus, I would hesitate to conclude that home-based patients had better disease-specific quality of life. Furthermore, patients who consented to participate in the original trial may be those who would tend to be compliant with rehabilitation programs. Thus, it may be important to screen for factors associated with adherence to rehabilitation treatment prior to deciding which type of rehabilitation approach should be used as home-based therapy.

D. E. Feldman, PT, PhD

Management of Tarsal Navicular Stress Fractures: Conservative Versus Surgical Treatment: A Meta-Analysis

Torg JS, Moyer J, Gaughan JP, et al (Temple Univ, Philadelphia, PA; et al)
Am J Sports Med 38:1048-1053, 2010

Purpose.—This study was conducted to provide a statistical analysis of previously reported tarsal navicular stress fracture studies regarding the outcomes and effectiveness of conservative and surgical management.

Study Design.—Systematic review.

Methods.—A systematic review of the published literature was conducted utilizing MEDLINE through Ovid, PubMed, ScienceDirect, and EBSCOhost. Reports of studies that provided the type of tarsal navicular stress fracture (ie, complete or incomplete), type of treatment, result of that treatment, and the time required to return to full activity were selected for analysis. Using a mixed generalized linear model with study as a random effect and treatment as a fixed effect, cases were separated and compared based on 3 different types of treatment: conservative, weightbearing permitted (WBR); conservative, non-weightbearing (NWB); and surgical treatment. The outcome of the treatment was recorded as either successful or unsuccessful based on radiographic and/or clinical healing of the fracture and time from onset of treatment to return to activity.

Results.—There was no statistically significant difference between NWB conservative treatment and surgical treatment regarding outcome ($P = .6441$). However, there is a statistical trend favoring NWB management (96% successful outcomes) over surgery (82% successful outcomes). Weightbearing as a conservative treatment was shown to be significantly less effective than either NWB ($P = .0001$) or surgical treatment ($P < .0003$).

Conclusion.—Non-weightbearing conservative management should be considered the standard of care for tarsal navicular stress fractures. The authors could find no advantage for surgical treatment compared with NWB immobilization. However, there is a statistical trend favoring NWB over surgery. Rest or immobilization with weightbearing was inferior to both other treatments analyzed. The authors concluded that conservative NWB management is the standard of care for initial treatment of both partial and complete stress fractures of the tarsal navicular.

▶ The management of tarsal navicular stress fractures is still somewhat controversial. One of the difficulties lies in the frequent delay in diagnosis of this problem. These authors have done a systematic review of the published literature looking at the type of fracture (ie, complete or incomplete), results of treatment, and time to return to full activity. As I have just finished managing exactly such an injury in a 16-year-old young soccer player, the results of this review were very helpful. Essentially, nonweightbearing (NWB) conservative management (ie, immobilization in a cast or cast boot) for at least 6 weeks should be considered standard of care for treatment of these difficult fractures. There is no documented advantage for surgical treatment compared with NWB immobilization; in fact, there is a statistical trend favoring the NWB over surgery. The most important takeaway message from this article is that simply rest or immobilization with weightbearing does not appear to lead to satisfactory outcomes. Another caveat that was not pointed out in this article is that NWB for any significant length of time tends to lead to regional osteopenia. Then with resumption of weightbearing, a repeat MRI scan will show evidence of stress patterns in the metatarsal bones, if done too soon. Therefore, it is better to clinically follow the patient for tenderness in the N or navicular spot when monitoring the result of return to activity.

C. Lebrun, MD

Shock Wave Therapy Compared with Intramedullary Screw Fixation for Nonunion of Proximal Fifth Metatarsal Metaphyseal-Diaphyseal Fractures
Furia JP, Juliano PJ, Wade AM, et al (SUN Orthopaedics and Sports Medicine, Lewisburg, PA; Penn State Milton S. Hershey Med Ctr, Hershey, PA; et al)
J Bone Joint Surg Am 92:846-854, 2010

Background.—The current "gold standard" for treatment of chronic fracture nonunion in the metaphyseal-diaphyseal region of the fifth metatarsal is intramedullary screw fixation. Complications with this procedure, however, are not uncommon. Shock wave therapy can be an effective treatment for fracture nonunions. The purpose of this study was to evaluate the safety and efficacy of shock wave therapy as a treatment of these nonunions.

Methods.—Twenty-three patients with a fracture nonunion in the metaphyseal-diaphyseal region of the fifth metatarsal received high-energy shock wave therapy (2000 to 4000 shocks; energy flux density per pulse, 0.35 mJ/mm^2), and twenty other patients with the same type of fracture nonunion were treated with intramedullary screw fixation. The numbers of fractures that were healed at three and six months after treatment in each group were determined, and treatment complications were recorded.

Results.—Twenty of the twenty-three nonunions in the shock wave group and eighteen of the twenty nonunions in the screw fixation group were healed at three months after treatment. One of the three nonunions that had not healed by three months in the shock wave group was healed by six months. There was one complication in the shock wave group (post-treatment petechiae) and eleven complications in the screw-fixation group (one refracture, one case of cellulitis, and nine cases of symptomatic hardware).

Conclusions.—Both intramedullary screw fixation and shock wave therapy are effective treatments for fracture nonunion in the metaphyseal-diaphyseal region of the fifth metatarsal. Screw fixation is more often associated with complications that frequently result in additional surgery.

▶ This is an interesting article; however, it should be noted that it is actually a retrospective cohort study, without any randomization of patients. Nevertheless, it describes a potentially useful management tool for nonunions: high-energy extracorporeal shock wave therapy (ESWT). ESWT has been used for some time now in the treatment of degenerative tendinopathies, such as for the Achilles and patellar tendons, and insertional tendinopathies of the wrist extensors or wrist flexors. It can sometimes be confusing for the reader, however, as there are several different types of ESWT. Some machines use low-energy shock waves only, which have mainly an analgesic effect, while others (such as in this study) use high-energy shock waves, which are thought to stimulate angiogenesis, release of growth factors, and healing (ie, osteogenic). The Dornier Epos Ultra machine additionally uses diagnostic ultrasound scanning to precisely visualize the focus of the shock waves. As most of the high-energy machines will also allow application of low-energy shock waves, sometimes it is possible to use the lower levels to create analgesia in the treated site and gradually increase the intensity of the shock waves to the desired therapeutic level. Some practitioners will alternatively use local anesthetic or a regional block to numb the area. The OssaTron machine (Fig 1 in the original article) is more frequently used in the operating room, with the patient under general anesthesia to avoid the associated discomfort. The shock waves are generated either with an electrohydraulic technology or through piezoelectric crystals.

Radial shock wave therapy is something else altogether, as the shock waves are generated in a totally different fashion and are distributed in a radial fashion to the site of treatment. This machine is currently quite popular in physiotherapy clinics. The shock waves omitted from this machine are clinically focused to the region of maximal tenderness, again providing mainly an analgesic rather than a healing effect.

The authors are quite right in that previous studies have looked at the effects of ESWT for treatment of nonunions of a variety of different fractures, using numerous different protocols. Some use multiple treatments (commonly up to 3) at various intervals and assess fracture healing by different methods. Further research on the utility of high-energy shock wave therapy to stimulate bone healing will benefit from exact documentation of the total energy flux density (which can be calculated by enumerating the exact number of shocks and the energy flux density per pulse) and standardizing the treatment regimens. It does remain as a viable option in patients with nonunions, eliminating the associated risks and costs of surgical management. Another potential challenge lies in getting the insurance companies to cover the expense of this treatment, something that will be facilitated by the publication of more high-quality studies documenting its effectiveness.

C. Lebrun, MD

Effect of Taping on Actual and Perceived Dynamic Postural Stability in Persons With Chronic Ankle Instability
Delahunt E, McGrath A, Doran N, et al (Univ College Dublin, Republic of Ireland)
Arch Phys Med Rehabil 91:1383-1389, 2010

Objective.—To investigate whether 2 different mechanisms of ankle joint taping ([1] lateral subtalar sling or [2] fibular repositioning) can enhance actual and perceived dynamic postural stability in participants with chronic ankle instability (CAI).

Design.—Laboratory-based repeated-measures study.

Setting.—University biomechanics laboratory.

Participants.—Participants (n = 16) with CAI.

Interventions.—Participants performed the Star Excursion Balance Test (SEBT) under 3 different conditions: (1) no tape, (2) lateral subtalar sling taping and (3) fibular repositioning taping.

Main Outcome Measures.—Reach distances in the anterior, posteromedial, and posterolateral directions on the SEBT. Participants' perceptions of stability, confidence, and reassurance when performing the SEBT under 2 different taping conditions.

Results.—Taping did not improve reach distance on the SEBT ($P>.05$). Feelings of confidence increased for 56% of participants ($P=.002$) under both tape conditions. Feelings of stability increased for 87.5% of participants ($P<.001$) using condition 2 (lateral subtalar sling taping) and 75% of participants ($P=.001$) using condition 3 (fibular repositioning taping). Feelings of reassurance increased for 68.75% of participants ($P=.001$) using condition 2 (lateral subtalar sling taping) and 50% of participants ($P=.005$) using condition 3 (fibular repositioning taping).

Conclusions.—No significant change in dynamic postural stability was observed after application of either taping mechanism; however, participants' perceptions of confidence, stability, and reassurance were significantly improved. Further research is necessary to fully elucidate the exact mechanisms by which taping may help reduce the incidence of repeated injury in subjects with CAI.

▶ Taping is often used for ankle sprains and for persons with chronic ankle instability. Although the results of this study do not support the efficacy of taping with respect to performance on the Star Excursion Balance Test because there were no differences between no tape and either of the 2 taping conditions, they do show that taping enhanced feelings of stability, confidence, and reassurance. There may be a placebo effect at play such that having the tape on (even the small amount of tape) produces such an effect. The authors argue that clinicians should emphasize the benefits of ankle joint taping "because this is likely to enhance feeling of confidence, stability, and reassurance." The statement adds credence to the placebo effect of taping. However, I do concur with the authors that further study is warranted. Specifically, it would be important to determine whether, in fact, there is a placebo effect or whether taping does produce the intended effects.

D. E. Feldman, PT, PhD

3 Biomechanics, Muscle Strength and Training

Kinesiology of the Hip: A Focus on Muscular Actions
Neumann DA (Marquette Univ, Milwaukee, WI)
J Orthop Sports Phys Ther 40:82-94, 2010

The 21 muscles that cross the hip provide both triplanar movement and stability between the femur and acetabulum. The primary intent of this clinical commentary is to review and discuss the current understanding of the specific actions of the hip muscles. Analysis of their actions is based primarily on the spatial orientation of the muscles relative to the axes of rotation at the hip. The discussion of muscle actions is organized according to the 3 cardinal planes of motion. Actions are considered from both femoral-on-pelvic and pelvic-on-femoral perspectives, with particular attention to the role of coactivation of trunk muscles. Additional attention is paid to the biomechanical variables that alter the effectiveness, force, and torque of a given muscle action. The role of certain muscles in generating compression force at the hip is also presented. Throughout the commentary, the kinesiology of the muscles of the hip are considered primarily from normal but also pathological perspectives, supplemented with several clinically relevant scenarios. This overview should serve as a foundation for understanding the assessment and treatment of musculo-skeletal impairments that involve not only the hip, but also the adjacent low back and knee regions.

► Understanding the action of a striated muscle crossing a human joint during activity is foundational clinical knowledge. During training, most clinicians are expected to learn the sagittal (flexion-extension), horizontal (internal-external rotation), and frontal (abduction-adduction) plane functions of the major muscles. Commonly, this knowledge is presented in tabular form listing the primary and secondary actions of the muscles that cross a joint. In this review article, Neumann tabulates this information for the hip joint. However, he also discusses why this information is simplistic and may mislead. The major concern is that the tabulated muscle actions are when the joint is in the anatomical position and muscle actions change when the joint deviates from the anatomical position. Neumann provides the example of the gluteus maximus action changing from an external to internal rotator as the hip is flexed. An additional concern is that muscles rarely act in isolation; muscles work synergistically at and across multiple joints. The synergistic action of the sagittal plane hip and pelvis muscles during the straight leg raise is discussed. This article is clinically relevant because it challenges some of the widely held beliefs regarding muscle action and questions the use of the commonly taught tables.

M. R. Pierrynowski, PhD

Three-Dimensional Scapular and Clavicular Kinematics and Scapular Muscle Activity During Retraction Exercises

Oyama S, Myers JB, Wassinger CA, et al (Univ of North Carolina at Chapel Hill; Univ of Otago, Dunedin, New Zealand; et al)
J Orthop Sports Phys Ther 40:169-179, 2010

Study Design.—Controlled laboratory study.

Objectives.—To describe and compare scapular and clavicular kinematics and muscle activity during 6 retraction exercises in young healthy adults (mean ± SD age, 23.2 ± 2.4 years).

Background.—Based on the association between shoulder injuries and scapular/clavicular movement, muscle activity during various exercises that target muscles surrounding the scapula have been investigated. However, the scapular and clavicular movements occurring during these exercises remain uninvestigated. Evaluation of the scapular and clavicular kinematics in addition to muscle activity provides additional information that allow clinicians to select exercises that best meet the patient's needs.

Methods.—Three-dimensional scapular and clavicular kinematics and scapular muscle activity data were collected while the participants performed 6 scapular retraction exercises. One-way repeated-measures ANOVA and post hoc analyses were used to determine differences in scapular/clavicular kinematics and activation levels of the upper, middle, and lower trapezius and serratus anterior muscles occurring during the exercises.

Results.—The general pattern of the kinematics observed during all retraction exercises was scapular external rotation, scapular upward rotation, scapular posterior tilting, clavicular retraction, and clavicular depression. However, the exercises resulted in varying amounts of scapular movement and muscle activity.

Conclusion.—Clinicians can select appropriate exercises for their patients based on their need to strengthen specific retractor muscles and to improve specific scapular and clavicular movement patterns, preexisting conditions, and available range of motion (Fig 1).

▶ Health care providers who treat patients with shoulder pain and altered scapular and clavicular motion (subacromial or posterior impingement, shoulder instability, and full-thickness rotator cuff tears) frequently prescribe shoulder retraction exercise to improve muscle force capacity, which is then thought to alter shoulder movement patterns and then reduce pain. Typically, these patients present with decreased scapular upward and external rotation and

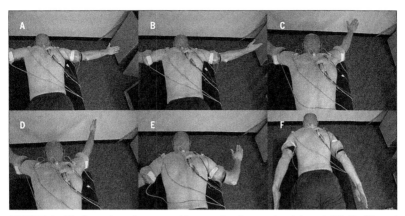

FIGURE 1.—The figure above shows a participant performing exercises 1 through 6 (A-F). All exercises were performed while the participant lay prone on the treatment table. During exercises 1 through 6, participant's upper limbs were positioned as follows: (A) exercise 1, 90° abduction and neutral humeral rotation (palm facing floor); (B) exercise 2, 90° abduction and external rotation (thumb pointing toward ceiling); (C) exercise 3, 120° abduction and neutral humeral rotation (palm facing floor); (D) exercise 4, 120° abduction and external rotation (thumb pointing toward ceiling); (E) exercise 5, abducted 45° with 90° of elbow flexion; (F) exercise 6, full extension. For all exercises, participants were instructed to lift the arms toward the ceiling and hold while squeezing the shoulder blades together. (Reprinted from Oyama S, Myers JB, Wassinger CA, et al. Three-dimensional scapular and clavicular kinematics and scapular muscle activity during retraction exercises. *J Orthop Sports Phys Ther.* 2010;40:169-179.)

posterior tilt. In this study, the authors compared the motion of the scapulae and clavicles in 23 volunteers performing 3 repetitions of 6 shoulder exercises. Each volunteer laid prone with their arms held in different postures (see Fig 1), then were asked to "lift the arms toward the ceiling and hold while squeezing the shoulder blades together." Each position was held for 6 seconds while bilateral scapular and clavicle positions and trapezius (upper, middle, and lower) and serratus muscle activations were measured. Results of the study suggest that if the health care provider wants to maximize scapular motion about multiple axes, they should prescribe exercise 2 and 5. If the goal of the exercise is to maximize trapezius muscle activation, they should prescribe exercise 4. Although the study only tested healthy volunteers, the findings provide some guidance for health care professionals when they select a shoulder retraction exercise to improve movement or activation.

M. R. Pierrynowski, PhD

Patellofemoral Joint Kinematics: The Circular Path of the Patella around the Trochlear Axis

Iranpour F, Merican AM, Baena FRY, et al (Imperial College, London, UK)
J Orthop Res 28:589-594, 2010

Differing descriptions of patellar motion relative to the femur have resulted from previous studies. We hypothesized that patellar kinematics would correlate to the trochlear geometry and that differing descriptions could be reconciled by accounting for differing alignments of measurement axes. Seven normal fresh-frozen knees were CT scanned, and their kinematics with quadriceps loading was measured by an optical tracker system. Kinematics was calculated in relation to the femoral epicondylar, anatomic, and mechanical axes. A novel trochlear axis was defined, between the centers of spheres best fitted to the medial and lateral trochlear articular surfaces. The path of the center of the patella was circular and uniplanar (root-mean-square error 0.3 mm) above $16 \pm 3°$ (mean $\pm$ SD) knee flexion. In the coronal plane, this circle was aligned $6 \pm 2°$ from the femoral anatomical axis, close to the mechanical axis alignment. It was $91 \pm 3°$ from the epicondylar axis, and $88 \pm 3°$ from the trochlear axis. In the transverse plane it was $91 \pm 3°$ and $88 \pm 3°$ from the epicondylar and trochlear axes, respectively. Manipulation of the data to different axis alignments showed that differing previously published data could be reconciled. The circular path of patellar motion around the trochlea, aligned with the mechanical axis of the leg, is easily visualized and understood.

▶ Joint kinematics is conventionally expressed as rotations and translations relative to a reference system comprised of the 3 orthogonal anatomical planes. As an example, flexion extension is considered a rotation about an axis perpendicular to the sagittal plane that bisects a joint when placed in the anatomical position. Flexion-extension motion of the tibia relative to the femur keeps the long axis of the tibia within the sagittal plane. However, if the motion is observed to have nonsagittal plane components, these secondary motions are frequently described as being independent of the primary flexion-extension motion. But if the axis of rotation is considered to be offset from the sagittal plane, the secondary motions can and often do diminish. In this study, the authors examined the rotation and translation of the patella relative to the femur (patellofemoral [PF] motion) during tibiofemoral flexion extension. Their major finding is that when the PF motion is described using a coordinate system offset from the conventional anatomical reference frame, the motion of the patella is (mostly) a simple circular arc. The new rotation axis intersects the spherical centers of the medial and lateral trochlear surfaces. This trochlear axis is offset from an axis perpendicular to the sagittal plane. This finding is important because it makes the description of PF motion relatively simple and, as the authors state, "... provides a clear datum when investigating the kinematic effects of surgical intervention." Deviations of the PF motion from a circular arc in patients with postknee replacement may indicate that the prosthesis was incorrectly aligned or translated or that the prosthesis geometry did not reproduce the natural geometry of the patient's knee. In either case, corrective interventions could then be examined to improve the PF motion.

M. R. Pierrynowski, PhD

Trunk Muscle Activity During Wheelchair Ramp Ascent and the Influence of a Geared Wheel on the Demands of Postural Control

Howarth SJ, Polgar JM, Dickerson CR, et al (Univ of Waterloo, Ontario, Canada; The Univ of Western Ontario, London, Canada)
Arch Phys Med Rehabil 91:436-442, 2010

Objectives.—To quantify levels of torso muscular demand during wheelchair ramp ascent and the ability of a geared wheel to influence trunk muscle activity.

Design.—Repeated-measures design. Each participant completed manual wheelchair ramp ascents for each combination of 4 ramp grades (1:12, 1:10, 1:8, and 1:6) and 3 wheel conditions (in gear, out of gear, and a standard spoked wheel) in a block randomized order by wheel condition.

Setting.—Biomechanics laboratory.

Participants.—Healthy novice wheelchair users (N = 13; 6 men) from a university student population.

Interventions.—Not applicable.

Main Outcome Measures.—Peak electromyographic activity, expressed as a percentage of maximal voluntary isometric contraction (MVIC) of the abdominals, latissimus dorsi, and erector spinae during ramp ascent. Temporal location of peak electromyographic activity (EMG) within a propulsive cycle and integrated electromyographic activity for a single propulsive cycle.

Results.—Abdominal peak activity increased 13.9% MVIC while peak posterior trunk muscle activity increased 4.9% MVIC between the shallowest and steepest ramp grades ($P<.05$). The geared wheel prevented increased peak activity of the rectus abdominis and external oblique ($P>.05$). Only peak electromyographic timing of the erector spinae was influenced during the push phase by increasing ramp slope.

Conclusions.—Increased trunk muscular demand as a result of increasing ramp slope is required to enhance stiffness of the spinal column and provide a stable base during manual propulsion. Manual wheelchair users with compromised activity capacity, compromised abdominal muscle strength, or both, may be able to navigate more difficult terrains while using a geared wheelchair wheel because of reduced demands from the abdominal musculature in the geared wheel condition.

▶ This biomechanical study of wheelchair ramp ascent highlights the trunk muscle activity required. Not surprisingly, there was an increase in abdominal peak activity and posterior trunk muscle activity with increasing ramp grades. Although tested on persons with no neurologic impairments (13 healthy university students with no history of pain or injury), the results of this study suggest that the use of a geared wheel may be helpful for those persons who have decreased abdominal muscle strength. This conclusion stems from their results that indicated that peak electromyographic activity in both rectus abdominus and external oblique muscles was reduced by using the geared wheelchair. The authors imply that studying a healthy population may provide a basis for comparison for those who have neurological impairments. Studying persons with neurological impairments with respect to use of a standard or geared wheelchair should be done to see whether the latter is beneficial for these persons.

D. E. Feldman, PT, PhD

Effect of Heel Lifts on Plantarflexor and Dorsiflexor Activity During Gait

Johanson MA, Allen JC, Matsumoto M, et al (Emory Univ School of Medicine, Atlanta, GA)
Foot Ankle Int 31:1014-1020, 2010

Background.—Previous investigators have shown that high heels decrease the muscle activity of the gastrocnemius muscle during gait. However, it is not known whether commonly used in-shoe heel lifts of lower heights will demonstrate similar effects on muscle activity. The aim of this study was to determine whether heel lifts alter the muscle activity of the ankle plantarflexors and dorsiflexors during the stance phase of gait among individuals with limited gastrocnemius extensibility.

Materials and Methods.—This study used a repeated measures design. Twentyfour healthy volunteers (12 males and 12 females) with less than 5 degrees of passive ankle dorsiflexion with the knee extended participated in the study. Electromyography (EMG), computerized motion analysis, and a force plate were used to measure mean muscle activity of the lateral gastrocnemius, medial gastrocnemius, soleus and tibialis anterior muscles during the stance phase of gait across three walking conditions. Muscle activity was measured as participants ambulated at a self-selected speed in athletic shoes alone and with heel lifts of 6 mm and 9 mm inserted in athletic shoes.

Results.—Between heel-strike and heel-off, the mean EMG amplitude of the medial gastrocnemius increased with both 6 and 9 mm heel lifts and the amplitude of the tibialis anterior increased with 9 mm heel lifts compared to shoes alone. Between heel-strike and heel-off, there were no significant differences in mean EMG amplitude of the lateral gastrocnemius or soleus muscles walking in heel lifts compared to shoes alone. Between heel-off and toe-off, there were no significant differences in mean EMG amplitude of the lateral gastrocnemius, medial gastrocnemius, soleus, or tibialis anterior muscles when walking in heel lifts compared to shoes alone.

Conclusion.—Heel lifts increase muscle activity of the medial gastrocnemius and tibialis anterior muscles between heel-strike and heel-off among individuals with limited gastrocnemius extensibility.

Clinical Relevance.—We were unable to confirm a decrease in muscle activity when using heel lifts.

▶ Patients with limited functional ankle dorsiflexion attributed to a tight gastrocnemius muscle are sometimes prescribed heel lifts to reduce the load within the Achilles tendon and the plantar fasciitis. The heel lift shifts the ankle's range of motion toward a plantarflexed posture thereby relaxing the passive and active structures within the gastrocnemius. It has been reported that during gait, the shifted ankle range of motion decreases the activity of the gastrocnemius muscle. In this study, Johanson et al tested 24 healthy volunteers with limited ankle dorsiflexion while they walked wearing different thickness heel lifts. Electromyographic evidence suggested that during early stance when one wears a heel lift, the gastrocnemius activity increases, not decreases as expected. Additionally, muscle activity in one of the ankle antagonist muscles, tibialis anterior muscle, was also increased. The clinical significance of this work is that heel lifts may not reduce ankle loading and it does not decrease gastrocnemius and tibialis anterior muscle activity during the early stance phase of gait.

M. R. Pierrynowski, PhD

Plantar Loading After Chevron Osteotomy Combined With Postoperative Physical Therapy
Schuh R, Adams S Jr, Hofstaetter SG, et al (Innsbruck Med Univ, Austria)
Foot Ankle Int 31:980-986, 2010

Background.—Recent pedobarographic studies have demonstrated decreased loading of the great toe region and the first metatarsal head at a short- and intermediate-term followup. The purpose of the present study was to determine if a postoperative rehabilitation program helped to improve weightbearing of the first ray after chevron osteotomy for correction of hallux valgus deformity.

Materials and Methods.—Twenty-nine patients with a mean age of 58 years with mild to moderate hallux valgus deformity who underwent a chevron osteotomy were included. Postoperatively, the patients received a multimodal rehabilitation program including mobilization, manual therapy, strengthening exercises and gait training. Preoperative and one year postoperative plantar pressure distribution parameters including maximum force, contact area and force-time integral were evaluated. Additionly the AOFAS score, ROM of the first MTP joint and plain radiographs were assessed. The results were compared using Student's t-test and level of significance was set at $p < 0.05$.

Results.—In the great toe, the mean maximum force increased from 72.2 N preoperatively to 106.8 N 1 year after surgery. The mean contact area increased from 7.6 cm^2 preoperatively to 8.9 cm^2 1 year after surgery and the mean force-time integral increased from 20.8 N* sec to 30.5 N* sec. All changes were statistically significant ($p < 0.05$). For the first metatarsal head region, the mean maximum force increased from 122.5 N preoperatively to 144.7 N one year after surgery and the mean force-time integral increased from 42.3 N* sec preoperatively to 52.6 N* sec 1 year postoperatively ($p = 0.068$ and $p = 0.055$, respectively). The mean AOFAS score increased from 61 points preoperatively to 94 points at final followup ($p < 0.001$). The average hallux valgus angle decreased from 31 degrees to 9 degrees and the average first intermetatarsal angle decreased from 14 degrees to 6 degrees ($p < 0.001$ for both).

Conclusion.—Our results suggest that postoperative physical therapy and gait training with a Chevron osteotomy may help to improve weight-bearing of the great toe and first ray. Therefore, we believe there is a restoration of more physiological gait patterns in patients who receive this postoperative regimen.

▶ The main limitation of this study is that there is no control group and patients may have improved with respect to the measured outcomes over time, without the postoperative physical therapy intervention. The authors compare their results with 4 previous studies in which patients did not receive physical therapy postsurgery and had decreased loading of the hallux region compared with preoperative level. The results of this study that indicate improved load distribution of the great toe following a physical therapy intervention program postsurgery suggest that perhaps the intervention is beneficial. Besides plantar pressure assessment, patient rated clinical outcome and radiographic measurements in terms of intermetatarsal angle, hallux valgus angle, and sesamoid position improved at the 1-year follow-up. The results of this observational study underscore the need to conduct a randomized controlled trial to be able to conclude that the intervention is in fact beneficial.

D. E. Feldman, PT, PhD

Body Composition and Strength Changes in Women with Milk and Resistance Exercise

Josse AR, Tang JE, Tarnopolsky MA, et al (McMaster Univ, Hamilton, Ontario, Canada; McMaster Univ Med Centre, Hamilton, Ontario, Canada)

Med Sci Sports Exerc 42:1122-1130, 2010

Purpose.—We aimed to determine whether women consuming fat-free milk versus isoenergetic carbohydrate after resistance exercise would see augmented gains in lean mass and reductions in fat mass similar to what we observed in young men.

Methods.—Young women were randomized to drink either fat-free milk (MILK: $n = 10$; age (mean ± SD) = 23.2 ± 2.8 yr; BMI = 26.2 ± 4.2 kg·m^{-2}) or isoenergetic carbohydrate (CON: $n = 10$; age = 22.4 ± 2.4 yr; BMI = 25.2 ± 3.8 kg·m^{-2}) immediately after and 1 h after exercise (2 × 500 mL). Subjects exercised 5 d·wk^{-1} for 12 wk. Body composition changes were measured by dual-energy x-ray absorptiometry, and subjects' strength and fasting blood were measured before and after training.

Results.—CON gained weight after training (CON: +0.86 ± 0.4 kg, $P < 0.05$; MILK: +0.50 ± 0.4 kg, $P = 0.29$). Lean mass increased with training in both groups ($P < 0.01$), with a greater net gain in MILK versus CON (1.9 ± 0.2 vs 1.1 ± 0.2 kg, respectively, $P < 0.01$). Fat mass decreased with training in MILK only (-1.6 ± 0.4 kg, $P < 0.01$; CON: -0.3 ± 0.3 kg, $P = 0.41$). Isotonic strength increased more in MILK than CON ($P < 0.05$) for some exercises. Serum 25-hydroxyvitamin D increased in both groups but to a greater extent in MILK than CON ($+6.5 \pm 1.1$ vs $+2.8 \pm 1.3$ nM, respectively, $P < 0.05$), and parathyroid hormone decreased only in MILK (-1.2 ± 0.2 pM, $P < 0.01$).

Conclusions.—Heavy, whole-body resistance exercise with the consumption of milk versus carbohydrate in the early postexercise period resulted in greater muscle mass accretion, strength gains, fat mass loss, and a possible reduction in bone turnover in women after 12 wk. Our results, similar to those in men, highlight that milk is an effective drink to support favorable body composition changes in women with resistance training.

▶ Relatively little is known about the potential for women to gain strength and lean mass in response to progressive resistance exercise training. One strategy to enhance the resistance training outcomes is to provide dietary protein immediately after each exercise session. Dietary protein and mechanical loading are potent stimuli for muscle protein synthesis. In young men, skeletal muscle fractional protein synthesis rate increased significantly when milk was consumed immediately after an acute bout of resistance exercise compared with the exercise stimulus alone.[1] In the study by Josse and colleagues, young women were randomly assigned to consume 500 mL of fat-free milk containing 18 grams of protein or a carbohydrate beverage immediately and 1 hour after resistance exercise (1 L of beverage each exercise day) in single-blinded fashion. The training intervention was supervised, moderate to high intensity (80%-90% of the single repetition maximum) resistance exercise for 5 days per week for 12 weeks. Participation in resistance or cardiovascular exercise training was exclusionary, as was the use of vitamin or mineral supplements. Five of the 10 women in each group were using oral contraceptives. The results were similar to those found previously in young men[2] that milk consumption was associated with greater loss of fat mass and increased fat-free mass than the carbohydrate drink. Total body mass increased in the carbohydrate group but not in the milk group. Significant strength improvements in the lower body were found in both groups, although women drinking milk became stronger with 2 upper body exercises. Because of the potential benefits of resistance exercise and milk for bone health in young women, the investigators evaluated serum markers of bone metabolism. Serum 25-hydroxyvitamin D increased more in the milk than in the carbohydrate group, whereas serum parathyroid hormone decreased more in the milk group. Markers of bone resorption (c-telopeptides) and formation (osteocalcin) increased in both groups in response to training. Together, these markers suggest a decrease in bone turnover in the women consuming milk after exercise. However, given the small sample size, these results are best considered preliminary. A longer intervention with measures of bone mineral density would be a logical follow-up study. Although young women tend to forgo milk in their diets, this study demonstrated favorable changes in body composition (decreased body fat and increased lean mass) and strength when 1 L of fat-free milk was consumed in close temporal association with resistance exercise.

C. M. Jankowski, PhD

References

1. Wilkinson SB, Tarnopolsky MA, Macdonald MJ, Macdonald JR, Armstrong D, Phillips SM. Consumption of fluid skim milk promotes greater muscle protein accretion after resistance exercise than does consumption of an isonitrogenous and isoenergetic soy-protein beverage. *Am J Clin Nutr.* 2007;85:1031-1040.
2. Hartman JW, Tang JE, Wilkinson SB, et al. Consumption of fat-free fluid milk after resistance exercise promotes greater lean mass accretion than does consumption of soy or carbohydrate in young, novice, male weightlifters. *Am J Clin Nutr.* 2007;86:373-381.

A Comparison of Elastic Tubing and Isotonic Resistance Exercises

Colado JC, Garcia-Masso X, Pellicer M, et al (Univ of Valencia, Spain; et al)
Int J Sports Med 31:810-817, 2010

The aim of this study was to assess effects of a short-term resistance program on strength in fit young women using weight machines/free weights or elastic tubing. 42 physically fit women (21.79 ± 0.7 years) were randomly assigned to the following groups: (i) the Thera-Band® Exercise Station Group (TBG); (ii) the weight machines/free weights group (MFWG); or (iii) the control group (CG). Each experimental group performed the same periodised training program that lasted for 8 weeks, with 2—4 sessions per week and 3—4 sets of 8—15 submaximal reps. A load cell (Isocontrol; ATEmicro, Madrid, Spain) was used to test the evolution of the Maximum Isometric Voluntary Contraction (MIVC) in 3 different exercises: Vertical Rowing (VR), Squat (S) and Back Extension (BE). A mixed model MANOVA [group (CG, TBG, MFWG) × testing time (pre-test, post-test)] was applied to determine the effect of the different resistance training devices on strength. The only groups to improve their MIVC ($p < 0.005$) were TBG and MFWG, respectively: VR 19.87% and 19.76%; S 14.07 and 28.88; BE 14.41% and 14.00%. These results indicate that resistance training using elastic tubing or weight machines/free weights have equivalent improvements in isometric force in short-term programs applied in fit young women (Figs 2A and 3A).

▶ There is a host of exercise equipment in the consumer market, but relatively little research has been done to compare outcomes in carefully controlled investigations. This study by Colado and colleagues is the first to compare changes in muscle strength in healthy young women who train using an elastic tubing system with a group using machines and free weights. Elastic tubing exercise has been used to improve strength in older adults, but the results could be explained partly by their deconditioned state before training. Young women who were physically active but not engaged in resistance training completed

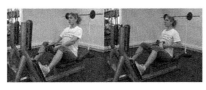
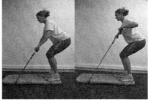

FIGURE 2.—Upper limb training exercises. Downwards: A, Inclined standing rowing. (Reprinted from Colado JC, Garcia-Masso X, Pellicer M, et al. A comparison of elastic tubing and isotonic resistance exercises. *Int J Sports Med*. 2010;31:810-817, with permission from Georg Thieme Verlag KG Stuttgart.)

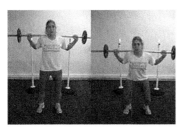
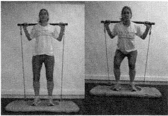

FIGURE 3.—Lower limb training exercises. *Downwards*: A, Squat. (Reprinted from Colado JC, Garcia-Masso X, Pellicer M, et al. A comparison of elastic tubing and isotonic resistance exercises. *Int J Sports Med*. 2010;31:810-817, with permission from Georg Thieme Verlag KG Stuttgart.)

15 exercises for the trunk, upper, and lower limbs using either the Thera-Band Exercise Station or a combination of free weights and resistance machines. They trained for 8 weeks, 2 to 3 days per week, and 3 to 4 sets per exercise. The investigators were careful to match movements (Figs 2A and 3A) and training intensity in the 2 exercise groups. The target for perceived exertion was between 7 and 9 using the OMNI-RES AM scale, whereby individuals choose a level of effort from 0 (no effort) to 10 (hardest effort) in the active muscle group for each exercise. This rating of perceived exertion for resistance exercise has been validated against blood lactate concentrations in young women and men.[1] Before and after the intervention, isometric strength was measured as maximal voluntary contraction using a load cell during vertical row, squat, and back extension movements. A no-exercise control group was included. There were significant increases in isometric strength for all 3 exercises in the exercise groups but not in the control group. The changes in strength were not significantly different between the 2 exercise groups, indicating that the elastic tubing system provided an effective training stimulus. Elastic tubing exercise provides an alternative training strategy that can be implemented in the home and at lower consumer cost than other equipment systems.

C. M. Jankowski, PhD

Reference

1. Robertson RJ, Goss FL, Rutkowski J, et al. Concurrent validation of the OMNI perceived exertion scale for resistance exercise. *Med Sci Sports Exerc*. 2003;35: 333-341.

Lower limb compression garment improves recovery from exercise-induced muscle damaged in young, active females

Jakeman JR, Byrne C, Eston RG (Univ of Exeter, UK)
Eur J Appl Physiol 109:1137-1144, 2010

This study aimed to investigate the efficacy of lower limb compression as a recovery strategy following exercise-induced muscle damage (EIMD). Seventeen female volunteers completed 10×10 plyometric drop jumps from a 0.6-m box to induce muscle damage. Participants were randomly allocated to a passive recovery $(n = 9)$ or a compression treatment $(n = 8)$ group. Treatment group volunteers wore full leg compression stockings for 12 h immediately following damaging exercise. Passive recovery group participants had no intervention. Indirect indices of muscle damage (muscle soreness, creatine kinase activity, knee extensor

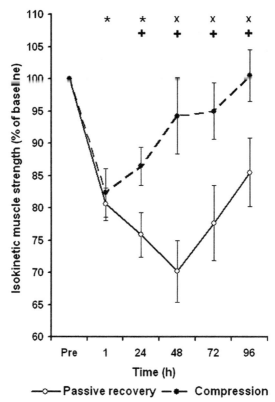

FIGURE 4.—Isokinetic muscle strength relative to baseline following exercise-induced muscle damage. *Asterisks* represent significant difference to baseline in both groups; *multiple symbols* represent significant difference to baseline in passive recovery group only; *plus symbols* represent significant difference between groups. (Reprinted from Jakeman JR, Byrne C, Eston RG. Lower limb compression garment improves recovery from exercise-induced muscle damaged in young, active females. *Eur J Appl Physiol.* 2010;109:1137-1144. With kind permission of Springer Science+Business Media.)

concentric strength, and vertical jump performance) were assessed prior to and 1, 24, 48, 72, and 96 h following plyometric exercise. Plyometric exercise had a significant effect ($p \leq 0.05$) on all indices of muscle damage. The compression treatment reduced decrements in countermovement jump performance (passive recovery 88.1 ± 2.8% vs. treatment 95.2 ± 2.9% of pre-exercise), squat jump performance (82.3 ± 1.9% vs. 94.5 ± 2%), and knee extensor strength loss (81.6 ± 3% vs. 93 ± 3.2%), and reduced muscle soreness (4.0 ± 0.23 vs. 2.4 ± 0.24), but had no significant effect on creatine kinase activity. The results indicate that compression clothing is an effective recovery strategy following exercise-induced muscle damage (Fig 4).

▶ Speedy recovery from exercise-induced muscle damage is an important goal in sports medicine, but unfortunately, currently used treatments such as cold-water immersion, massage, and active recovery are all of doubtful efficacy.[1-5] There has thus been growing interest in the potential of compressive clothing to support and splint the injured muscle and/or reduce the associated edema that may cause much of the soreness, although not all of these reports have shown much benefit from compression therapy.[6-10] The present small-scale randomized controlled trial shows a dramatic decrease in muscle soreness in the first 4 days after eccentric exercise among subjects who wore lower limb compression tights for 12 hours immediately following injury, with even larger gains in muscle strength (Fig 4) and physical performance relative to controls. This approach thus seems to merit further consideration, with exploration of possible mechanisms on a larger sample of subjects; however, 1 negative aspect of the data is the absence of any effect on the most objective indicator of injury: creatine kinase levels.

R. J. Shephard, MD (Lond), PhD, DPE

References

1. Gill ND, Beaven CM, Cook C. Effectiveness of post-match recovery strategies in rugby players. *Br J Sports Med.* 2006;40:260-263.
2. Bailey DM, Erith SJ, Griffin PJ, et al. Influence of cold water immersion on indices of muscle damage following prolonged intermittent shuttle running. *J Sports Sci.* 2007;25:1163-1170.
3. Jakeman JR, Macrae R, Eston R. A single 10-min bout of cold-water immersion therapy after strenuous plyometric exercise has no beneficial effect on recovery from the symptoms of exercise-induced muscle damage. *Ergonomics.* 2009;52: 456-460.
4. Farr T, Nottle C, Nosaka K, Sacco P. The effects of therapeutic massage on delayed onset muscle soreness and muscle function following downhill walking. *J Sci Med Sport.* 2002;5:297-306.
5. Mancinelli CA, Davis DS, Aboulhosn L, Brady M, Eisenhofer J, Foutty S. The effects of massage on delayed onset muscle soreness and physical performance in female collegiate athletes. *Phys Ther Sport.* 2006;7:5-13.
6. Kraemer WJ, Bush JA, Wickham RB, et al. Influence of compression therapy on symptoms following soft tissue injury from maximal eccentric exercise. *J Orthop Sports Phys Ther.* 2001;31:282-290.
7. Ali A, Caine MP, Snow BG. Graduated compression stockings: physiological and perceptual responses during and after exercise. *J Sports Sci.* 2007;25:413-419.

8. Trenell MI, Rooney KB, Sue CM, Thompson CH. Compression garments and recovery from eccentric exercise: a ^{31}P-MRS study. *J Sport Sci Med*. 2006;5:106-114.
9. Duffield R, Portus M. Comparison of three types of full-body compression garments on throwing and repeat-sprint performance in cricket players. *Br J Sports Med*. 2007;41:409-414.
10. French DN, Thompson KG, Garland SW, et al. The effects of contrast bathing and compression therapy on muscular performance. *Med Sci Sport Exerc*. 2008;40:1297-1306.

Cryotherapy Impairs Knee Joint Position Sense

Oliveira R, Ribeiro F, Oliveira J (Jean Piaget Inst, Vila Nova de Gaia, Portugal; Health School of Vale do Sousa, Gandra PRD, Portugal; Univ of Porto, Portugal)

Int J Sports Med 31:198-201, 2010

The effects of cryotherapy on joint position sense are not clearly established; however it is paramount to understand its impact on peripheral feedback to ascertain the safety of using ice therapy before resuming exercise on sports or rehabilitation settings. Thus, the aim of the present study was to determine the effects of cryotherapy, when applied over the quadriceps and over the knee joint, on knee position sense. This within-subjects repeated-measures study encompassed fifteen subjects. Knee position sense was measured by open kinetic chain technique and active positioning at baseline and after cryotherapy application. Knee angles were determined by computer analysis of the videotape images. Twenty-minute ice bag application was applied randomly, in two sessions 48 h apart, over the quadriceps and the knee joint. The main effect for cryotherapy application was significant ($F_{1.14} = 7.7$, $p = 0.015$) indicating an increase in both absolute and relative angular errors after the application. There was no significant main effect for the location of cryotherapy application, indicating no differences between the application over the quadriceps and the knee joint. In conclusion, cryotherapy impairs knee joint position sense in normal knees. This deleterious effect is similar when cryotherapy is applied over the quadriceps or the knee joint.

▶ This is yet another in a series of studies that show that cryotherapy impairs joint position sense in normal knees. The novelty in this study is that it does not matter where the ice pack is placed—that is, over the quadriceps or knee joint itself—the results are the same in terms of joint position sense. The small sample is a problem, but the results do concur with previous studies regarding joint sense after cryotherapy. As the authors state, it would be important to conduct further research to determine how long the negative effect of cryotherapy on joint proprioception might last in injured subjects (past research indicates that it is normalized in healthy subjects at 15 minutes postcooling). This information would be important in terms of when it would be safe to return athletes onto the field after the application of ice to the injury site.

D. E. Feldman, PT, PhD

Low level laser therapy before eccentric exercise reduces muscle damage markers in humans

Baroni BM, Leal ECP Jr, De Marchi T, et al (Federal Univ of Rio Grande do Sul (UFRGS), Porto Alegre, Brazil; Univ of Bergen, Norway; Univ of Caxias do Sul (UCS), RS, Brazil)
Eur J Appl Physiol 110:789-796, 2010

The purpose of the present study was to determine the effect of low level laser therapy (LLLT) treatment before knee extensor eccentric exercise on indirect markers of muscle damage. Thirty-six healthy men were randomized in LLLT group ($n = 18$) and placebo group ($n = 18$). After LLLT or placebo treatment, subjects performed 75 maximal knee extensors eccentric contractions (five sets of 15 repetitions; velocity $= 60°$ seg^{-1}; range of motion $= 60°$). Muscle soreness (visual analogue scale—VAS), lactate dehydrogenase (LDH) and creatine kinase (CK) levels were measured prior to exercise, and 24 and 48 h after exercise. Muscle function (maximal voluntary contraction—MVC) was measured before exercise, immediately after, and 24 and 48 h post-exercise. Groups had no difference on kineanthropometric characteristics and on eccentric exercise performance. They also presented similar baseline values of VAS (0.00 mm for LLLT and placebo groups), LDH (LLLT $= 186$ IU/l; placebo $= 183$ IU/l), CK (LLLT $= 145$ IU/l; placebo $= 155$ IU/l) and MVC (LLLT $= 293$ Nm; placebo $= 284$ Nm). VAS data did not show group by time interaction ($P = 0.066$). In the other outcomes, LLLT group presented (1) smaller increase on LDH values 48 h postexercise (LLLT $= 366$ IU/l; placebo $= 484$ IU/l; $P = 0.017$); (2) smaller increase on CK values 24 h (LLLT $= 272$ IU/l; placebo $= 498$ IU/l; $P = 0.020$) and 48 h (LLLT $= 436$ IU/l; placebo $= 1328$ IU/l; $P < 0.001$) postexercise; (3) smaller decrease on MVC immediately after exercise (LLLT $= 189$ Nm; placebo $= 154$ Nm; $P = 0.011$), and 24 h (LLLT $= 249$ Nm; placebo $= 205$ Nm; $P = 0.004$) and 48 h (LLLT $= 267$ Nm; placebo $= 216$ Nm; $P = 0.001$) post-exercise compared with the placebo group. In conclusion, LLLT treatment before eccentric exercise was effective in terms of attenuating the increase of muscle proteins in the blood serum and the decrease in muscle force (Table 2).

▶ Sports physicians have tried varied approaches for reducing the muscle damage that follows eccentric muscle training; they have shown benefit from improved nutrition and the administration of antioxidant drugs and less certain gains from massage and cryotherapy.[1,2] Low-level laser therapy has previously been suggested as promoting the regeneration of rat muscle,[3] and there is thus some logic in testing its efficacy against eccentric muscle damage. The present controlled trial evaluated a THOR 810-nm laser containing 5 diodes, applying the apparatus (switched off for the control subjects) at 5 sites on the leg for a total energy input of 180 J. This level of treatment appears to have caused a marked reduction in visual analog and biochemical indicators of muscle damage 48 hours after the eccentric exercise (75 maximal knee extensor contractions) (Table 2), with corresponding gains in the individual's postexercise

TABLE 2.—Indirect Markers of Exercise-Induced Muscle Damage (mean ± SD)

	Baseline	Immediately After	24 h	48 h
VAS (mm)				
LLLT	0.00 ± 0.00	–	21.39 ± 20.31[a,d]	29.78 ± 30.75[a,c]
Placebo	0.00 ± 0.00	–	32.17 ± 19.92[a,d]	50.78 ± 29.79[a,c]
LDH (IU/l)				
LLLT	186.02 ± 44.92	–	296.93 ± 99.98[a,d]	366.06 ± 84.46* [a,c]
Placebo	182.59 ± 43.84	–	290.10 ± 87.54[a,d]	483.85 ± 180.29* [a,c]
CK (IU/l)				
LLLT	144.69 ± 59.01	–	271.70 ± 146.31* [a,d]	435.95 ± 238.04* [a,c]
Placebo	155.16 ± 51.27	–	497.75 ± 362.97* [a,d]	1327.58 ± 949.82* [a,c]
MVC (Nm)				
LLLT	292.92 ± 42.93	188.93 ± 43.04* [a,c,d]	249.43 ± 42.61* [a,b,d]	267.09 ± 37.40* [a,b,c]
Placebo	283.98 ± 47.07	154.03 ± 34.57* [a,c,d]	205.09 ± 43.52* [a,b]	216.14 ± 50.17* [a,b]

*Different from the other group.
[a]Different from baseline.
[b]Different from immediately after.
[c]Different from 24 h.
[d]Different from 48 h.

performance. Possible explanations of benefit include an anti-inflammatory action,[4] a reduction in the release of reactive oxygen species,[5] and an increase of antioxidant capacity.[6] I am always a little suspicious of devices such as this laser, but on the evidence that is presented in this article, further trials certainly seem warranted.

R. J. Shephard, MD (Lond), PhD, DPE

References

1. Cheung K, Hume P, Maxwell L. Delayed onset muscle soreness—treatment strategies and performance factors. *Sports Med.* 2003;33:145-164.
2. Howatson G, van Someren KA. The prevention and treatment of exercise-induced muscle damage. *Sports Med.* 2008;38:483-503.
3. Cressoni MD, Dib Giusti HH, Casarotto RA, Anaruma CA. The effects of a 785-nm AlGaInP laser on the regeneration of rat anterior tibialis muscle after surgically-induced injury. *Photomed Laser Surg.* 2008 10.1089/pho.2007.2150 [published online ahead of print September 18, 2008].
4. Yamaura M, Yao M, Yaroslavsky I, Cohen R, Smotrich M, Kochevar IE. Low level light effects on inflammatory cytokine production by rheumatoid arthritis synoviocytes. *Lasers Surg Med.* 2009;41:282-290.
5. Rizzi CF, Mauriz JL, Freitas Corrêa DS, et al. Effects of low-level laser therapy (LLLT) on the nuclear factor (NF)-kappaB signaling pathway in traumatized muscle. *Lasers Surg Med.* 2006;38:704-713.
6. Avni D, Levkovitz S, Maltz L, Oron U. Protection of skeletal muscles from ischemic injury: low-level laser therapy increases antioxidant activity. *Photomed Laser Surg.* 2005;23:273-277.

Cardiovascular safety of non-steroidal anti-inflammatory drugs: network meta-analysis

Trelle S, Reichenbach S, Wandel S, et al (Univ of Bern, Switzerland; et al)
BMJ 342:c7086, 2011

Objective.—To analyse the available evidence on cardiovascular safety of non-steroidal anti-inflammatory drugs.

Design.—Network meta-analysis.

Data Sources.—Bibliographic databases, conference proceedings, study registers, the Food and Drug Administration website, reference lists of relevant articles, and reports citing relevant articles through the Science Citation Index (last update July 2009). Manufacturers of celecoxib and lumiracoxib provided additional data.

Study Selection.—All large scale randomised controlled trials comparing any non-steroidal anti-inflammatory drug with other non-steroidal anti-inflammatory drugs or placebo. Two investigators independently assessed eligibility.

Data Extraction.—The primary outcome was myocardial infarction. Secondary outcomes included stroke, death from cardiovascular disease, and death from any cause. Two investigators independently extracted data.

Data Synthesis.—31 trials in 116 429 patients with more than 115 000 patient years of follow-up were included. Patients were allocated to naproxen, ibuprofen, diclofenac, celecoxib, etoricoxib, rofecoxib, lumiracoxib, or placebo. Compared with placebo, rofecoxib was associated with the highest risk of myocardial infarction (rate ratio 2.12, 95% credibility interval 1.26 to 3.56), followed by lumiracoxib (2.00, 0.71 to 6.21). Ibuprofen was associated with the highest risk of stroke (3.36, 1.00 to 11.6), followed by diclofenac (2.86, 1.09 to 8.36). Etoricoxib (4.07, 1.23 to 15.7) and diclofenac (3.98, 1.48 to 12.7) were associated with the highest risk of cardiovascular death.

Conclusions.—Although uncertainty remains, little evidence exists to suggest that any of the investigated drugs are safe in cardiovascular terms. Naproxen seemed least harmful. Cardiovascular risk needs to be taken into account when prescribing any non-steroidal anti-inflammatory drug (Fig 2).

► Athletes, like many patients,[1,2] frequently consume nonsteroidal anti-inflammatory drugs (NSAIDs). However, there has been growing concern that NSAIDs can provoke cardiovascular events, and in 2004 the cyclo-oxygenase-2 specific selective inhibitor rofecoxib was withdrawn from the market because of concerns that it was provoking myocardial infarction.[3] The recent article of Trelle and associates makes a helpful meta-analysis of the risks of myocardial infarction, stroke, and cardiovascular death associated with each of the various available NSAIDs (Fig 2), looking at data from 31 trials on 7 drugs. Perhaps the most striking feature is the wide range of confidence limits for most drugs and outcomes. This is in part because the search is for rare events. None of the 7 drugs tested can be given a clear bill of health on the basis of the available data,

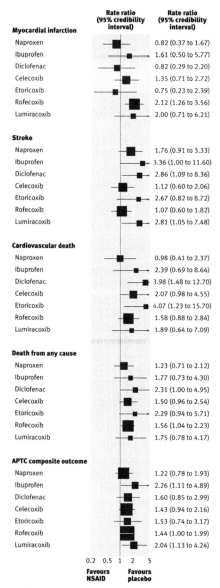

FIGURE 2.—Estimates of rate ratios for non-steroidal anti-inflammatory drugs compared with placebo. NSAID=nonsteroidal anti-inflammatory drug; APTC=Antiplatelet Trialists' Collaboration. (Reprinted from Trelle S, Reichenbach S, Wandel S, et al. Cardiovascular safety of non-steroidal anti-inflammatory drugs: network meta-analysis. *BMJ.* 2011;342:c7086, reproduced with permission from the BMJ Publishing Group Ltd.)

but ibuprofen seemed associated with a high risk of stroke. Naproxen at present seems to be the least harmful choice.

R. J. Shephard, MD (Lond), PhD, DPE

References

1. Dai C, Stafford RS, Alexander GC. National trends in cyclooxygenase-2 inhibitor use since market release: nonselective diffusion of a selectively cost-effective innovation. *Arch Intern Med.* 2005;165:171-177.
2. Kaufman DW, Kelly JP, Rosenberg L, Anderson TE, Mitchell AA. Recent patterns of medication use in the ambulatory adult population of the United States: the Slone survey. *JAMA.* 2002;287:337-344.
3. Bresalier RS, Sandler RS, Quan H, et al. Cardiovascular events associated with rofecoxib in a colorectal adenoma chemoprevention trial. *N Engl J Med.* 2005; 352:1092-1102.

Use of NSAIDs in triathletes: prevalence, level of awareness and reasons for use

Gorski T, Cadore EL, Pinto SS, et al (Federal Univ of Rio Grande do Sul, Porto Alegre, Brazil; et al)

Br J Sports Med 45:85-90, 2011

Objective.—To determine the level of awareness regarding nonsteroidal anti-inflammatory drugs (NSAIDs) and the prevalence and reasons for their consumption among athletes competing at the 2008 Brazil Ironman Triathlon (3.8 km swim, 180 km cycle and 42.2 km run).

Design.—Survey study.

Setting.—2008 Brazil Ironman Triathlon, Florianópolis, Brazil, May 2008.

Participants.—327 Of the 1250 athletes competing at the 2008 Brazil Ironman Triathlon were enrolled in the study.

Main Outcome Measures.—Athletes answered a questionnaire about NSAID effects, side effects and consumption at the bike checkout or awards lunch.

Results.—196 (59.9%) Athletes reported using NSAIDs in the previous 3 months; of these, 25.5% (n=50), 17.9% (n=35) and 47.4% (n=93) consumed NSAIDs the day before, immediately before and during the race, respectively. Among NSAID users, 48.5% (n=95) consumed them without medical prescription. The main reason given for NSAID consumption in the previous 3 months was the treatment of injuries, while the main reason given for consuming NSAIDs during the race was pain prevention. Despite anti-inflammatory and analgesic effects, most athletes were unaware of the effects of NSAIDs, and the only adverse effects known by most athletes were the gastrointestinal complications.

Conclusions.—This study found a high prevalence of NSAID consumption, limited awareness of the effects and side effects of them and a high rate of nonprescribed use. It is suggested that long-distance triathlon events include in their programmes educational devices such as talks or folders about NSAID use, effects and side effects (Table 3).

▶ The article of Gorski et al on 327 Ironman competitors adds to much existing evidence on the overuse of nonsteroidal anti-inflammatory drugs (NSAIDs) by

TABLE 3.—Medical Complication During the Race (NSAIDs, Nonsteroidal Anti-Inflammatory Drugs)

Medical Complication During the Race	NSAIDs Consumption During the Race Yes (n=93)	No (n=234)
Dehydration	1.1% (n=1)	0.4% (n=1)
Hyponatremia	2.2% (n=2)	0% (n=0)
Gastrointestinal problems	7.5% (n=7)	5.1% (n=12)
Cramps	5.4% (n=5)	2.1% (n=5)
Tendinopathies	0% (n=0)	0.9% (n=2)
Asthma	0% (n=0)	0.4% (n=1)
Hypothermia	0% (n=0)	0.4% (n=1)
Hypotension	0% (n=0)	0.4% (n=1)
Headache	0% (n=0)	0.4% (n=1)
Hyperventilation	0% (n=0)	0% (n=0)
Bone fractures and orthopaedic problems	2.2% (n=2)	2.1% (n=5)
Muscular spasms	0% (n=0)	0% (n=0)
None	84.9% (n=79)	88.5% (n=207)

athletes in various sports disciplines; inappropriately large doses are often taken over long periods.[1-6] Since not all athletes agreed to participate, NSAIDs use may have been even higher than the reported prevalence of 60%. Sometimes such medications are self-administered to allow training to continue in the face of minor injuries or even in the hope of enhancing performance by blocking the pain associated with delayed-onset muscle soreness[7], on other occasions, their use is proposed by coaches, as a means of speeding recuperation following training sessions.[8] In more than half of the present individuals, the drugs were not medically prescribed. The greater prevalence of NSAIDs use on the day of competition supports the view that these drugs are being used in part with the hope of improving performance. However, side effects such as changes in thermoregulation are plainly undesirable for an endurance competitor, and the findings from this study suggest performance was actually poorer, with a greater incidence of medical complications reported by users both during and immediately following the event (Table 3). Physicians increasingly recognize the major problems that can result from the prolonged use of NSAIDs, but unfortunately, most athletes are unaware of issues other than gastrointestinal symptoms. Furthermore, it seems undesirable that athletes who are in serious pain from musculoskeletal injuries should be competing in ultramarathon events. Plainly, more education is needed on the dangers associated with excessive use of these readily available medications.

R. J. Shephard, MD (Lond), PhD, DPE

References

1. Corrigan B, Kazlauskas R. Medication use in athletes selected for doping control at the Sydney Olympics (2000). *Clin J Sport Med.* 2003;13:33-40.
2. Reid SA, Speedy DB, Thompson JM, et al. Study of hematological and biochemical parameters in runners completing a standard marathon. *Clin J Sport Med.* 2004; 14:344-353.

3. Nieman DC, Dumke CL, Henson DA, McAnulty SR, Gross SJ, Lind RH. Muscle damage is linked to cytokine changes following a 160-km race. *Brain Behav Immun.* 2005;19:398-403.
4. Huang SH, Johnson K, Pipe AL. The use of dietary supplements and medications by Canadian athletes at the Atlanta and Sydney Olympic Games. *Clin J Sport Med.* 2006;16:27-33.
5. Wharam PC, Speedy DB, Noakes TD, Thompson JM, Reid SA, Holtzhausen LM. NSAID use increases the risk of developing hyponatremia during an Ironman triathlon. *Med Sci Sports Exerc.* 2006;38:618-622.
6. Alaranta A, Alaranta H, Heliövaara M, Airaksinen M, Helenius I. Ample use of physician-prescribed medication in Finnish elite athletes. *Int J Sports Med.* 2006;27:919-925.
7. Warner DC, Schnepf G, Barrett MS, Dian D, Swigonski NL. Prevalence, attitudes, and behaviors related to the use of nonsteroidal anti-inflammatory drugs (NSAIDs) in student athletes. *J Adolesc Health.* 2002;30:150-153.
8. Martin DE, Coe PN. *Better Training for Distance Runners.* 2nd ed. Champaign, IL: Human Kinetics; 1997.

4 Physical Activity, Cardiorespiratory Physiology and Immune Function

Energy expenditure in adults living in developing compared with industrialized countries: a meta-analysis of doubly labeled water studies

Dugas LR, Harders R, Merrill S, et al (Loyola Univ Chicago, Maywood, IL, et al)

Am J Clin Nutr 93:427-441, 2011

Background.—There is an assumption that people in developing countries have a higher total energy expenditure (TEE) and physical activity level (PAL) than do people in developed nations, but few objective data for this assertion exist.

Objective.—We conducted a meta-analysis of TEE and PAL by using data from countries that have a low or middle human development index (HDI) compared with those with a high HDI to better understand how energy-expenditure variables are associated with development status and population differences in body size.

Design.—We performed a literature search for studies in which energy expenditure was measured by using doubly labeled water. Mean data on age, weight, body mass index (BMI; in kg/m^2), TEE, and PAL were extracted, and HDI status was assessed. Pooled estimates of the mean effect by sex were obtained, and the extent to which age, weight, HDI status, and year of publication explained heterogeneity was assessed.

Results.—A total of 98 studies (14 studies from low- or middle-HDI countries) that represented 183 cohorts and 4972 individuals were included. Mean ($\pm$ SE) BMI was lower in countries with a low or middle HDI than in those with a high HDI for both men and women (22.7 $\pm$ 1.0 compared with 26.0 $\pm$ 0.7, respectively, in men and 24.3 $\pm$ 0.7 compared with 26.6 $\pm$ 0.4, respectively, in women). In meta-regression models, there was an inverse association of age ($P < 0.001$) and a positive association of weight ($P < 0.001$) with TEE for both sexes; there was an association of age only in men with PAL ($P < 0.001$). There was no association of HDI status with either TEE or PAL.

TABLE 1.—Results of Meta-Analysis by Sex, Human Development Index (HDI) Status, and Age Group[1]

	Men				Women			
	All	Low or Middle HDI	High HDI	High HDI ≤65 y of Age[2]	All	Low or Middle HDI	High HDI	High HDI <65 y of Age[2]
No. of studies	53	9	44	35	81	12	69	62
No. of cohorts	68	10	58	42	115	13	102	87
No. of subjects	1719	144	1575	1135	3253	339	2914	2462
Age (y)	43.2 ± 2.3[3]	32.5 ± 3.3	45.0 ± 2.6	44.5 ± 1.7	39.3 ± 1.9	33.2 ± 2.7	40.1 ± 2.1	35.1 ± 1.3
Weight (kg)	78.1 ± 1.5	66.1 ± 2.7	80.0 ± 1.6	81.3 ± 2.0	70.4 ± 2.8	59.3 ± 2.0	71.8 ± 3.0	72.6 ± 3.2
BMI (kg/m^2)	25.5 ± 0.4	22.7 ± 1.0	26.0 ± 0.7	26.0 ± 0.6	26.3 ± 0.4	24.3 ± 0.7	26.6 ± 0.4	26.6 ± 0.4
Total energy expenditure (MJ/d)	12.7 ± 0.2	12.3 ± 0.4	12.7 ± 0.3	13.5 ± 0.3	9.9 ± 0.1	9.3 ± 0.2	10.0 ± 0.1	10.3 ± 0.1
Physical activity level	1.80 ± 0.03	1.88 ± 0.06	1.79 ± 0.02	1.81 ± 0.03	1.71 ± 0.01	1.70 ± 0.03	1.71 ± 0.02	1.72 ± 0.02

[1]HDI is a composite statistic developed by the United Nations Development Program to rank countries by level of development. In our model, HDI status values were 0 (low or middle HDI) and 1 (high HDI).
[2]Cohorts were restricted to those in which the mean age of participants was <65 y of age.
[3]Mean ± SE (all such values).

Conclusion.—TEE adjusted for weight and age or PAL did not differ significantly between developing and industrialized countries, which calls into question the role of energy expenditure in the cause of obesity at the population level (Table 1).

▶ When comparing health outcomes in various parts of the world, epidemiologists sometimes make sweeping assumptions about regional differences in lifestyle that are difficult to substantiate on closer examination. One such myth has been that those living in developing countries invariably have a larger daily energy expenditure than those living in western countries. Sometimes, this may be true. For instance, we have documented very high rates of energy expenditure among Inuit who were undertaking traditional forms of hunting.[1] However, a careful analysis of energy expenditures among !Kung bushmen in the Kalahari desert found that they were able to meet their limited needs for subsistence by working no more than 2.5 days per week.[2] Much depends on the harshness of the habitat and the perceived minimum requirements for survival in a given community. The meta-analysis of Dugas and associates is based on the gold standard for the estimation of total daily energy expenditure (doubly labeled water). This is both a strength and a weakness in the article; because the technique is very costly, the number of subjects tested in each of the 98 studies is relatively small (an average of about 50 subjects), and it is difficult to be certain that they are representative of the countries considered. In many countries, tests are likely to be performed mainly on the urban rich, and it is only the very occasionally dedicated group of investigators who are able to make effective contact with those who are living a traditional lifestyle. However, in this study, there also seems to be a problem of selection in developed countries, and it is hard to accept that a daily energy of 13.5 MJ (Table 1) is typical of the average man in western society. This is the dilemma of the epidemiologist, as precise methods of measurement lead to misleading conclusions because they cannot be applied to enough people to obtain representative information, and it is difficult to accept the conclusion of this report that lower daily energy expenditures make no contribution to the wider prevalence of obesity in Western society.

R. J. Shephard, MD (Lond), PhD, DPE

References

1. Shephard RJ, Rode A. *The Health Consequences of "Modernization": Evidence From Circumpolar Peoples.* London, UK: Cambridge University Press; 1995.
2. Lee RB. !Kung Bushmen subsistence: an input output analysis. In: Vayda AP, ed. *Environment and Cultural Behavior.* New York, NY: Natural History Press; 1969:47-79.

Economic Analysis of Physical Activity Interventions

Wu S, Cohen D, Shi Y, et al (RAND Corporation, Santa Monica, CA)
Am J Prev Med 40:149-158, 2011

Background.—Numerous interventions have been shown to increase physical activity but have not been ranked by effectiveness or cost.

Purpose.—This study provides a systematic review of physical activity interventions and calculates their cost-effectiveness ratios.

Methods.—A systematic literature review was conducted (5579 articles) and 91 effective interventions promoting physical activity were identified, with enough information to translate effects into MET-hours gained. Cost-effectiveness ratios were then calculated as cost per MET-hour gained per day per individual reached. Physical activity benefits were compared to U.S. guideline—recommended levels (1.5 MET-hours per day for adults and 3.0 MET-hours per day for children, equivalent to walking 30 and 60 minutes, respectively).

Results.—The most cost-effective strategies were for point-of-decision prompts (e.g., signs to prompt stair use), with a median cost of $0.07/MET-hour/day/person; these strategies had tiny effects, adding only 0.2% of minimum recommended physical activity levels. School-based physical activity interventions targeting children and adolescents ranked well with a median of $0.42/MET-hour/day/person, generating an average of 16% of recommended physical activity. Although there were few interventions in the categories of "creation or enhanced access to places for physical activity" and "community campaigns," several were cost effective. The least cost-effective categories were the high-intensity "individually adapted behavior change" and "social support" programs, with median cost-effectiveness ratios of $0.84 and $1.16 per MET-hour/day/person. However, they also had the largest effect sizes, adding 35%–43% of recommended physical activity, respectively. Study quality was variable, with many relying on self-reported outcomes.

Conclusions.—The cost effectiveness, effect size, and study quality should all be considered when choosing physical activity (Table 4).

▶ Many of those engaged in health promotion have recognized that persuading people to become more active is an uphill task, but this is probably the first article to make a systematic analysis of the cost-effectiveness of comparing various approaches with this task. Ideally, a cost-effectiveness analysis would look at benefits in terms of quality-adjusted life years, include all costs (including the opportunity cost associated with the time commitment of the exerciser), and discount long-term costs and outcomes. Unfortunately, published information on physical activity programs is not yet at a point where such a sophisticated analysis can be undertaken. Effectiveness is thus assessed simply in terms of the increase of physical activity achieved (measured in metabolic equivalent of task [MET]-hours), and the cost estimate neglects opportunity cost (which can be quite high if a person chooses to drive to a distant gymnasium to undertake an hour of exercise). Another factor yet to be included

TABLE 4.—Physical Activity Interventions that Meet Seven or More Quality Criteria

Study	Intervention	Cost of Intervention/ Pop reached ($)	MET-Hours Gained/Day/ Person	Cost Per MET-Hour Gained ($)/ Person
Objectively measured				
Sallis (2003)[24]	School-based PE intervention, nutrition intervention (provide low-fat foods) and environmental, policy, and social marketing interventions (effect on boys only)	508,913/13,308 boys	0.42	0.50
Stratton (2005)[23]	Environmental change—Playgrounds painted with multicolored markings	5779/1139 children	0.98	0.17
Verstraete (2006)[25]	Provide game equipment to children in school during recess	1840/122 children	0.62	0.40
Subjectively measured				
Aittasalo (2006)[26]	Physical activity self-monitoring using pedometer and physical activity log for 5 consecutive days	3427/62 adults	0.18	5.95
Aittasalo (2006)[26]	Physician individual counseling (one time)	8334/130 adults	0.28	1.71
Arao (2007)[27]	Individual counseling for 15 minutes at the goal-setting session and 5 sessions monthly individual consultations for 10 minutes, plus environmental and social support	8073/84 adults	0.82	0.70
Haerens (2006)[28]	School-based intervention combining environmental changes with computer-tailored feedback (plus parental involvement)	1,106/2232 boys	0.29	0.11
Haerens (2007)[29]	School-based computer-tailored intervention to increase physical activity provided by CDs	525/139 youth	0.23	0.27
Halbert (2000)[30]	20-minute individualized physical activity advice by an exercise specialist in general practice, reinforced at 3 and 8 months	4771/149 seniors	0.79	0.14
Kolt (2007)[31]	8 telephone counseling sessions	5578/93 seniors	0.59	0.3
Manios (2005)[32]	School-based health education, school physical education, parental involvement	534,300/4171 youth	1.25	0.05
Marshall (2003)[33]	Mailed stage-targeted print intervention, consisted of a single mailing of a letter and full-color stage-targeted booklets	1192/227 adults	0.20	0.17
McKenzie (1996)[34]	School-based CATCH intervention included school policy changes, food service intervention, a physical education program, cardiovascular health and tobacco curriculum, home/family component	400,113/5,352 children	1.37	0.33
Pazoki (2007)[35]	Community-based lifestyle modification: audiotaped activity instructions with music and practical usage of the educational package were given in weekly home visits	1919/179 women	0.76	0.24
Rhudy (2007)[36]	20 personal phone calls from a nurse	5336/70 veterans	0.21	1.17
Rhudy (2007)[36]	10 randomly interspersed personal and 10 automated phone calls	3818/70 veterans	0.21	0.84

(Continued)

TABLE 4. (*continued*)

Study	Intervention	Cost of Intervention/ Pop reached ($)	MET-Hours Gained/Day/ Person	Cost Per MET Hour Gained ($)/ Person
Shirazi (2007)[37]	Home-based exercise prescription consisted of strength and balance training that was rogressive, individually tailored, and included a walking program	4962/61 Iranian women	0.95	0.94

CATCH, The Child and Adolescent Trial for Cardiovascular Health; CD, compact disc; pop, population.
Editor's Note: Please refer to original journal article for full references.

in the analysis is the persistence of the change in behavior because this is essential to achieve the posited health gains; in the analysis of Wu et al, persistence for 1 year was assumed. These authors assume that the annual US health costs associated with sedentary behavior are in the range $184 to $384 and that if all of this cost could be averted by meeting the currently recommended minimum levels of physical activity (390 MET-hour per year in adults and 1095 MET-hour per year in children), it would be reasonable to spend equivalent amounts in achieving these objectives. Such expenditures can be expressed as $0.50 to $1.00 per MET-hour and $0.17 to $0.35 per MET-hour in adults and children, respectively. By no means, all of the currently available options meet these standards of effectiveness (Table 4). Factors other than cost-effectiveness that public health decision makers may need to evaluate when choosing between options are the number of individuals reached, the distribution of costs and benefits within the community, perceptions of fairness, and political support.[1]

R. J. Shephard, MD (Lond), PhD, DPE

Reference

1. Grosse SD, Teutsch SM, Haddix AC. Lessons from cost-effectiveness research for United States public health policy. *Annu Rev Public Health*. 2007;28:365-391.

Dog Ownership and Adolescent Physical Activity

Sirard JR, Patnode CD, Hearst MO, et al (Univ of Virginia, Charlottesville; Kaiser Permanente Northwest, Portland, OR; Univ of Minnesota, Minneapolis)
Am J Prev Med 40:334-337, 2011

Background.—Positive associations between dog ownership and adult health outcomes have been observed, but research involving youth is lacking.

Purpose.—The purpose of this study was to assess the relationship of family dog ownership to adolescent physical activity.

Methods.—Data were collected on dog ownership in 618 adolescent/ parent pairs between 9/2006 and 6/2008 and analyzed in 2010. Adolescent physical activity was assessed by ActiGraph accelerometers.

Results.—Adolescents' mean age was 14.6 ± 1.8 years and 49% were male. White and higher-SES adolescents were more likely to own a dog. In models adjusted for age, puberty, gender, race, total household members, and SES, adolescent physical activity (mean counts·$\min^{-1}$day^{-1}) remained significantly associated with dog ownership ($\beta=24.3$, SE$=12.4$, $p=0.05$), whereas the association with minutes of moderate to vigorous physical activity per day became nonsignificant ($\beta=2.2$, SE$=1.2$, $p=0.07$). No significant results were observed for other adolescent characteristics.

Conclusions.—Dog ownership was associated with more physical activity among adolescents. Further research using longitudinal data will help clarify the role that dog ownership may have on adolescent physical activity (Table 1).

▶ In his popular lectures, the Swedish exercise physiologist Dr Per-Olof Åstrand frequently commended the purchase of a dog as a practical means of sustaining motivation for regular physical activity. He even went so far as to suggest that those who did not have a dog should pretend that they had one! A number of authors have documented the very logical association between habitual physical activity and dog ownership in adults[1-6] and an increase of activity after acquiring a pet.[7-9] The article of Sirard and associates examines the influence of dog ownership on the behavior of adolescents, using the relatively incontrovertible evidence of accelerometer counts. After adjusting for other pertinent variables, the influence of dog ownership on moderate to vigorous activity was remarkably small (Table 1). Several factors are at play. The choice of dog ownership usually reflects a certain minimum of income and often implies living in an area that facilitates dog walking and other forms of outdoor physical activity. The individuals thus identified have a greater liability to be active, even if they do not have a dog. Moreover, dog walking is

TABLE 1.—Participant Health-Related Physiologic and Behavioral Measures by Dog Ownership ($n=618$); M (SD) or %

Characteristics	Full Sample	0 Dogs (47.4%)	≥1 Dogs (52.6%)	p-Value
Gender, % male	49.0	45.4	52.3	0.09
Age (years)	14.6 (1.8)	14.5 (1.8)	14.7 (1.8)	0.72
Race, % white	84.6	81.6	87.4	0.05
Eligible to receive free or reduced-price lunch	11.5	15.4	8.0	0.003
Puberty ($n=687$)	2.9 (0.7)	2.9 (0.7)	2.9 (0.8)	0.65
Counts/minute/day	383.7 (160.3)	373.5 (163.3)	392.8 (157.3)	0.14
MVPA minutes/day	30.9 (16.9)	29.5 (15.8)	32.1 (17.8)	0.04
Sedentary minutes/day	570.5 (92.7)	573.3 (95.2)	566.1 (90.2)	0.22
Screen time, minutes/day	322.0 (225.9)	330.5 (234.7)	314.3 (217.7)	0.19

MVPA, moderate to vigorous physical activity.

now commonly entrusted to companies that provide this service. Finally, the speed of dog walking may improve the health of an older person but is unlikely to be of great benefit to a teenager.

R. J. Shephard, MD (Lond), PhD, DPE

References

1. Bauman AE, Russell SJ, Furber SE, Dobson AJ. The epidemiology of dog walking: an unmet need for human and canine health. *Med J Aust.* 2001;175:632-634.
2. Ham S, Epping J. Dog walking and physical activity in the U.S. *Prev Chronic Dis.* 2006;3, www.cdc.gov/pcd/issues/2006/apr/pdf/05_0106.pdf.
3. Coleman KJ, Rosenberg DE, Conway TL, et al. Physical activity, weight status, and neighborhood characteristics of dog walkers. *Prev Med.* 2008;47:309-312.
4. Brown SG, Rhodes RE. Relationships among dog ownership and leisure-time walking in Western Canadian adults. *Am J Prev Med.* 2006;30:131-136.
5. Cutt H, Giles-Corti B, Knuiman M, Burke V. Dog ownership, health and physical activity: a critical review of the literature. *Health Place.* 2007;13:261-272.
6. Thorpe RJ Jr, Simonsick EM, Brach JS, et al. Dog ownership, walking behavior, and maintained mobility in late life. *J Am Geriatr Soc.* 2006;54:1419-1424.
7. Cutt H, Knuiman MW, Giles-Corti B. Does getting a dog increase recreational walking? *Int J Behav Nutr Phys Act.* 2008;5:17.
8. Schofield G, Mummery K, Steele R. Dog ownership and human health-related physical activity: an epidemiological study. *Health Promot J Austr.* 2005;16:15-19.
9. Serpell J. Beneficial effects of pet ownership on some aspects of human health and behavior. *J R Soc Med.* 1991;84:717-720.

Family Dog Ownership and Levels of Physical Activity in Childhood: Findings From the Child Heart and Health Study in England

Owen CG, Nightingale CM, Rudnicka AR, et al (St George's, Univ of London, UK; et al)

Am J Public Health 100:1669-1671, 2010

Dog ownership is associated with higher physical activity levels in adults; whether this association occurs in children is unknown. We used accelerometry to examine physical activity levels in 2065 children aged 9 to 10 years. Children from dog-owning families spent more time in light or moderate to vigorous physical activity and recorded higher levels of activity counts per minute (25; 95% confidence interval [CI] = 6,44) and steps per day (357; 95% CI = 14, 701) than did children without dogs.

▶ Dr Kenneth H Cooper, the father of the modern-day aerobics movement, once quipped that individuals "should take their dog for a walk every day whether they own one or not." Several studies with adults indicate that those who own dogs are more physically active and take approximately 25% more steps per day than are those who do not own dogs.[1,2] Adults who get dogs become more physically active.[3] In this study, children with a dog spent more time in light, moderate to vigorous, and vigorous physical activity and recorded more overall activity counts, counts per minute, and steps compared with nondog owners. Thus, promoting dog ownership and dog walking among children and as a family are potential strategies for increasing physical activity.

D. C. Nieman, DrPH

References

1. Brown SG, Rhodes RE. Relationships among dog ownership and leisure-time walking in Western Canadian adults. *Am J Prev Med.* 2006;30:131-136.
2. Cutt H, Giles-Corti B, Knuiman M, Timperio A, Bull F. Understanding dog owners' increased levels of physical activity: results from RESIDE. *Am J Public Health.* 2008;98:66-69.
3. Cutt HE, Knuiman MW, Giles-Corti B. Does getting a dog increase recreational walking? *Int J Behav Nutr Phys Act.* 2008;5:17.

Better with a Buddy: Influence of Best Friends on Children's Physical Activity

Jago R, Macdonald-Wallis K, Thompson JL, et al (Univ of Bristol, UK)

Med Sci Sports Exerc 43:259-265, 2011

Purpose.—The purpose of this study was to examine the extent to which the physical activity modeling and physical activity actions of best friends are associated with the physical activity of 10- to 11-yr-old children.

Methods.—Data were collected from 986 children of whom 472 provided complete physical activity and best friend data. Participants identified their "best friend" within the school and answered how often they took part in physical activity with the friend and if the friend had encouraged them to be active. Physical activity was assessed via accelerometer for all children and friends. Mean minutes of moderate-to-vigorous physical activity per day (MVPA) and mean accelerometer counts per minute (CPM) were obtained for all children and best friends. Regression models were run separately for boys and girls and used to examine associations between child and best friend physical activity.

Results.—For girls, mean MVPA was associated with frequency of activity of the best friend ($P \leq 0.02$ for all categories) and engaging in physical activity at home or in the neighborhood ($t = 2.27$, $P = 0.030$), with similar patterns for mean CPM. Boys' mean MVPA was associated with their best friend's mean MVPA ($t = 3.68$, $P = 0.001$) and being active at home or in the local neighborhood ($t = 2.52$, $P = 0.017$).

Conclusions.—Boys who have active friends spend more minutes in MVPA. Girls who frequently take part in physical activity with their best friend obtain higher levels of physical activity. Boys and girls who take part in physical activity with their best friend at home or in the neighborhood where they live engage in higher levels of physical activity.

▶ Most children and adolescents do not engage in the recommended 60 minutes of physical activity per day, and interventions efforts to increase physical activity are largely ineffectual.[1-3] A relatively underexplored factor is how friends influence children's physical activity levels. The data from this study of 10- and 11-year-old boys and girls indicate that those who have best friends who are physically active engage in greater amounts of physical activity. The authors emphasize that taken together, "these findings indicate that interventions that focus on building support for physical activity among friendship groups and encouraging friends to be active together, particularly outside of school, may yield important changes to children's physical activity."

D. C. Nieman, DrPH

References

1. Riddoch CJ, Mattocks C, Deere K, et al. Objective measurement of levels and patterns of physical activity. *Arch Dis Child.* 2007;92:963-969.
2. Jago R, Anderson C, Baranowski T, Watson K. Adolescent patterns of physical activity: differences by gender, day and time of day. *Am J Prev Med.* 2005;28: 447-452.
3. van Sluijs EM, McMinn AM, Griffin SJ. Effectiveness of interventions to promote physical activity in children and adolescents: systematic review of controlled trials. *BMJ.* 2007;335:703.

Sisters in Motion: A Randomized Controlled Trial of a Faith-Based Physical Activity Intervention

Duru OK, Sarkisian CA, Leng M, et al (David Geffen School of Medicine, Los Angeles, CA; Univ of California at Los Angeles)
J Am Geriatr Soc 58:1863-1869, 2010

Objectives.—To evaluate a faith-based intervention (Sisters in Motion) intended to increase walking in older, sedentary African-American women.

Design.—Randomized controlled trial using within-church randomization.

Setting.—Three Los Angeles churches.

Participants.—Sixty-two African-American women aged 60 and older who reported being active less than 30 minutes three times per week and walked less than 35,000 steps per week as measured using a baseline pedometer reading.

Intervention.—Intervention participants received a multicomponent curriculum including scripture readings, prayer, goal-setting, a community resource guide, and walking competitions. Intervention and control participants both participated in physical activity sessions.

Measurements.—The primary outcome was change in weekly steps walked as measured using the pedometer. Secondary outcomes included change in systolic blood pressure (SBP). Outcomes were assessed at baseline and 6 months after the intervention.

Results.—Eighty-five percent of participants attended at least six of eight sessions. Intervention participants averaged 12,727 steps per week at baseline, compared with 13,089 steps in controls. Mean baseline SBP was 156 mmHg for intervention participants and 147 mmHg for controls

($P = .10$). At 6 months, intervention participants had increased their weekly steps by 9,883 on average, compared with an increase of 2,426 for controls ($P = .02$); SBP decreased on average by 12.5 mmHg in intervention participants and only 1.5 mmHg in controls ($P = .007$).

Conclusion.—The Sisters in Motion intervention led to an increase in walking and a decrease in SBP at 6 months. This is the first randomized controlled trial of a faith-based physical activity program to increase physical activity in older African-American women and represents an attractive approach to stimulate lifestyle change in this population (Table 1).

▶ The Sisters in Motion study is the first randomized controlled trial to evaluate a faith-based approach to increasing physical activity in overweight African American women. African American women have a greater risk of being overweight or obese and are less physically active than women of other races. This population is also very active in church activities. The study was conducted in 3 churches in the Los Angeles area. Randomization was within church. The intervention and control groups met on separate days once a week for 8 weeks

TABLE 1.—Details of the Intervention and Control Group Protocols Implemented at Each Site

	Intervention Group (8-week program)	Control Group (8-week program)
Group Structure	Participants self-selected into small groups of 3-4 women	One large group
Curriculum/Lectures (45 minutes)	1) Faith-based component • Scripture reading, with a discussion of how the spiritual message related to physical activity, overall health, and mutual group support • Group prayers to close each session 2) Goal-setting and reinforcement Each participant set 2 weekly goals: • personal goals for physical activity • goals to assist other members of their small group with initiating and maintaining physical activity The research assistant led a discussion each week of the prior week's goals, including a conversation about strategies to overcome any barriers to PA 3) Pedometer competition • Each week, the step counts of each participant were averaged to calculate a group score. The group with the greatest mean increase in steps from the pre-study baseline received a "win" for that week. Participants who did not attend for a given week were assigned a value of zero steps.	Lectures on topics unrelated to physical activity (e.g., memory loss, advance directives, identity theft)
Physical Activity Session (45 minutes)	Classes led by fitness instructor or research assistant. Activities included walking, resistance and balance exercises, as well as line dancing, praise dancing to spiritual music, and basic yoga.	Same as intervention group

and then monthly for the next 6 months (Table 1) Each 90-minute group session included 45 minutes of instructor-led exercise. The intervention group used a cognitive behavioral approach combined with faith practices to increase physical activity measured as pedometer step counts (steps taken during the group exercise class were excluded). The control group discussed topics unrelated to physical activity. The faith-based approach showed promise, with a significantly greater increase in step counts in the intervention group compared with control group. The 7500—steps per day increase found in the intervention group is roughly equivalent to 3 miles of walking. There was a trend for decreased systolic blood pressure (-12 ± 1.5 mm Hg; $P < .007$, adjusted for baseline) in the intervention group. A larger study will be needed to confirm this trend in blood pressure, determine other health outcomes, and evaluate long-term adherence to the physical activity plan. This study demonstrates creativity in reaching out to a high-risk population that has been marginalized from exercise intervention studies by recognizing cultural preferences for faith-based activities.

C. M. Jankowski, PhD

Interventions to promote cycling: systematic review
Yang L, Sahlqvist S, McMinn A, et al (Med Res Council Epidemiology Unit and UK Clinical Res Collaboration Centre for Diet and Activity Res (CEDAR), Cambridge, UK)
BMJ 341:c5293, 2010

Objectives.—To determine what interventions are effective in promoting cycling, the size of the effects of interventions, and evidence of any associated benefits on overall physical activity or anthropometric measures.

Design.—Systematic review.

Data Sources.—Published and unpublished reports in any language identified by searching 13 electronic databases, websites, reference lists, and existing systematic reviews, and papers identified by experts in the field.

Review Methods.—Controlled "before and after" experimental or observational studies of the effect of any type of intervention on cycling behaviour measured at either individual or population level.

Results.—Twenty five studies (of which two were randomised controlled trials) from seven countries were included. Six studies examined interventions aimed specifically at promoting cycling, of which four (an intensive individual intervention in obese women, high quality improvements to a cycle route network, and two multifaceted cycle promotion initiatives at town or city level) were found to be associated with increases in cycling. Those studies that evaluated interventions at population level reported net increases of up to 3.4 percentage points in the population prevalence of cycling or the proportion of trips made by bicycle. Sixteen studies assessing individualised marketing of "environmentally friendly" modes of transport to interested households reported modest but consistent net effects equating to an average of eight additional cycling trips per person per year in the local population. Other interventions that targeted travel behaviour in general were not associated with a clear increase in cycling. Only two studies assessed effects of interventions on physical activity; one reported a positive shift in the population distribution of overall physical activity during the intervention.

Conclusions.—Community-wide promotional activities and improving infrastructure for cycling have the potential to increase cycling by modest amounts, but further controlled evaluative studies incorporating more precise measures are required, particularly in areas without an established cycling culture. Studies of individualised marketing report consistent positive effects of interventions on cycling behaviour, but these findings should be confirmed using more robust study designs. Future research should also examine how best to promote cycling in children and adolescents and through workplaces. Whether interventions to promote cycling result in an increase in overall physical activity or changes in anthropometric measures is unclear (Table 1).

▶ Debate has continued for a number of years on the question whether the encouragement of active commuting (by bicycle or on foot) is an effective path to community health.[1] Answers can be sought in terms of the likely impact of walking and cycling on body physiology (influenced by the commuter's age, the terrain to be covered, and the pace of commuting) or in terms of more practical issues, such as the number of people who can be persuaded to engage in active transportation, irrespective of whether this activity has the desired health effects or not. The systematic review of Yang and associates looks at the effectiveness of trials designed to promote cycling and/or walking as a normal mode of urban transportation. As their analysis shows, such data have usually been collected on the dubious basis of self-report, and it has often been difficult to conduct a carefully controlled and randomized trial; there have rarely been formal statistical tests of the significance of any apparent changes in behavior. Nevertheless, Yang et al concluded that the reports they examined pointed to very limited success in promoting active transportation. Six interventions intended to encourage cycling increased the annual number of such trips by only 0% to 3.4% (Table 1), and in 16 other studies, the professional marketing of environmentally friendly modes of transport resulted in an average of only 8 additional cycle trips per person per year. Moreover, it was generally unclear whether the initiatives had recruited new active commuters or whether they had merely persuaded existing cyclists and pedestrians to make small increases in their daily activities, with little potential impact upon overall population health.

Do these findings imply that there is little point in continuing to encourage active commuting? Of the studies cited by Yang et al,[1] most were propaganda efforts based on the stage of change model, an approach that rarely seems successful in changing the physical activity patterns of a community. Only 2 of the articles considered the effects of changes of urban design. These reports

TABLE 1.—Characteristics of the Included Studies of Interventions Primarily to Promote Cycling

Study	Country	Setting	Intervention	Control	Study Population	Study Design	Period of Follow-up	Sample Size*
Hemmingsson et al, 2009[25]	Sweden	Community	Intensive individual intervention, based on the transtheoretical model of behaviour change, that included free bikes	Low intensity group support programme that included pedometers	Women with abdominal obesity	Randomised controlled trial	6 months[†]	99
Groesz, 2007[26]	USA	School	BikeTexas Safe Routes to School, consisting of both educational and motivational activities by teachers based on social cognitive theory, theory of reasoned action, theory of planned behaviour, and social ecological models	Waiting list schools that received no intervention	Children in primary schools	Cluster randomised controlled trial	5 months[†]	107
Wilmink and Hartman, 1987[27]	Netherlands	City	Cycle route network extended and improved	Comparison area of city that received no intervention	City residents	Controlled repeat cross sectional study	3 years[‡]	2000
Troelsen et al, 2004-5[28,29]	Denmark	City	Multifaceted urban initiative (Danish National Cycle City project)	Comparison areas that received no intervention	City residents	Controlled repeat cross sectional study	3 years[‡]	~1000
Sloman et al, 2009[30]	England	Towns	Various combinations of town-wide media campaigns, personalised travel planning, cycle repair and cycle training services, and improvements to cycle infrastructure	Comparison local authority areas that received no intervention	Adult residents	Controlled repeat cross sectional study	2 years[‡]	710
Rissel et al, 2010[31]	Australia	Community	Social marketing of cycle infrastructure based on transtheoretical model of behaviour change	Comparison area that received no intervention	Adult residents	Controlled cohort study	2 years[‡]	909

Editor's Note: Please refer to original journal article for full references.

*Total number of participants in intervention and control groups combined at follow-up.

[†]Period of follow-up after completion of intervention.

[‡]Period of follow-up after inception of intervention (period of follow-up after completion either not reported or not applicable).

were from Holland[2] and Denmark,[3] 2 countries where the number of cyclists is already very high and cycle paths and walkways already make good provision for the safety and convenience of both cyclists and pedestrians. Much more benefit might accrue if similar initiatives were to be adopted in North America or other European countries. Other factors that point to a need for continued study of the merits of encouraging active commuting include the rather brief time frame of observations and limited information on the climate and the typical commuting distance in the cities studied.

Many of the adverse health effects of cigarette smoking were already known in the early 1960s, but it took 40 to 50 years for the associated public health messages to hit home. Fortunately, the advocates of regular physical activity do not face such powerful misinformation as was the case for tobacco products (although the advertising budgets of car manufacturers are far from negligible). Nevertheless, it may well take several decades to see the full benefits from an encouragement of active commuting; the present group of studies (lasting 5 months to 3 years) is unlikely to give a true impression of the long-term effectiveness of initiatives to promote active commuting.

The weather also has an important bearing upon the acceptability of active commuting. In many countries, summer heat may deter workers from cycling unless showers are available at their place of employment. And in winter, walking and cycling can be hazardous in northern climates, unless municipalities make a specific point of regularly clearing snow and ice from sidewalks and cycle paths.

Finally, what is the maximum acceptable duration of a regular active commute? Thirty minutes in each direction seems a likely ceiling. Novitiate cyclists are unlikely to exceed a speed of 16 to 20 km/h (less in a city with many controlled intersections). Thus, a cycling campaign is likely to be ineffective if the average commuting distance is more than 8 to 10 km. Unfortunately, workers must travel much farther than this in many North American cities. In such environments, the emphasis should shift to encouraging walking from stations and bus depots, and the provision of increased facilities to transport cycles on buses or trains, and/or the installation of a convenient method of borrowing bicycles at major commuter terminals.

Plainly, encouraging the widespread adoption of active commuting requires a multifaceted and innovative approach from both municipalities and public health agencies, and if efforts are to be effective, they must likely be maintained for many years.

R. J. Shephard, MD (Lond), PhD, DPE

References

1. Shephard RJ. Is active commuting the answer to population health? *Sports Med.* 2008;38:751-758.
2. Wilmink A, Hartman J. *Evaluation of the Delft bicycle Network Plan: Final Summary Report.* Netherlands: Ministry of Transport and Public Works; 1987.
3. Troelsen J. [Transport and health: Odense—The National Cycling City of Denmark, 1999-2002]. *Ugeskr Laeger.* 2005;167:1164-1166.

The Built Environment and Location-Based Physical Activity

Troped PJ, Wilson JS, Matthews CE, et al (Purdue Univ, West Lafayette, IN; Indiana Univ–Purdue Univ Indianapolis; Natl Cancer Inst, Rockville, MD; et al)
Am J Prev Med 38.429-438, 2010

Background.—Studies of the built environment and physical activity have implicitly assumed that a substantial amount of activity occurs near home, but in fact the location is unknown.

Purpose.—This study aims to examine associations between built environment variables within home and work buffers and moderate-to-vigorous physical activity (MVPA) occurring within these locations.

Methods.—Adults ($n = 148$) from Massachusetts wore an accelerometer and GPS unit for up to 4 days. Levels of MVPA were quantified within 50-m and 1-km home and work buffers. Multiple regression models were used to examine associations between five objective built environment variables within 1-km home and work buffers (intersection density, land use mix, population and housing unit density, vegetation index) and MVPA within those areas.

Results.—The mean daily minutes of MVPA accumulated in all locations $= 61.1 \pm 32.8$, whereas duration within the 1-km home buffers $= 14.0 \pm 16.4$ minutes. Intersection density, land use mix, and population and housing unit density within 1-km home buffers were positively associated with MVPA in the buffer, whereas a vegetation index showed an inverse relationship (all $p < 0.05$). None of these variables showed associations with total MVPA. Within 1 km of work, only population and housing unit density were significantly associated with MVPA within the buffer.

Conclusions.—Findings are consistent with studies showing that certain attributes of the built environment around homes are positively related to physical activity, but in this case only when the outcome was location-based. Simultaneous accelerometer–GPS monitoring shows promise as a method to improve understanding of how the built environment influences physical activity behaviors by allowing activity to be quantified in a range of physical contexts and thereby provide a more explicit link between physical activity outcomes and built environment exposures (Fig 2).

▶ Most previous epidemiological studies have focused simply on determining the amount of physical activity performed by an individual. This has been true not only of investigations looking at associations between physical activity and chronic disease but also of articles relating such activity to the built environment. However, the built environment may differ substantially between a person's residence and the place of work, making it difficult to evaluate the impact of a combination of physical milieus on how much overall physical activity an individual chooses to take. The concept of combining accelerometer and global positioning system (GPS) data to see where a person is most active (Fig 2) is a novel approach, and in the future it may offer interesting information

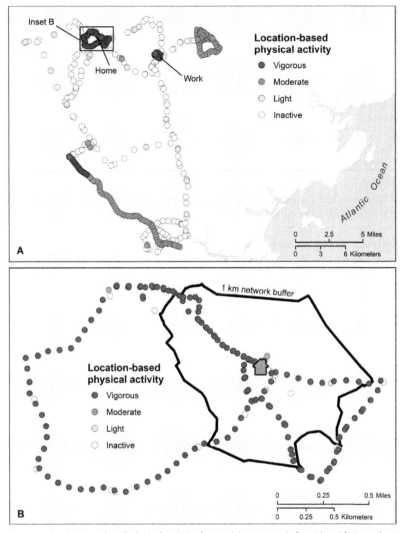

FIGURE 2.—Location-based physical activity for participant over 4 days (A) with inset showing activity around home (B). (Reprinted from Troped PJ, Wilson JS, Matthews CE, et al. The built environment and location-based physical activity. *Am J Prev Med.* 2010;38:429-438.)

about relationships to the local built environment. However, right now, the authors are only able to explain a small fraction of the interindividual variation in physical activity in terms of local environmental characteristics, with housing density being the dominant term. One of the challenges to future investigators seems to be loss of the GPS signal when subjects enter buildings. There may also be a reactive effect upon the amount of physical activity undertaken because the GPS pack weighs about 0.5 kg and must be carried in a small backpack. Finally, the published data were obtained on regular trail users and are not representative of the general population.

R. J. Shephard, MD (Lond), PhD, DPE

The Effect of Light Rail Transit on Body Mass Index and Physical Activity
MacDonald JM, Stokes RJ, Cohen DA, et al (Univ of Pennsylvania, Philadelphia; Drexel Univ, Philadelphia, PA; RAND Corporation, Los Angeles, CA)
Am J Prev Med 39:105-112, 2010

Background.—The built environment can constrain or facilitate physical activity. Most studies of the health consequences of the built environment face problems of selection bias associated with confounding effects of residential choice and transportation decisions.

Purpose.—To examine the cross-sectional associations between objective and perceived measures of the built environment; BMI; obesity (BMI>30 kg/m^2); and meeting weekly recommended physical activity (RPA) levels through walking and vigorous exercise. To assess the effect of using light rail transit (LRT) system on BMI, obesity, and weekly RPA levels.

Methods.—Data were collected on individuals before (July 2006—February 2007) and after (March 2008—July 2008) completion of an LRT system in Charlotte NC. BMI, obesity, and physical activity levels were calculated for a comparison of these factors pre- and post-LRT construction. A propensity score weighting approach adjusted for differences in baseline characteristics among LRT and non-LRT users. Data were analyzed in 2009.

Results.—More-positive perceptions of one's neighborhood at baseline were associated with a −0.36 ($p<0.05$) lower BMI; 15% lower odds (95% CI = 0.77, 0.94) of obesity; 9% higher odds (95% CI = 0.99, 1.20) of meeting weekly RPA through walking; and 11% higher odds (95% CI = 1.01, 1.22) of meeting RPA levels of vigorous exercise. The use of LRT to commute to work was associated with an average −1.18 reduction in BMI ($p<0.05$) and an 81% reduced odds (95% CI = 0.04, 0.92) of becoming obese over time.

Conclusions.—The results of this study suggest that improving neighborhood environments and increasing the public's use of LRT systems could provide improvements in health outcomes for millions of individuals (Table 3).

▶ It seems logical that use of a mass transit system will increase physical activity and be of help in controlling obesity,[1,2] but in most cross-sectional studies, it is difficult to rule out socioeconomic differences related to living within reach of mass transit. The collection of data before and after installation of a light rail system allowed the present authors to circumvent this problem, and the data that were collected certainly support an impact upon both physical

TABLE 3.—Effects of Using LRT on Changes in BMI and Physical Activity

	Estimate	*p*-Value
	B (95% CI)	
BMI (change T2—T1)	−1.18 (−2.22, −0.13)	0.015
	OR (95% CI)	
Obesity (change T2—T1)	0.19 (0.04, 0.92)	0.039
Met walking physical activity (change T2—T1)	1.36 (0.39, 4.73)	0.48
Met vigorous physical activity (change T2—T1)	3.32 (0.81, 13.63)	0.094

Note: Baseline plans to use LRT (=1) and race (black = 1) were controlled for.
B, linear coefficient; LRT, light rail transit.

activity and body mass index (Table 3). Unfortunately, the number of residents opting to use the new transit system was relatively small, giving quite wide confidence limits to the supposed benefits. It is also unfortunate that the key variables were not measured at the same time of the year because in many communities, there are appreciable seasonal variations in both body build and habitual physical activity.[3] It is amazing to realize how far the United States has to go in providing mass transit for its population. The figure of 200 million trips per year for the entire nation of some 300 million, as cited here, must be contrasted with the city of London, where there are more than 3 million subway users per day.

R. J. Shephard, MD (Lond), PhD, DPE

References

1. Besser LM, Danneberg AL. Walking to public transit: steps to help meet physical activity recommendations. *Am J Prev Med.* 2005;29:273-280.
2. Wener RE, Evans GW. A morning stroll: levels of physical activity in car and mass transit commuting. *Environ Behav.* 2007;39:62-74.
3. Shephard RJ, Aoyagi Y. Seasonal variations in physical activity and implications for human health. *Eur J Appl Physiol.* 2009;107:251-271.

Physical activity of Canadian adults: Accelerometer results from the 2007 to 2009 Canadian Health Measures Survey
Colley RC, Garriguet D, Janssen I, et al (Children's Hosp of Eastern Ontario Res Inst and the Health Analysis Division at Statistics Canada, Ontario; Health Analysis Division, Ontario, Canada; Queen's Univ, Kingston, Ontario, Canada; et al)
Health Reports 22:2011

Background.—Rising obesity rates and declining fitness levels have increased interest in understanding what underlies these trends. This article presents the first directly measured data on physical activity and sedentary behaviour on a nationally representative sample of Canadians aged 20 to 79 years.

Data and Methods.—Data are from the 2007 to 2009 Canadian Health Measures Survey (CHMS). Physical activity was measured using accelerometry. Data are presented as time spent in sedentary, light, moderate and vigorous intensity movement as well as steps accumulated per day.

Results.—An estimated 15% of Canadian adults accumulate 150 minutes of moderate-to-vigorous physical activity (MVPA) per week; 5% accumulate 150 minutes per week as at least 30 minutes of MVPA on 5 or more days a week. Men are more active than women and MVPA declines with increasing age and adiposity. Canadian adults are sedentary for approximately 9.5 hours per day (69% of waking hours). Men accumulate an average of 9,500 steps per day and women, 8,400 steps per day. The 10,000-steps-per-day target is achieved by 35% of adults.

Interpretation.—Before the CHMS, objective measures of physical activity and sedentary behaviour were not available for a representative sample of Canadians. The findings indicate that 85% of adults are not active enough to meet Canada's new physical activity recommendation (Table 5).

▶ I have for a long time been very skeptical about reports describing the physical activity of large populations in Canada and elsewhere.[1] A glance out of the office window or down the street has been enough to convince me that the numbers of active individuals were far fewer than usually reported. The problem lies mainly

TABLE 5.—Percentage Attaining Selected Physical Activity Criteria, by Age Group and Sex, Household Population Aged 20 to 79 Years, Canada, March 2007 to February 2009

Criterion/ Age Group (Years)	Total %	Total 95% Confidence Interval From	Total To	Men %	Men 95% Confidence Interval From	Men To	Women %	Women 95% Confidence Interval From	Women To
At least 30 minutes of moderate-to-vigorous physical activity, accumulated in bouts of at least 10 minutes, on at least 5 out of 7 days									
Total	4.8	3.2	6.3	5.5	3.6	7.5	4.0^E	2.5	5.5
20 to 39[†]	4.5^E	2.6	6.4	5.7^E	3.3	8.2	3.3^E	1.4	5.2
40 to 59	5.1^E	2.9	7.3	5.5^E	2.4	8.5	4.7^E	2.6	6.8
60 to 79	4.5	3.1	6.0	5.3^E	2.2	8.4	3.8^E	2.0	5.6
More than 150 minutes a week of moderate-to-vigorous physical activity accumulated in bouts of at least 10 minutes									
Total	15.4	10.9	19.8	17.1	11.3	23.0	13.7	10.1	17.3
20 to 39[†]	17.4	11.2	23.7	21.1^E	11.7	30.4	13.8^E	7.8	19.8
40 to 59	14.6	9.4	19.8	15.1^E	7.9	22.3	14.1	9.1	19.1
60 to 79	13.1	9.0	17.3	13.7^E	8.1	19.3	12.6	8.3	16.9
Average more than 10,000 steps a day									
Total	34.5	30.5	38.4	39.0*	33.0	45.0	30.0	25.4	34.6
20 to 39[†]	36.2	29.2	43.2	38.3	28.8	47.9	34.0	22.8	45.3
40 to 59	40.0	34.0	45.9	46.9*	36.8	56.9	33.1	27.8	38.5
60 to 79	$20.3^‡$	14.0	26.7	$24.1^‡$	16.5	31.7	$17.0^{‡,E}$	10.7	23.2

Source: 2007 to 2009 Canadian Health Measures Survey.
[†]reference category.
*significantly different from estimate for women (p<0.05).
[‡]significantly different from estimate for reference category (p<0.05).
[E]use with caution.

with the inaccuracy of questionnaires[2] and the tendency of people to exaggerate their activity patterns—whether from poor memory, inclusion of travel and changing time into estimates, or simply a wish to conform with popular views about appropriate behavior. The difficulty is highlighted by the recent report of Colley and associates; they used a simple Actical accelerometer to assess the activity of 2832 representative Canadians for a nominal 7 days (satisfactory records were obtained from some subjects for only 4 days, and some studies have suggested that longer periods of observation are needed for totally reliable records[3,4]). They found that the proportion of people meeting even a modest definition of minimum physical activity (150 minutes per week) was about 15%, much lower than the 52.5% questionnaire estimate for the same population (Table 5). These findings raise at least 2 questions. First, how accurate are the older epidemiological studies of health benefit, based largely on questionnaire data, that suggested a need to develop a gross weekly expenditure of at least 4 MJ?[5] Second, given that most people take so little activity, should health agencies follow the lead of Canada[6] and the World Health Organization[7] in reducing minimum recommendations, on the basis that any activity is better than none and demanding targets may have a negative effect on motivation?

R. J. Shephard, MD (Lond), PhD, DPE

References

1. Craig CL, Russell SJ, Cameron C, Bauman A. Twenty-year trends in physical activity among Canadian adults. *Can J Public Health*. 2004;95:59-63.
2. Shephard RJ. Limits to the measurement of habitual physical activity by questionnaires. *Br J Sports Med*. 2003;37:197-206.
3. Togo F, Watanabe E, Park H, et al. How many days of pedometer use predict the annual activity of the elderly reliably? *Med Sci Sports Exerc*. 2008;40:1058-1064.
4. Shephard RJ, Aoyagi Y. Objective monitoring of physical activity in older adults: clinical and practical implications. *Phys Therap Rev*. 2010;15:170-182.
5. Paffenbarger R, Hyde RT, Wing AL, et al. Some interrelations of physical activity, physiological fitness, health, and longevity. In: Bouchard C, Shephard RJ, Stephens T, eds. *Physical Activity, Fitness and Health*. Champaign, IL: Human Kinetics; 1994:119-133.
6. Warburton DER, Charlesworth S, Ivey A, Nettlefold L, Bredin SS. A systematic review of the evidence for Canada's Physical Activity Guidelines for Adults. *Int J Behav Nutr Phys Act*. 2010;7:39.
7. World Health Organization. *Global Recommendations on Physical Activity for Health. Geneva, World Health Organization*. Geneva, Switzerland: World Health Organization; 2010.

Compensation or displacement of physical activity in middle-school girls: the Trial of Activity for Adolescent Girls

Baggett CD, Stevens J, Catellier DJ, et al (Univ of North Carolina at Chapel Hill; et al)

Int J Obes 34:1193-1199, 2010

Objective.—The 'activitystat' hypothesis suggests that increases in moderate-to-vigorous physical activity (MVPA) are accompanied by a compensatory reduction in light physical activity (LPA) and/or an increase in inactivity to maintain a consistent total physical activity level (TPA). The purpose of this study was to identify the evidence of compensation in middle-school girls.

Subjects.—Participants were 6916, 8th grade girls from the Trial of Activity for Adolescent Girls (TAAG).

Design.—Inactivity and physical activity were measured over 6- consecutive days using accelerometry (MTI Actigraph). A within-girl, repeated measures design was used to assess associations between physical activity and inactivity using general linear mixed models.

Results.—Within a given day, for every one MET-minute more of inactivity, there was 3.18 MET-minutes (95% confidence interval (CI): -3.19, -3.17) less of TPA (activity > 2 METS) on the same day. Daily inactivity was also negatively associated with TPA on the following day. Each additional minute of MVPA was associated with 1.85 min less of inactivity on the same day (95% CI: -1.89, -1.82). Daily MVPA was also negatively associated with inactivity the following day.

Conclusion.—Our results, based on 6 days of observational data, were not consistent with the 'activitystat' hypothesis, and instead indicated that physical activity displaced inactivity, at least in the short term. Longer intervention trials are needed, nevertheless our findings support the use of interventions to increase physical activity over discrete periods of time in middle-school girls (Table 3)

▶ One of the problems in treating obesity has seemed that the body adjusts for a therapeutically induced negative energy balance by a reduction in daily energy expenditure of as much as 15%; it is less clear whether this reflects a reduction in physical activity or a decrease in resting metabolism. The existence of an "activitystat"[1] might negate attempts to gain other health benefits through required programs of daily physical activity. Baggett and associates cite several previous experimental studies in primary school students that cast doubt on the "activitystat" hypothesis,[2-4] but they overlook an important

TABLE 3.—Associations Between Selected Physical Activity Measures for Analyses Comparing Variables on the Same Day in Selected 8th Grade TAAG Participants, 2005–2006*

| | MET-Minutes[a] | | Minutes[a] | | % of Monitored Time[b] | |
	β	95% CI	β	95% CI	β	95% CI
Total PA = inactivity	-3.18	$-3.19, -3.17$	-1		-1	
Inactivity = MVPA	-0.25	$-0.25, -0.24$	-1.85	$-1.89, -1.82$	-1.85	$-1.89, -1.82$
LPA = MVPA	0.38	$0.36, 0.39$	0.85	$0.82, 0.89$	0.85	$0.82, 0.89$

Abbreviations: LPA, light physical activity; MET, metabolic equivalent; MVPA, moderate-to-vigorous physical activity; TAAG, Trial of Activity for Adolescent Girl; Total PA, total physical activity; 95% CI, 95% confidence interval.

*$P < 0.01$ for all associations.

[a]Linear mixed model: dependent variable = independent variable + monitored time + day of week + sample + race/ethnicity + (field center + school within field center + girl within school within field center included as random effects).

[b]Linear mixed model: dependent variable = independent variable + day of week + sample + race/ethnicity + (field center + school within field center + girl within school within field center included as random effects).

quasi-experimental study of primary school students that we undertook many years ago.[5] Our study was based on a large sample (n = 546) and was continued over 6 years. Experimental students were required to take an additional 5 hours of required physical education per week relative to control students who attended other classes at the same schools; nevertheless, questionnaires indicated that they developed no compensatory reduction of physical activity during their leisure time. This study complements this information in that measurements were made in older students (eighth grade girls) and activity patterns were assessed by accelerometers; accelerometers offer objective rather than subjective data, although they underrecord some activities of adolescents, particularly bicycle riding. Baggett and associates found a negative association between both total and moderately vigorous physical activity and inactivity, contrary to the "activitystat" hypothesis (Table 3). This article thus adds to a growing body of information indicating that fears of compensatory reductions in leisure activity have little substance. Nevertheless, from the viewpoint of controlling obesity, it would be interesting to test how far an increase of physical activity is compensated by an increase in the amount of food ingested.

R. J. Shephard, MD (Lond), PhD, DPE

References

1. Rowland TW. The biological basis of physical activity. *Med Sci Sports Exerc.* 1998;30:392-399.
2. Cooper AR, Page AS, Foster LJ, Qahwaji D. Commuting to school: are children who walk more physically active? *Am J Prev Med.* 2003;25:273-276.
3. Blaak EE, Westerterp KR, Bar-Or O, Wouters LJ, Saris WH. Total energy expenditure and spontaneous activity in relation to training in obese boys. *Am J Clin Nutr.* 1992;55:777-782.
4. Dale D, Corbin CB, Dale KS. Restricting opportunities to be active during school time: do children compensate by increasing physical activity levels after school? *Res Q Exerc Sport.* 2000;71:240-248.
5. Shephard RJ, Jéquier JC, Lavallée H, La Barre R, Rajic M. Habitual physical activity: effects of sex, milieu, season and required activity. *J Sports Med Phys Fitness.* 1980;20:55-66.

Pedometer counts superior to physical activity scale for identifying health markers in older adults

Ewald B, McEvoy M, Attia J (Univ of Newcastle, New South Wales, Australia)
Br J Sports Med 44:756-761, 2010

Objective.—Measuring physical activity is a key part of studying its health effects. Questionnaires and pedometers each have weaknesses but are the cheapest and easiest to use measurement methods for large-scale studies. We examined their capacity to detect expected associations between physical activity and a range of surrogate health measures.

Design.—Cross-sectional analysis of 669 community-dwelling participants (mean age 63.3 (7.7) years) who completed the Physical Activity Scale for the Elderly (PASE) questionnaire and who, within 2 weeks, wore a pedometer for 7 days.

TABLE 2.—Output from Regression Models Adjusted for Age, Sex, Smoking and Alcohol Intake

	Step Models			PASE Models			Both Adj r² PASE and Steps
	Change Attributed to 1 SD Increase (95% CI)	p Value	Adj r²	Change Attributed to 1 SD Increase (CI)	p Value	Adj r²	
HDL, women (mmol)	0.109 (0.050 to 0.167)	0.000	0.055	0.034 (−0.033 to 0.101)	0.323	0.009	0.052
HDL, men (mmol)	0.040 (0.001 to 0.079)	0.008	0.025	0.022 (−0.017 to 0.062)	0.264	−0.004	0.007
BMI, women	−2.03 (−2.68 to −1.37)	0.000	0.113	−0.999 (−1.760 to −0.237)	0.01	0.018	0.113
BMI, men	−0.98 (−1.51 to −0.45)	0.000	0.048	−0.41 (−0.94 to 0.12)	0.128	0.008	0.047
Waist, women (mm)	−45.4 (−6.16 to −2.91)	0.000	0.086	−31.4 (−4.99 to −1.28)	0.001	0.027	0.097
Waist, men (mm)	−25.3 (−3.91 to −1.16)	0.000	0.040	−12.5 (−2.62 to 0.12)	0.073	0.004	0.041
Waist-to-hip ratio	−0.010 (−0.016 to −0.005)	0.000	0.501	−0.007 (−0.012 to −0.001)	0.022	0.494	0.503
Fasting glucose (mmol)	−0.252 (−0.395 to −0.109)	0.001	0.059	−0.093 (−0.250 to 0.064)	0.243	0.032	0.057
White cell count (cells/mm³)	−327 (−471 to −184)	0.000	0.104	−119 (−273 to 35)	0.130	0.071	0.103
Fibrinogen (mmol)	−0.079 mmol (−0.137 to −0.021)	0.008	0.061	−0.036 (−0.098 to 0.026)	0.248	0.050	0.059
Systolic BP (mm Hg)	0.386 (−1.25 to 2.03)	0.644	0.077	−0.110 (−1.81 to 1.59)	0.899	0.076	0.075
Diastolic BP	0.468 (−0.37 to 1.31)	0.273	0.034	0.640 (−0.23 to 1.51)	0.148	0.035	0.035

Adj, adjusted; BMI, body mass index; BP, blood pressure; HDL, high-density lipoprotein.

Results.—PASE score and step count were only poorly correlated ($r = 0.37$ in women, $r = 0.30$ in men). Of 12 expected associations examined between activity and surrogate markers of health, 10 were detected as statistically significant by step counts but only 3 by PASE scores. Significant associations in the expected direction were found between step counts and high-density lipoprotein, body mass index, waist circumference, waist-to-hip ratio, blood glucose level, white cell count and fibrinogen. There was no association with either systolic or diastolic blood pressure. The association between PASE score and these markers was detected as significant only for body mass index and waist circumference in women and waist-to-hip ratio in both sexes. Associations were stronger for steps multiplied by stride length than for raw step count.

Conclusions.—Pedometer-derived step counts are a more valid measurement of overall physical activity in this sample than PASE score. Researchers should use objective measures of physical activity whenever possible (Table 2).

▶ There is now widespread agreement that pedometer data are more reliable than questionnaire assessments of physical activity.[1] This is particularly true in the elderly, where the main form of regular and deliberate physical activity is walking—the activity that is best recorded by a pedometer or uniaxial accelerometer. Questionnaire responses also become progressively more dubious in the elderly because of memory loss and problems of cognition. One aspect of the weakness of questionnaire information is demonstrated by the poor correlation of the estimated physical activity with that determined by step test results; a correlation of 0.30 to 0.37 implies that little more than 10% of the pedometer data is captured by a questionnaire. Questionnaires also show a correlation of only about 0.3 with the gold standard of energy expenditures: doubly labeled water sampling.[2] Devotees of the questionnaire might argue that at least a part of the problem lies with the pedometer score; however, the respective abilities of the 2 types of measurement to indicate the ill effects of physical inactivity (Table 2) plainly show the superiority of the objective data. The 12-item questionnaire used in this study[3] was adapted for elderly individuals, yet it identified only 3 of 12 accepted surrogate markers of health; in contrast, the simple and inexpensive Yamax DW200 pedometer identified 10 of 12 markers (although with both types of assessment, the measures accounted for a relatively small fraction of the total variance in the regression model). This study underlines the importance of using objective data when assessing associations between physical activity and health; nevertheless, it is important to allow a period of habituation if a pedometer is used, to avoid a reactive response to wearing of the instrument.[4]

R. J. Shephard, MD (Lond), PhD, DPE

References

1. Shephard RJ, Vuillemin A. Limits to the measurement of habitual physical activity by questionnaires. *Br J Sports Med.* 2003;37:197-206.

2. Neilson HK, Robson PJ, Freidenreich CM, Csizmadi I. Estimating activity energy expenditure: how valid are physical activity questionnaires? *Am J Clin Nutr.* 2008; 87:279-291.

3. Washburn RA, Smith KW, Jette AM, Janney CA. The Physical Activity Scale for the Elderly (PASE): development and evaluation. *J Clin Epidemiol.* 1993;46: 153-162.

4. Clemes SA, Matchett N, Wane SL. Reactivity: an issue for short term pedometer studies? *Br J Sports Med.* 2008;42:68-70.

Pedometer-Measured Physical Activity and Health Behaviors in U.S. Adults

Bassett DR Jr, Wyatt HR, Thompson H, et al (Univ of Tennessee Obesity Res Ctr, Knoxville; Univ of Colorado, Denver; et al)
Med Sci Sports Exerc 42:1819-1825, 2010

Purpose.—The purpose of this study was to provide descriptive, epidemiological data on the average number of steps per day estimated to be taken by U.S. adults and to identify predictors of pedometer-measured physical activity on the basis of demographic characteristics and self-reported behavioral characteristics.

Methods.—The America On the Move study was conducted in 2003. Individuals (N = 2522) aged 13 yr and older consented to fill out a survey, including 1921 adults aged 18 yr and older. Valid pedometer data were collected on 1136 adults with Accusplit AE120 pedometers. Data were weighted to reflect the general U.S. population according to several variables (age, gender, race/ethnicity, education, income, level of physical activity, and number of 5- to 17-yr-old children in the household). Differences in steps per day between subgroups were analyzed using unpaired t-tests when only two subgroups were involved or one-way ANOVA if multiple subgroups were involved.

Results.—Adults reported taking an average of 5117 steps per day. Male gender, younger age, higher education level, single marital status, and lower body mass index were all positively associated with steps per day. Steps per day were positively related to other self-reported measures of physical activity and negatively related to self-reported measures on physical inactivity. Living environment (urban, suburban, or rural) and eating habits were not associated with steps per day.

Conclusions.—In the current study, men and women living in the United States took fewer steps per day than those living in Switzerland, Australia, and Japan. We conclude that low levels of ambulatory physical activity are contributing to the high prevalence of adult obesity in the United States (Fig 1).

▶ This study measured physical activity through pedometers and found that US adults averaged 5117 steps per day, with men taking about 400 more daily steps than women (Fig 1), older adults about 1800 fewer steps than younger adults, and obese individuals about 1500 fewer steps than those who were not overweight or obese.

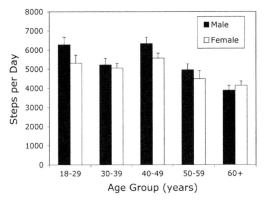

FIGURE 1.—Pedometer-determined physical activity (steps per day) for men and women by age categories. (Reprinted from Bassett DR Jr, Wyatt HR, Thompson H, et al. Pedometer-measured physical activity and health behaviors in U.S. adults. *Med Sci Sports Exerc.* 2010;42:1819-1825, with permission from the American College of Sports Medicine.)

This sample of US adults was less active than those from Switzerland (10 400 steps per day in men and 8900 in women), Australia (10 221 in men and 9178 in women), and Japan (7575 in men and 6821 in women).[1] This is undoubtedly one reason why the prevalence of obesity in the United States is higher than that in other countries.

D. C. Nieman, DrPH

Reference

1. Sequeira MM, Rickenbach M, Wietlisbach V, Tullen B, Schutz Y. Physical activity assessment using a pedometer and its comparison with a questionnaire in a large population survey. *Am J Epidemiol.* 1995;142:989-999.

Validity of Armband Measuring Energy Expenditure in Overweight and Obese Children

Bäcklund C, Sundelin G, Larsson C (Umeå Univ, Sweden)
Med Sci Sports Exerc 42:1154-1161, 2010

Purpose.—The purpose of this study was to examine the ability of the SenseWear Pro2 Armband (SWA) to accurately assess energy expenditure in free-living overweight or obese children during a 2-wk period by comparison with energy expenditure measured using the doubly labeled water (DLW) method. A second aim was to examine which software version, Innerview Professional 5.1 or Sensewear Professional 6.0, is the most appropriate for use together with SWA in overweight and obese children.

Methods.—A random sample of 22 healthy, overweight, or obese children (11 girls and 11 boys) aged 8—11 yr were recruited from an ongoing intervention study. Energy expenditure in free-living conditions was simultaneously assessed with the SWA and DLW methods during a 14-d period. All data from the SWA were analyzed using InnerView Professional software versions 5.1 (SWA 5.1) and 6.1 (SWA 6.1).

Results.—An accurate estimation in energy expenditure was obtained when SWA 5.1 was used, showing a nonstatistically significant difference corresponding to 17 (1200) kJ·d^{-1} compared with the energy expenditure measured using the DLW method. However, when SWA 6.1 was used, a statistically significant (18%) underestimation of energy expenditure was obtained, corresponding to 1962 (1034) kJ·d^{-1} compared with the DLW method.

Conclusions.—The SWA together with software version 5.1, but not 6.1, is a valid method for accurately measuring energy expenditure at group level of free-living overweight and obese children (Fig 1).

▶ The accurate monitoring of physical activity remains a major problem for epidemiologists. One possibility is to combine several indices of physical activity into a single measure of energy expenditure. In the armband tested in this study, a thermal signal is combined with accelerometry. The algorithm used to estimate energy expenditure is secret, which inevitably arouses some suspicion, and confidence is not increased when the results of an improved instrument seem worse than its predecessor. The authors' claim that their device is valid must be tempered by the wide interindividual errors (to around 25%) relative to the gold standard estimate of energy expenditure over a 14-day period obtained from doubly labeled water (Fig 1). Errors are presumably even larger when attempts are made to distinguish intensities of physical

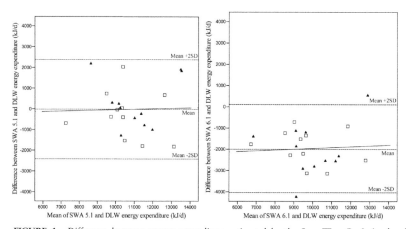

FIGURE 1.—Difference between energy expenditure estimated by the SenseWear Pro2 Armband, software versions 5.1 (SWA 5.1) and 6.1 (SWA 6.1), respectively, and energy expenditure measured using the doubly labeled water (DLW) method plotted against the mean of the two variables, for 22 overweight and obese children, 11 boys (▲) and 11 girls (□). Correlation coefficient for SWA 5.1 was 0.03 ($P = 0.90$), and the linear regression equation was $y = -268 + 0.23x$. Correlation coefficient for SWA 6.1 was 0.06 ($P = 0.80$), and the linear regression equation was $y = -2338 + 0.038x$. (Reprinted from Bäcklund C, Sundelin G, Larsson C. Validity of Armband measuring energy expenditure in overweight and obese children. *Med Sci Sports Exerc.* 2010;42:1154-1161.)

activity over shorter periods. The price of around $400 is not noted in this report, but it is high relative to simpler accelerometers; this inevitably limits applicability of the instrument in epidemiological work. It seems that the perfect indicator of human activity patterns remains to be found.

R. J. Shephard, MD (Lond), PhD, DPE

Accelerometer Output and MET Values of Common Physical Activities
Kozey SL, Lyden K, Howe CA, et al (Univ of Massachusetts, Amherst)
Med Sci Sports Exerc 42:1776-1784, 2010

Purpose.—This article 1) provides the calibration procedures and methods for metabolic and activity monitor data collection, 2) compares measured MET values to the MET values from the compendium of physical activities, and 3) examines the relationship between accelerometer output and METs for a range of physical activities.

Methods.—Participants ($N = 277$) completed 11 activities for 7 min each from a menu of 23 physical activities. Oxygen consumption ($\dot{V}O_2$) was measured using a portable metabolic system, and an accelerometer was worn. MET values were defined as measured METs ($\dot{V}O_2$/measured resting metabolic rate) and standard METs ($\dot{V}O_2$/3.5 mL·kg^{-1}·min^{-1}). For the total sample and by subgroup (age [young < 40 yr], sex, and body mass index [normal weight < 25 kg·m^{-2}]), measured METs and standard METs were compared with the compendium, using 95% confidence intervals to determine statistical significance ($\alpha = 0.05$). Average counts per minute for each activity and the linear association between counts per minute and METs are presented.

Results.—Compendium METs were different than measured METs for 17/21 activities (81%). The number of activities different than the compendium was similar between subgroups or when standard METs were used. The average counts for the activities ranged from 11 counts per minute (dishes) to 7490 counts per minute (treadmill: 2.23 m·s^{-1}, 3%). The r^2 between counts and METs was 0.65.

Conclusions.—This study provides valuable information about data collection, metabolic responses, and accelerometer output for common physical activities in a diverse participant sample. The compendium should be updated with additional empirical data, and linear regression models are inappropriate for accurately predicting METs from accelerometer output (Table 3).

▶ Compendia[1] showing the energy costs of various physical activities (usually expressed in metabolic equivalents or METs) are commonly used in exercise prescription. However, there are many problems in using such documents. The energy expenditure varies dramatically with the pace of the activity, and with the commonest form of activity (walking), it is also strongly affected by terrain and ground conditions (for instance, snow). Changes in equipment

TABLE 3.—Measured MET Values for Study Activities Compared with the MET Values from the Compendium of Physical Activities

		Measured METs			Compendium
	N	Mean	SD	95% CI	MET Value
Ascend stairs	215	10.3*	1.89	10.00, 10.51	5
Shooting baskets	39	9.3*	1.96	8.70, 9.93	4.5
Moving a box	271	5.0*	1.05	4.88, 5.13	4
Descending stairs	231	4.4*	1.03	4.28, 4.54	3
Washing dishes	42	2.1	0.40	2.01, 2.26	2.3
Dusting	39	2.8*	0.66	2.62, 3.04	2.5
Gardening	38	4.0*	1.25	3.59, 4.39	4.5
2.23 m·s^{-1}, 3% grade	189	10.4	1.49	10.14, 10.56	N/A
1.56 m·s^{-1}, 3% grade	266	6.2*	0.94	6.07, 6.29	6
1.34 m·s^{-1}, 3% grade	268	5.2	0.79	5.11, 5.30	N/A
Folding laundry	39	2.4*	0.30	2.32, 2.51	2
2.23 m·s^{-1}, 0% grade	227	9.2*	1.36	9.03, 9.38	8
1.56 m·s^{-1}, 0% grade	267	5.0*	0.83	4.92, 5.12	3.8
1.34 m·s^{-1}, 0% grade	270	4.2*	0.69	4.13, 4.30	3.3
Mopping	38	3.9*	0.77	3.67, 4.16	3.5
Mowing	37	5.9	1.36	5.42, 6.29	5.5
Painting	38	3.3*	0.85	3.03, 3.58	4.5
Raking	39	4.7*	1.35	4.26, 5.11	4
Organizing a room	37	5.2*	1.11	4.87, 5.58	3
Sweeping	40	3.4	0.71	3.17, 3.61	3.3
Tennis	39	9.5*	1.61	9.04, 10.06	7
Trimming lawn	38	3.6	0.78	3.34, 3.83	3.5
Vacuuming	38	3.5	0.66	3.28, 3.70	3.5

Measured METs (measured $\dot{V}O_2$/measured RMR).
n = number of participants that completed that activity.
*If the compendium MET value is outside the 95% confidence interval (CI) for the measured MET, the values are considered statistically different at $\alpha = 0.05$.

are also constantly modifying the energy cost of many sports and household activities. Interest is thus strong in obtaining more objective evidence of the intensity of the prescribed activity, using small portable accelerometers[2-4]; these are now relatively inexpensive and can store detailed data for 60 days or longer. Such devices have commonly been correlated against direct measurements of oxygen consumption. The assumption underlying such calibrations of a linear relationship between accelerometer output and oxygen cost remains debatable, although in this study the linear model accounted for a substantial 65% of the variance in this relationship. The article of Kozey and colleagues underlines the potentially wide gap between actual MET values and those obtained from the compendium (Table 3), as seen in a sample of healthy and moderately active subjects aged 20 to 60 years (drawn mainly from a university community) and performing the required activities in a laboratory. The practical implication is that epidemiological estimates of the volume of activity needed to sustain health that are based on the compendia may be seriously flawed and should be replaced by objective accelerometer estimates as soon as possible.

R. J. Shephard, MD (Lond), PhD, DPE

References

1. Ainsworth BE, Haskell WL, Whitt MC, et al. Compendium of physical activities: an update of activity codes and MET intensities. *Med Sci Sports Exerc.* 2000;32: S498-S504.
2. Shephard RJ, Aoyagi Y. Objective monitoring of physical activity in older adults: clinical and practical implications. *Phys Ther Rev.* In press.
3. Pober DM, Staudenmayer J, Raphael C, Freedson PS. Development of novel techniques to classify physical activity mode using accelerometers. *Med Sci Sports Exerc.* 2006;38:1626-1634.
4. Troiano RP, Berrigan D, Dodd KW, Mâsse LC, Tilert T, McDowell M. Physical activity in the United States measured by accelerometer. *Med Sci Sports Exerc.* 2008;40:181-188.

Ethnic Differences in Physiological Cardiac Adaptation to Intense Physical Exercise in Highly Trained Female Athletes

Rawlins J, Carre F, Kervio G, et al (King's College Hosp, London, UK; Univ of Rennes, France; et al)
Circulation 121:1078-1085, 2010

Background.—Ethnicity is an important determinant of cardiovascular adaptation in athletes. Studies in black male athletes reveal a higher prevalence of electric repolarization and left ventricular hypertrophy than observed in white males; these frequently overlap with those observed in cardiomyopathy and have important implications in the preparticipation cardiac screening era. There are no reports on cardiac adaptation in highly trained black females, who comprise an increasing population of elite competitors.

Methods and Results.—Between 2004 and 2009, 240 nationally ranked black female athletes (mean age 21 ± 4.6 years old) underwent 12-lead ECG and 2-dimensional echocardiography. The results were compared with 200 white female athletes of similar age and size participating in similar sports. Black athletes demonstrated greater left ventricular wall thickness (9.2 ± 1.2 versus 8.6 ± 1.2 mm, $P<0.001$) and left ventricular mass (187.2 ± 42 versus 172.3 ± 42 g, $P=0.008$) than white athletes. Eight black athletes (3%) exhibited a left ventricular wall thickness >11 mm (12 to 13 mm) compared with none of the white athletes. All athletes revealed normal indices of systolic and diastolic function. Black athletes exhibited a higher prevalence of T-wave inversions (14% versus 2%, $P<0.001$) and ST-segment elevation (11% versus 1%, $P<0.001$) than white athletes. Deep T-wave inversions (-0.2 mV) were observed only in black athletes and were confined to the anterior leads (V_1 through V_3).

Conclusions.—Systematic physical exercise in black female athletes is associated with greater left ventricular hypertrophy and higher prevalence of repolarization changes than in white female athletes of similar age and size participating in identical sporting disciplines. However, a maximal left ventricular wall thickness >13 mm or deep T-wave inversions in the inferior and lateral leads are rare and warrant further investigation (Fig 2).

▶ This is the first study to examine cardiac adaptations in response to sport participation in elite black female athletes. Black male athletes are known to have a greater prevalence of repolarization changes and left ventricular hypertrophy compared with white male athletes. Standard electrocardiogram (ECG) guidelines for screening white male athletes may lead to false positives in black males and potentially black female athletes. Healthy athletes may thus be excluded from sport participation. Race-specific guidelines may be required to correctly identify black athletes with pathological, as opposed to physiological, cardiac adaptations. A battery of cardiac function and structure tests were administered to more than 400 black and white female athletes in England and France competing on the national team level. They participated in team (basketball, football [soccer], and netball) and individual (judo, track, and wrestling) sports. All the athletes were asymptomatic, normotensive, and free of family history of cardiomyopathy or premature sudden cardiac death. The black athletes' hearts demonstrated significant structural and conduction differences than white athletes. The black athletes had greater left ventricular wall thickness (LVWT), LV mass, and left atrial diameter than white athletes. The prevalence of ECG anomalies was greater in black athletes than in white athletes (Fig 2). Using multiple linear regression analyses, race was the strongest predictor of LVWT and ST-segment elevation. Although further comparisons must be made with athletes representing a broader spectrum of sport disciplines, this study suggests that black female athletes will present cardiac anomalies more often than their white peers. Longitudinal studies will be needed to determine

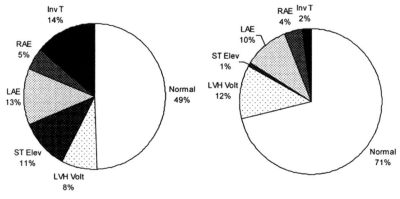

Black Athletes   **White Athletes**

FIGURE 2.—Pie charts comparing ECG anomalies between black athletes and white athletes. Black athletes exhibited a higher prevalence of ST-segment elevation and T-wave inversions than white athletes. LAE indicates voltage criterion for left atrial enlargement; RAE, voltage criterion for right atrial enlargement; LVH volt, voltage criterion for LVH; ST Elev, ST-segment elevation; and Inv T, T-wave inversion. (Reprinted from Rawlins J, Carre F, Kervio G, et al. Ethnic differences in physiological cardiac adaptation to intense physical exercise in highly trained female athletes. *Circulation.* 2010;121:1078-1085.)

the changes in cardiac structure and function that occur over the course of sport training and competition.

C. M. Jankowski, PhD

Longitudinal Examination of Age-Predicted Symptom-Limited Exercise Maximum HR

Zhu N, Suarez-Lopez JR, Sidney S, et al (Univ of Minnesota, Minneapolis; Kaiser Permanente Med Care Program, Oakland, CA; et al)
Med Sci Sports Exerc 42:1519-1527, 2010

Purpose.—To estimate the association of age with maximal HR (MHR).

Methods.—Data were obtained from the Coronary Artery Risk Development in Young Adults (CARDIA) study. Participants were black and white men and women aged 18–30 yr in 1985–1986 (year 0). A symptom-limited maximal graded exercise test was completed at years 0, 7, and 20 by 4969, 2583, and 2870 participants, respectively. After exclusion, 9622 eligible tests remained.

Results.—In all 9622 tests, estimated MHR (eMHR, bpm) had a quadratic relation to age in the age range of 18–50 yr, eMHR = $179 + 0.29 \times age - 0.011 \times age^2$. The age–MHR association was approximately linear in the restricted age ranges of consecutive tests. In 2215 people who completed tests of both years 0 and 7 (age range = 18–37 yr), eMHR = $189 - 0.35 \times age$; and in 1574 people who completed tests of both years 7 and 20 (age range = 25–50 yr), eMHR = $199 - 0.63 \times age$. In the lowest baseline body mass index (BMI) quartile, the rate of decline was 0.24 bpm·yr^{-1} between years 0 and 7 and 0.51 bpm·yr^{-1} between years 7 and 20, whereas in the highest baseline BMI quartile, there was a linear rate of decline of approximately 0.7 bpm·yr^{-1} for the full age range of 18–50 yr.

Conclusions.—Clinicians making exercise prescriptions should be aware that the loss of symptom-limited MHR is much slower in young adulthood and more pronounced in later adulthood. In particular, MHR loss is very slow in those with the lowest BMI younger than 40 yr (Fig 1).

▶ The maximal heart rate is a central variable in many areas of sports medicine, particularly when prescribing exercise and regulating the intensity of training. It is thus important to know how maximal values change with age. Various factors are thought to cause a progressive decrease in maxima as a person becomes older, including a decrease in responsiveness to β-adrenergic stimulation, a decrease in the reactivity of baroreceptors and chemoreceptors, and hypoxia or apoptosis in the pacemaker.[1-3] At first sight, the promise of longitudinal data on age-related changes of maximal heart rate in a large population sample thus seems an attractive source of new information. The main points argued from this study are that the change of maximal heart rate is curvilinear rather than linear (Fig 1) and that previous authors have tended to miss this point either because their samples were not representative of the general population

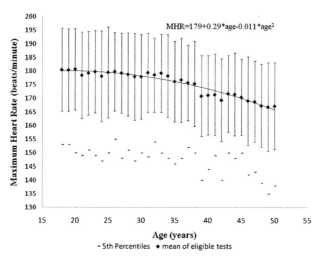

FIGURE 1.—Distribution of MHR (1 SD *error bars* and age-specific fifth percentiles) of eligible tests across a 20-yr follow-up by age at examination (9622 tests in 4844 participants). (Reprinted from Zhu N, Suarez-Lopez JR, Sidney S, et al. Longitudinal examination of age-predicted symptom-limited exercise maximum HR. *Med Sci Sports Exerc.* 2010;42:1519-1527.)

or because they used cross-sectional rather than longitudinal data. This sample itself is hardly representative of the US population because the participants were enrolled either in the Kaiser Permanente health program or a research program. However, a much bigger criticism is that the tests were self-limited, with the initial end points of supposedly maximal treadmill tests of young adults falling 20 to 30 beats/min short of commonly observed true maximal values. It thus seems misleading of the authors to categorize their data as maximal. Given such poor motivation even when the participants were young adults, the curve in peak heart rate that is reported may reflect a further age-related deterioration in motivation, rather than any physiological or pathological phenomenon.

R. J. Shephard, MD (Lond), PhD, DPE

References

1. Cheitlin MD. Cardiovascular physiology-changes with aging. *Am J Geriatr Cardiol.* 2003;12:9-13.
2. Rodeheffer RJ, Gerstenblith G, Becker LC, Fleg JL, Weisfeldt ML, Lakatta EG. Exercise cardiac output is maintained with advancing age in healthy human subjects: cardiac dilatation and increased stroke volume compensate for a diminished heart rate. *Circulation.* 1984;69:203-213.
3. Salvadori A, Fanari P, Palmulli P, et al. Cardiovascular and adrenergic response to exercise in obese subjects. *J Clin Basic Cardiol.* 1999;2:229-236.

Near-infrared spectroscopy and indocyanine green derived blood flow index for noninvasive measurement of muscle perfusion during exercise

Habazettl H, Athanasopoulos D, Kuebler WM, et al (Inst of Physiology, Berlin, Germany; Natl and Kapodistrian Univ of Athens, Greece; et al)

J Appl Physiol 108:962-967, 2010

Near-infrared spectroscopy (NIRS) with the tracer indocyanine green (ICG) may be used for measuring muscle blood flow (MBF) during exercise, if arterial ICG concentration, is measured simultaneously. Although pulse dye densitometry allows for noninvasive measurement of arterial dye concentration, this technique is sensitive to motion, and may not be applicable during exercise. The aim of this study was to evaluate a noninvasive blood flow index (BFI), which is derived solely from the muscle ICG concentration curve. In 10 male cyclists 5 mg ICG were injected into an antecubital vein at rest and during cycling at 30, 60, 70, 80, 90, and 100% of previously determined maximal work load. Simultaneously blood was withdrawn through a photodensitometer at 20 ml/min from the radial artery to measure arterial ICG concentration. To measure muscle tissue ICG concentrations, two sets of NIRS optodes were positioned on the skin, one over the left seventh intercostal space and the other over the left vastus lateralis muscle. MBF was calculated from the arterial and muscle concentration data according to Fick's principle. BFI was calculated solely from the muscle concentration curve as ICG concentration difference divided by rise time between 10 and 90% of peak. During exercise mean BFI values changed similarly to MBF in both intercostal and quadriceps muscles and showed excellent correlations with MBF: $r = 0.98$ and 0.96, respectively. Individual data showed some scattering among BFI and MBF values but still reasonable correlations of BFI with MBF: $r = 0.73$ and 0.72 for intercostal and quadriceps muscles, respectively. Interobserver variability, as analyzed by Bland-Altman. plots, was considerably less for BFI than MBF. These data suggest that BFI can be used for measuring changes in. muscle perfusion from rest to maximal exercise. Although absolute blood flow cannot be determined, BFI has the advantages of being essentially noninvasive and having low interobserver variability (Fig 4).

▶ A knowledge of local muscle blood flow is fundamental to our understanding of exercise, yet its determination is by no means an easy matter. I still have memories of trying to exercise with heated needle thermocouples inserted into my leg and of measuring the clearance of radioactive substances from muscles following bouts of exercise; the yield of scientific information was very limited, and neither of these procedures attracted a great number of volunteers! The Fick principle can be applied locally after injection of a bolus of an appropriate marker dye,[1] but this requires cannulation of the local artery and vein, again not too popular with volunteers, and it does not distinguish the blood flow to active muscle from the flow to inactive muscle and other limb tissues. Recently, there has been interest in applying near infrared

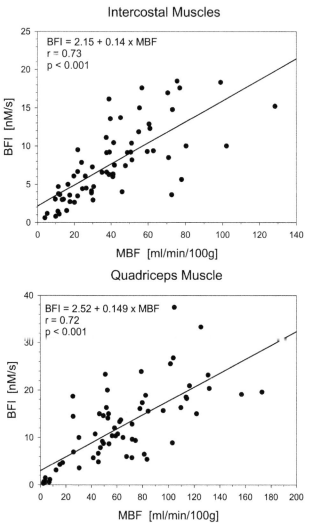

FIGURE 4.—Regression analyses of individual BFI vs. MBF values for intercostal muscles (*top*) and quadriceps muscle (*bottom*). Linear regression equations, regression coefficients, and significance levels are given in the figure. (Reprinted from Habazettl H, Athanasopoulos D, Kuebler WM, et al. Near-infrared spectroscopy and indocyanine green derived blood flow index for noninvasive measurement of muscle perfusion during exercise. *J Appl Physiol.* 2010;108:962-967, Used with permission.)

spectroscopy to the well-accepted dye indocyanine green. Wavelengths in the range 700 to 1000 nm can penetrate deeply into the limb tissue, measuring the concentrations of light-absorbing chromophores.[1] Although this methodology avoids the need for local blood sampling, it is still necessary to collect arterial blood for several seconds to assess the input profile of the injected dye. This article evaluates a method of getting around this problem by calculating the ratio of the peak dye concentration to the time needed to reach this peak; this has recently been suggested as providing an index of relative blood flow rates under various conditions.[2] A comparison with direct Fick measurements of local blood flow (Fig 4) shows a moderate correspondence of the 2 data sets, although unfortunately there is also a considerable interindividual scatter. The method may have some current value in looking at within-group blood flow responses, but it needs to be improved before it can have great value for studies of individual subjects. Future research may possibly improve correspondence between the index and direct measurements of local blood flow by taking account of the subject's blood volume and the kinetics of dye injection.

R. J. Shephard, MD (Lond), PhD, DPE

References

1. Boushel R, Langberg H, Olesen J, et al. Regional blood flow during exercise in humans measured by near-infrared spectroscopy and indocyanine green. *J Appl Physiol.* 2000;89:1868-1878.
2. Reekers M, Simon MJ, Boer F, et al. Cardiovascular monitoring by pulse dye densitometry or arterial indocyanine green dilution. *Anesth Analg.* 2009;109:441-446.

Impaired left and right ventricular function following prolonged exercise in young athletes: influence of exercise intensity and responses to dobutamine stress

Banks L, Sasson Z, Busato M, et al (Univ of Toronto, Ontario, Canada; Mt Sinai Hosp, Toronto, Ontario, Canada)

J Appl Physiol 108:112-119, 2010

We examined the effect of intensity during prolonged exercise (PE) on left (LV) and right ventricular (RV) function. Subjects included 18 individuals (mean ± SE: age = 28.1 ± 1.1 yr, maximal aerobic power = 55.1 ± 1.6 ml · kg^{-1} · min^{-1}), who performed 150 min of exercise at 60 and 80% maximal aerobic power on two separate occasions. Transthoracic echocardiography assessed systolic and diastolic performance, and blood sampling assessed hydration status and noradrenaline levels before (pre), during (15 and 150 min), and 60 min following (post) PE. β-Adrenergic sensitivity pre- and post-PE was assessed by dobutamine stress. High-intensity PE (15 vs. 150 min) induced reductions in LV ejection fraction (69.3 ± 1.3 vs. 63.5 ± 1.3%, $P = 0.000$), LV strain (−23.5 ± 0.6 vs. −22.3 ± 0.6%, $P = 0.034$), and RV strain (−26.3 ± 0.6 vs. −23.0 ± 0.6%, $P < 0.01$). Both exercise intensities induced diastolic reductions (pre vs. post) in the ratio of septal early wave of annular tissue velocities to late/atrial wave of annular tissue velocities (2.15 ± 0.15 vs. 1.62 ± 0.09; 2.21 ± 0.15 vs. 1.48 ± 0.10), ratio of lateral early wave of annular tissue velocities to late/atrial wave of annular tissue velocities (3.84 ± 0.42 vs. 2.49 ± 0.20; 3.56 ± 0.32 vs. 2.08 ± 0.18), ratio of early to late LV strain rate (2.42, ± 0.16 vs. 1.97 ± 0.13; 2.30 ± 0.15 vs. 1.81 ± 0.11), and ratio of early to late RV strain rate (2.03 ± 0.17 vs. 1.51 ± 0.09;

2.16 ± 0.16 vs. 1.44 ± 0.11) ($P < 0.001$). Evidence of β-adrenergic sensitivity was supported by a decreased strain, strain rate, ejection fraction, and systolic pressure-volume ratio response to dobutamine ($P < 0.05$) with elevated noradrenaline ($P < 0.01$). PE-induced reductions in LV and RV systolic function were related to exercise intensity and β-adrenergic desensitization. The clinical significance of exercise-induced cardiac fatigue warrants further research.

▶ Evidence continues to grow that extended sports play may impair myocardial function. All studies to date have indicated that this is a transient phenomenon, with no immediate clinical risks. These observations have both applied significance and importance to understanding how and why heart muscle fatigues with extended work. Is the process the same as identified in skeletal muscle? Despite the apparent benign nature of these responses, could there exist implications for arrhythmogenesis and sudden death? Mild increases in circulating biomarkers of cardiac damage (ie, troponins) are also observed after sustained endurance events. Physicians, particularly those working in emergency room settings, need to be aware that such abnormalities in echocardiographic findings and mild elevations in blood levels of these biomarkers may reflect athletic participation and not ischemic myocardial events. The phenomenon is now well described. What we need to know now is more about mechanisms and possible clinical implications of myocardial fatigue with sports play.

T. Rowland, MD

Acute cardiac effects of marathon running

Trivax JE, Franklin BA, Goldstein JA, et al (William Beaumont Hosp, Royal Oak, MI)
J Appl Physiol 108:1148-1153, 2010

We sought to clarify the significance of cardiac dysfunction and to assess its relationship with elevated biomarkers by using cardiovascular magnetic resonance imaging in healthy, middle-aged subjects immediately after they ran 26.2 miles. Cardiac dysfunction and elevated blood markers of myocardial injury have been reported after prolonged strenuous exercise. From 425 volunteers, 13 women and 12 men were randomly selected, provided medical and training history, and underwent baseline cardiopulmonary exercise testing to exhaustion. Blood biomarkers, cardiovascular magnetic resonance imaging, and 24-h ambulatory electrocardiography were performed 4 wk before and immediately after the race. Participants were 38.7 ± 9.0 yr old, had baseline peak oxygen consumption of 52.9 ± 5.6 ml·kg^{-1}·min^{-1}, and completed the marathon in 256.2 ± 43.5 min. Cardiac troponin I and B-type natriuretic peptide increased following the race ($P = 0.001$ and $P < 0.0001$, respectively). Cardiovascular magnetic resonance-determined pre- and postmarathon left ventricular ejection fractions were comparable, $57.7 \pm 4.1\%$ and $58.7 \pm 4.3\%$,

TABLE 3.—Cardiovascular Magnetic Resonance Imaging Data Before and After Marathon

Variable	Baseline	Postmarathon	Change in Value	P Value
LVEF, %	57.7 ± 4.1	58.7 ± 4.3	1.0 ± 4.9	0.32
LVEDV index, ml/m^2	79.1 ± 13.7	78.8 ± 11.5	0.3 ± 1.7	0.88
LVESV index, ml/m^2	33.5 ± 6.7	32.6 ± 6.0	0.9 ± 1.0	0.36
LA volume index, ml/m^2	48.0 ± 9.4	49.8 ± 9.8	1.8 ± 10.2	0.38
RVEF, %	53.6 ± 7.1	45.5 ± 8.5	8.1 ± 7.5	<0.0001
RVEDV index, ml/m^2	101.7 ± 17.8	104.2 ± 19.7	2.5 ± 14.3	0.40
RVESV index, ml/m^2	47.4 ± 11.2	57.0 ± 14.5	9.6 ± 11.3	<0.0001
RA volume index, ml/m^2	46.7 ± 14.4	57.0 ± 14.5	10.3 ± 11.3	<0.0001

Values are means ± SD. LA, left atrium; LVEDV, left ventricular end-diastolic volume; LVEF, left ventricular ejection fraction; LVESV, left ventricular end-systolic volume; RA, right atrium; RVEDV, right ventricular end-diastolic volume; RVEF, right ventricular ejection fraction; RVESV, right ventricular end-systolic volume.

respectively $(P = 0.32)$. Right atrial volume index increased from 46.7 ± 14.4 to 57.0 ± 14.5 ml/m^2 $(P < 0.0001)$. Similarly, right ventricular end-systolic volume index increased from. 47.4 ± 11.2 to 57.0 ± 14.6 ml/m^2 $(P < 0.0001)$ whereas the right ventricular ejection fraction dropped from 53.6 ± 7.1 to $45.5 \pm 8.5\%$ $(P < 0.0001)$. There were no morphological changes observed in the left atrium or ventricle or evidence of ischemic injury to any chamber by late gadolinium enhancement. There were no significant arrhythmias. Marathon running causes dilation of the right atrium and right ventricle, reduction of right ventricular ejection fraction, and release of cardiac troponin I and B-type natriuretic peptide but does not appear to result in ischemic injury to any chamber (Table 3).

▶ Debate continues on the clinical significance of the creatine kinase MB isoenzyme, cardiac troponin, and B-type natriuretic peptide released after participation in marathon and ultramarathon events.[1] There have been reports of associated temporary alterations in left ventricular function.[2] A small number of participants (6 to 8 per year in the United States)[3] also die following marathon running, but it is likely that most of these individuals had preexisting cardiac disease. This report is based on a small group of middle-aged runners with relatively slow race times. Using the technically superior approach of cardiovascular magnetic resonance imaging (CMR) rather than echocardiography, these individuals showed no evidence of left ventricular dysfunction immediately after the race, despite the release of the biomarkers seen in previous studies. On the other hand, there was a substantial decrease in the right ventricular ejection fraction, accompanied by an increase of right atrial volume (Table 3). The authors concluded that there was some myonecrosis induced by strain on the right side of the heart, although this did not follow the time course expected with a myocardial infarction.[4] Furthermore, CMR should have detected the presence of even a small infarct. They point out that prolonged endurance exercise is thought to increase pulmonary arterial pressures, thus causing a greater increase of workload on the right than on the left side of the heart. Changes in cardiac function are probably short term in nature, but further studies are needed to define the precise time course of the alterations in right ventricular function and to assess any long-term consequences.

R. J. Shephard, MD (Lond), PhD, DPE

References

1. Scharhag J, George K, Shave R, Urhausen A, Kindermann W. Exercise-associated increases in cardiac biomarkers. *Med Sci Sports Exerc.* 2008;40:1408-1415.
2. Douglas PS, O'Toole ML, Hiller WD, Hackney K, Reichek N. Cardiac fatigue after prolonged exercise. *Circulation.* 1987;76:1206-1213.
3. USA Marathoning. Overview, http://www.marathonguide.com/features/Articles/2008RecapOverview.cfm; 2007.
4. Mair J, Artner-Dworzak E, Lechleitner P, et al. Cardiac troponin T in diagnosis of acute myocardial infarction. *Clin Chem.* 1991;37:845-852.

Diagnosing overtraining in athletes using the two-bout exercise protocol
Meeusen R, Nederhof E, Buyse L, et al (Vrije Universiteit Brussel, Belgium; et al)
Br J Sports Med 44:642-648, 2010

Objective.—In this work, whether a two-bout exercise protocol can be used to make an objective, immediately available distinction between non-functional over reaching (NFO) and overtraining syndrome (OTS) was studied.

Design.—Underperforming athletes who were diagnosed with the suspicion of NFO or OTS were included in the study. Recovery of the athletes was monitored by a sports physician to retrospectively distinguish NFO from OTS.

Setting.—Sports medicine laboratory.

Participants.—The protocol was started and completed by 10 underperforming athletes. NFO was retrospectively diagnosed in five athletes, and OTS was diagnosed in five athletes.

Interventions.—A two-bout maximal exercise protocol was used to measure physical performance and stress-induced hormonal reactions.

Main Outcome Measurements.—Exercise duration, heart rate and blood lactate concentration were measured at the end of both exercise tests. Venous concentrations cortisol, adrenocorticotrophic hormone (ACTH), prolactin and growth hormone were measured both before and after both exercise tests.

Results.—Maximal blood lactate concentration was lower in OTS compared with NFO, while resting concentrations of cortisol, ACTH and prolactin concentrations were higher. However, sensitivity of these measures was low. The ACTH and prolactin reactions to the second exercise bout were much higher in NFO athletes compared with OTS and showed the highest sensitivity for making the distinction.

Conclusions.—NFO might be distinguished from OTS based on ACTH and prolactin reactions to a two-bout exercise protocol. This protocol

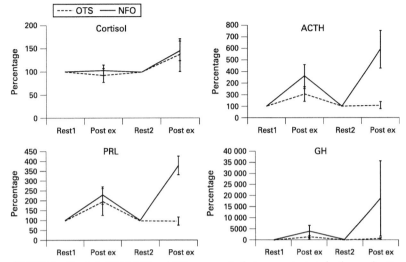

FIGURE 4.—Cortisol, ACTH, PRL and GH responses to the two exercise tests for the non-functional over-reached (NFO) group (solid lines) and the OTS group (dashed lines). Data are presented as percentage increase from both baseline values (SE) of the mean. (Reprinted from Meeusen R, Nederhof E, Buyse L, et al. Diagnosing overtraining in athletes using the two-bout exercise protocol. *Br J Sports Med.* 2010;44:642-648 and reproduced with permission from the BMJ Publishing Group.)

could be a useful tool for diagnosing NFO and OTS; however, more data should be collected before this test can be used as the gold standard (Fig 4).

▶ Sports physicians have long sought a reliable indicator of athletes who are affected by the overtraining syndrome. The question is difficult to examine experimentally as it is not ethically appropriate to deliberately induce overtraining in a healthy athlete. To date, the best measures of overtraining have seemed to be the decline in physical performance and simple assessments of current mood state.[1] The article of Meeusen and associates suggests that a simple double exercise test with determinations of relative changes in prolactin and adrenocorticotropic hormone concentrations may offer a new hormonal indication of problems (Fig 4). It is important to underline that there were only 5 subjects arbitrarily classed as nonfunctional overreaching and 5 classed as overtraining; nevertheless, the differences observed in this study seem large enough to merit further investigation.

R. J. Shephard, MD (Lond), PhD, DPE

Reference

1. Verde T, Thomas S, Shephard RJ. Potential markers of heavy training in highly trained distance runners. *Br J Sports Med.* 1992;26:167-175.

Effects of Recovery Method After Exercise on Performance, Immune Changes, and Psychological Outcomes

Stacey DL, Gibala MJ, Martin Ginis KA, et al (Fowler Kennedy Sports Medicine Clinic, London, Ontario, Canada; McMaster Univ, Hamilton, Ontario, Canada)
J Orthop Sports Phys Ther 40:656-665, 2010

Study Design.—Randomized controlled trial using a repeated-measures design.

Objectives.—To examine the effects of commonly used recovery interventions on time trial performance, immune changes, and psychological outcomes.

Background.—The use of cryotherapy is popular among athletes, but few studies have simultaneously examined physiological and psychological responses to different recovery strategies.

Methods.—Nine active men performed 3 trials, consisting of three 50-kJ "all out" cycling bouts, with 20 minutes of recovery after each bout. In a randomized order, different recovery interventions were applied after each ride for a given visit: rest, active recovery (cycling at 50 W), or cryotherapy (cold tub with water at 10°C). Blood samples obtained during each session were analyzed for lactate, IL-6, total leukocyte, neutrophil, and lymphocyte cell counts. Self-assessments of pain, perceived exertion, and lower extremity sensations were also completed.

Results.—Time trial performance averaged 118 ± 10 seconds (mean ± SEM) for bout 1 and was 8% and 14% slower during bouts 2 (128 ± 11 seconds) and 3 (134 ± 11 seconds), respectively, with no difference between interventions (time effect, $P \leq .05$). Recovery intervention did not influence lactate or IL-6, although greater mobilization of total leukocytes and neutrophils was observed with cryotherapy. Lymphopenia during recovery was greater with cryotherapy. Participants reported that their lower extremities felt better after cryotherapy (mean ± SEM, 6.0 ± 0.7 out of 10) versus active recovery (4.8 ± 0.9) or rest (2.8 ± 0.6) (trial effect, $P \leq .05$).

Conclusion.—Common recovery interventions did not influence performance, although cryotherapy created greater immune cell perturbation and the perception that the participants' lower extremities felt better.

▶ Although the sample size is small ($n = 9$), Stacey et al designed a nice repeated measure study where they examined the effect of three 20-minute recovery strategies on exercise performance. These 3 strategies were rest (lying on a bed), active recovery (cycling at 50 W), and cryotherapy (sitting in a hydrotherapy tub submerged to the neck with a water temperature of 10°C). Their findings revealed that there were no significant differences in cycling performance, blood lactate, and interleukin-6. They also assessed participant perception (pain, exertion, and whether the intervention made their legs feel better). Although there were no differences in quadriceps pain or rating of perceived exertion, participants indicated that their lower extremities felt better during cryo (as compared with the other recovery strategies). This study is definitely underpowered (as admitted by the authors). However, it should be replicated in a larger sample to answer this important question regarding optimal recovery strategies for athletic performance.

D. E. Feldman, PT, PhD

The effects of the 5-HT$_{2C}$ agonist *m*-chlorophenylpiperazine on elite athletes with unexplained underperformance syndrome (overtraining)
Budgett R, Hiscock N, Arida R, et al (Northwick Park Hosp, Watford, UK; Univ of Oxford, UK)
Br J Sports Med 44:280-283, 2010

A possible link between the neurotransmitter, 5-hydroxytryptamine (5-HT), plasma tryptophan, and branched chain amino acids concentration and exercise-induced fatigue is described by the central fatigue hypothesis. 5-HT receptors and neuroendocrine "challenge" tests, using prolactin release as an indirect measure of 5-HT activity were studied by recent investigations. In the present study, the original hypothesis about the role of amino acids in increasing brain 5-HT with a neuroendocrine challenge test on elite athletes diagnosed with unexplained, underperformance syndrome (UUPS) was combined. There was an apparent increased sensitivity of 5-HT receptors in athletes with UUPS compared with fit, well-trained controls, as measured via increased prolactin release following a bolus dose of *m*-chlorophenylpiperazine, a 5-HT agonist. No changes were observed in plasma amino acid concentrations in either group. There is evidence that well-trained athletes have a reduced sensitivity of 5-HT receptors. The present study suggests that this adaptation may be lost in athletes with UUPS: this might explain some of their observed symptoms (Fig 1).

▶ Overtraining is an important problem for high-performance athletes, possibly affecting as many as 5% to 10% of competitors per year. However, we still know relatively little about either its cause or its treatment,[1] in part because ethical considerations force observers to use observational rather than experimental techniques when studying overtraining. Biochemical and immunological changes associated with the syndrome are inconsistent, and the problem is most consistently identified in terms of a decrease in performance associated with a deterioration of mood state[2] plus feelings of increased effort and fatigue.[3,4] Central fatigue (emanating from the brain rather than the muscles and involving the neurotransmitter 5-hydroxytryptamine [5-HT]) may be an important component of the syndrome. The passage of tryptophan across the blood/brain barrier and thus the synthesis of 5-HT in the cerebrospinal fluid depend on the plasma ratio of free tryptophan to branch-chained amino acids (BCAA), and some studies have suggested that the feeding of BCAA can reduce fatigue by altering the plasma tryptophan/BCAA balance.[5] Well-trained athletes appear to develop a decreased sensitivity to 5-HT.[6] Conversely, patients with chronic fatigue syndrome seem to have an increase in the

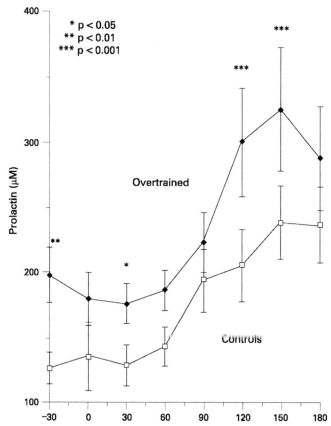

FIGURE 1.—Plasma prolactin concentration (μM) (SE). Time (min) before and after administration of a bolus dose of mCPP at 0. p Denotes significance between control (n = 12) and UUPS (n = 19) groups. (Reprinted from Budgett R, Hiscock N, Arida R, et al. The effects of the 5-HT$_{2C}$ agonist *m*-chlorophenylpiperazine on elite athletes with unexplained underperformance syndrome (overtraining). *Br J Sports Med.* 2010;44:280-283, with permission from BMJ Publishing Group Ltd.)

sensitivity of their 5-HT receptors.[7] This study used prolactin release as an index of 5-HT activity and the drug m-chlorophenylpiperazine as a 5-HT agonist. This stimulus was applied to resting athletes; in those with symptoms suggestive of overtraining, the 5-HT agonist consistently led to greater prolactin levels than in those without such symptoms (Fig 1), supporting the view that 5-HT is involved in the overtraining syndrome. However, 5-HT is not the entire story because it does not explain some manifestations of overtraining, such as an increased vulnerability to upper respiratory infections. Possibly, a monitoring of prolactin levels might be helpful in identifying athletes who are overtrained, and a countering of increased 5-HT levels might form a useful component of treatment.

R. J. Shephard, MD (Lond), PhD, DPE

References

1. Shephard RJ. *Physical activity, Training and the Immune Response.* Carmel, IN: Cooper Publications; 1997.
2. Verde T, Thomas S, Shephard RJ. Potential markers of heavy training in highly trained distance runners. *Br J Sports Med.* 1992;26:167-175.
3. Budgett R. Fatigue and underperformance in athletes: the overtraining syndrome. *Br J Sports Med.* 1998;32:107-110.
4. Derman W, Schwellnus MP, Lambert MI, et al. The 'worn-out athlete': a clinical approach to chronic fatigue in athletes. *J Sports Sci.* 1997;15:341-351.
5. Newsholme EA, Leech AR. *Biochemistry for the Medical Sciences.* Chichester: Wiley; 1983.
6. Struder HK, Hollman W, Platen P, Wöstmann R, Weicker H, Molderings GJ. Effect of acute and chronic exercise on plasma amino acids and prolactin concentrations and on [3H]ketanserin binding to serotonin2A receptors on human platelets. *Eur J Appl Physiol.* 1999;79:318-324.
7. Cleare AJ, Bearn J, Allain T, et al. Contrasting neuroendocrine responses in depression and chronic fatigue syndrome. *J Affect Disord.* 1995;34:283-289.

Association between physical activity energy expenditure and inflammatory markers in sedentary overweight and obese women

Lavoie M-E, Rabasa-Lhoret R, Doucet É, et al (Université de Montréal, Québec, Canada; Univ of Ottawa, Ontario, Canada; et al)
Int J Obes 34:1387-1395, 2010

Objective.—Chronic subclinical inflammation and regular physical activity have opposing relationships to obesity-related metabolic diseases. Yet, the association between chronic inflammation and physical activity has rarely been examined in obese subjects. We examined the association between physical activity energy expenditure (PAEE), total (TEE) and resting energy expenditure (REE) and cardiorespiratory fitness (VO$_2$peak) with inflammatory markers in overweight/obese women.

Design.—Cross-sectional study.

Methods.—The study included 152 overweight/obese postmenopausal women who were sedentary and free of chronic/inflammatory diseases (mean age: 57.5 (95% confidence interval (CI) 56.7−58.3) years, body mass index (BMI): 32.5 (95% CI 31.8−33.2) kg m^{-2}). The following parameters were measured: TEE (doubly labeled water), REE (indirect calorimetry), PAEE (as (TEE × 0.90)−REE), VO$_2$peak (ergocycle) and serum high-sensitive C-reactive protein (hsCRP), haptoglobin, soluble tumor necrosis factor-α receptor 1 (sTNFR1), interleukin-6, orosomucoid and white blood cells.

Results.—Sedentary women with the highest tertile of PAEE (1276 (1233−1319) kcal day^{-1}) had lower concentrations of hsCRP and haptoglobin than those in the lowest tertile (587 (553−621) kcal day^{-1}) after adjustment for fat mass ($P < 0.05$). Soluble TNFR1 was positively correlated with VO$_2$peak, TEE and REE ($P < 0.05$), and hsCRP and orosomucoid were positively associated with REE ($P < 0.01$), whereas haptoglobin was negatively associated with PAEE ($P < 0.05$). In stepwise regression analyses that examined the concomitant associations of components of energy expenditure with inflammatory markers, PAEE remained the only predictor of hsCRP and haptoglobin ($P < 0.05$), explaining 14 and 5%, respectively, of their variation, whereas REE was the only predictor of orosomucoid ($r^2 = 0.05$, $P = 0.02$) after adjustment for fat mass. Adding leptin to the regression models results in similar relationships between inflammatory markers and components of energy expenditure.

Conclusion.—PAEE is an independent predictor of hsCRP and haptoglobin in sedentary overweight/obese postmenopausal women free of chronic disease. Our data support the role of physical activity in reducing

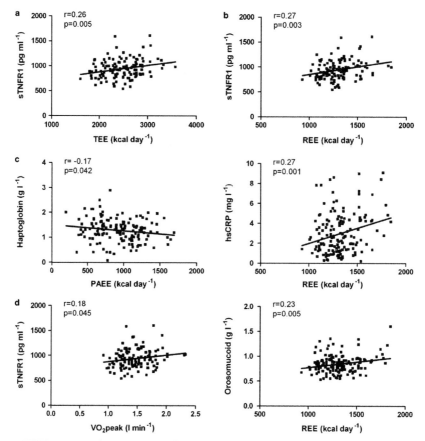

FIGURE 1.—Correlations between inflammatory markers and components of energy expenditure. (a) TEE correlated with sTNFR1 ($r = 0.26$, $P = 0.005$), (b) REE correlated with sTNFR1 ($r = 0.27$, $P = 0.003$), hsCRP ($r = 0.27$, $P = 0.001$), orosomucoid ($r = 0.23$, $P = 0.005$), (c) PAEE correlated with haptoglobin ($r = -0.17$, $P = 0.04$) and (d) VO₂peak correlated with sTNFR1 ($r = 0.18$, $P = 0.045$). (Reprinted from Lavoie M-E, Rabasa-Lhoret R, Doucet É, et al. Association between physical activity energy expenditure and inflammatory markers in sedentary overweight and obese women. *Int J Obes.* 2010;34:1387-1395, with permission from Macmillan Publishers Limited.)

subclinical inflammation and risk of metabolic and cardiovascular diseases (Fig 1).

▶ Inflammation underlies most of the chronic diseases that are prevalent causes of morbidity and mortality in modern society. Other cross-sectional studies established a linkage between physical activity and/or physical fitness and reduced chronic inflammation.[1,2] This study is unique in that physical activity was measured using the gold standard doubly labeled water (DLW) technique in overweight/obese postmenopausal sedentary women. Higher levels of physical activity, even among these women with low cardiovascular fitness, were related to reduced subclinical chronic inflammation (Fig 1). These findings stand in contrast to several randomized exercise training studies that indicate no independent influence on inflammation.[3,4] One explanation is that the change in aerobic fitness is often small in these exercise intervention studies, the duration of training seldom extends beyond 6 months, and the number of subjects is relatively small. In large, community-based, observational studies, the difference in exercise frequency and physical fitness levels far exceeds changes that are attainable in the training studies.

D. C. Nieman, DrPH

References

1. Beavers KM, Brinkley TE, Nicklas BJ. Effect of exercise training on chronic inflammation. *Clin Chim Acta*. 2010;411:785-793.
2. Abramson JL, Vaccarino V. Relationship between physical activity and inflammation among apparently healthy middle-aged and older US adults. *Arch Intern Med*. 2002;162:1286-1292.
3. Church TS, Earnest CP, et al. Exercise without weight loss does not reduce C-reactive protein: the INFLAME Study. *Med Sci Sports Exerc*. 2010;42:708-716.
4. Kelley GA, Kelley KS. Effects of aerobic exercise on C-reactive protein, body composition, and maximum oxygen consumption in adults: a meta-analysis of randomized controlled trials. *Metabolism*. 2006;55:1500-1507.

Associations of physical activity, cardiorespiratory fitness and fatness with low-grade inflammation in adolescents: the AFINOS Study

Martinez-Gomez D, for the AFINOS Study Group (Spanish Natl Res Council (CSIC), Madrid, Spain; et al)
Int J Obes (Lond) 34:1501-1507, 2010

Objective.—To examine the independent associations of objectively measured physical activity (PA), cardiorespiratory fitness (CRF) and fatness with low-grade inflammatory markers in adolescents.

Design.—Cross-sectional study in Spain.

Subjects.—A sample of 192 adolescents aged 13—17 years.

Measurements.—PA was assessed with an accelerometer for 7 days. A 20-m shuttle-run test was used to assess CRF. Skinfold thicknesses at six sites and WCs were measured. BMI was calculated from measured height and weight. C-reactive protein (CRP), interleukin-6 (IL-6) and

TABLE 4.—Associations Between PA, Fitness and Fatness with Inflammatory Markers in Adolescents ($n = 192$)

Model	Predictor Variables	C-Reactive Protein (mg l⁻¹)[a]			Interleukin-6 (pg ml⁻¹)[b]			C3 (g l⁻¹)[b]			C4 (g l⁻¹)[b]		
		β	P	R²	β	P	R²	β	P	R²	β	P	R²
1	Total PA (c.p.m.)[a]	0.037	0.648	0.009	0.016	0.346	0.012	−0.023	0.772	0.025	0.037	0.475	0.051
2	CRF (laps)[a]	−0.199	0.033	0.014	0.041	0.136	0.011	−0.427	<0.001	0.137	−0.312	<0.001	0.110
3	Body fat (mm)[a]	0.241	0.002	0.040	−0.016	0.342	0.005	0.491	<0.001	0.232	0.250	<0.001	0.113
4	Total PA (c.p.m.)[a]	0.085	0.314		0.006	0.748		0.070	0.352		0.108	0.167	
	CRF (laps)[a]	−0.121	0.277		0.045	0.191		−0.227	0.022		−0.163	0.113	
	Body fat (mm)[a]	0.198	0.027	0.038	−0.004	0.764	0.016	0.403	<0.001	0.245	0.337	<0.001	0.187

Abbreviations: CRF, cardiorespiratory fitness; PA, physical activity. Data were adjusted for age, sex, pubertal status and homeostasis model assessment of insulin resistance.
[a]Values were natural log-transformed before analysis.
[b]Values were square-root-transformed before analysis.

complement factors C3 and C4 were assayed. The homeostasis model assessment of insulin resistance (HOMA-IR) was calculated from glucose and insulin. Regression analysis adjusted for potential confounders and HOMA-IR was used to determine the associations between PA, CRF and fatness with low-grade inflammatory markers.

Results.—Total PA, vigorous PA and MVPA were positively associated with CRF ($r = 0.25–0.48$), whereas vigorous PA was negatively associated with skinfolds ($r = -0.27$). CRF was inversely associated with fatness, ($r = -0.30$ to -0.48). CRF and fatness were inversely and positively associated with HOMA-IR ($r = -0.16$ and 0.21, respectively). PA variables were not independently associated with inflammatory markers. CRF and fatness were inversely and positively associated with CRP, C3 and C4, respectively. Only body fat explained a relevant amount of the variance of the model in CRP (4%) and C4 (19%), whereas CRP and body fat jointly explained the variance in C3 (25%). All these observations were independent of HOMA-IR.

Conclusions.—These findings support the key role of CRF and fatness on low-grade inflammation, as well as the possible indirect role of habitual PA through CRF and body fat in adolescents (Table 4).

▶ Evidence of low-grade inflammation in the adolescent is important in part because it is a harbinger of subsequent atherosclerosis[1] and in part because chronic inflammation also predisposes to subsequent carcinogenesis. C-reactive protein (CRP), complement factors C3 and C4, and interleukin-6 seem among the most powerful markers of such inflammation.[2-4] This relatively large cross-sectional study of adolescents from Madrid shows that inflammatory markers are negatively associated with fitness (as assessed by a shuttle run score) and positively associated with obesity (as indicated by 6 skinfolds and waist circumference measurements), not only in adults but also in teenagers. The independent effects of physical activity (probably acting through modulation of CRP levels) were demonstrated by actigraph measurements, as opposed to earlier negative studies, most of which relied upon rather uncertain questionnaire assessments of physical activity (Table 4). The present data reinforce pleas to encourage adolescents to sustain a sufficient level of physical activity to maintain a healthy body mass.

R. J. Shephard, MD (Lond), PhD, DPE

References

1. Hansson GK. Inflammation, atherosclerosis, and coronary artery disease. *N Engl J Med.* 2005;352:1685-1695.
2. Ridker PM, Stampfer MJ, Rifai N. Novel risk factors for systemic atherosclerosis: a comparison of C-reactive protein, fibrinogen, homocysteine, lipoprotein(a), and standard cholesterol screening as predictors of peripheral arterial disease. *JAMA.* 2001;285:2481-2485.
3. Järvisalo MJ, Harmoinen A, Hakanen M, et al. Elevated serum C-reactive protein levels and early arterial changes in healthy children. *Arterioscler Thromb Vasc Biol.* 2002;22:1323-1328.
4. Oksjoki R, Kovanen PT, Pentikäinen MO. Role of complement activation in atherosclerosis. *Curr Opin Lipidol.* 2003;14:477-482.

Exercise without Weight Loss Does Not Reduce C-Reactive Protein: The INFLAME Study

Church TS, Earnest CP, Thompson AM, et al (Louisiana State Univ System, Baton Rouge; et al)
Med Sci Sports Exerc 42:708-716, 2010

Purpose.—Numerous cross-sectional studies have observed an inverse association between C-reactive protein (CRP) and physical activity. Exercise training trials have produced conflicting results, but none of these studies was specifically designed to examine CRP. The objective of the Inflammation and Exercise (INFLAME) study was to examine whether aerobic exercise training without dietary intervention can reduce CRP in individuals with elevated CRP.

Methods.—The study was a randomized controlled trial of 162 sedentary men and women with elevated CRP (≥ 2.0 mg·L^{-1}). Participants were randomized into a nonexercise control group or an exercise group that trained for 4 months. The primary outcome was change in CRP.

Results.—The study participants had a mean (SD) age of 49.7 (10.9) yr and a mean body mass index of 31.8 (4.0) kg·m^{-2}. The median (interquartile range (IQR)) and mean baseline CRP levels were 4.1 (2.5–6.1) and 4.8 (3.4) mg·L^{-1}, respectively. In the exercise group, median exercise compliance was 99.9%. There were no differences in median (IQR) change in CRP between the control and exercise groups (0.0 (−0.5 to 0.9) vs 0.0 (−0.8 to 0.7) mg·L^{-1}, $P = 0.4$). The mean (95% confidence interval) change in CRP adjusted for gender and baseline weight was similar in the control and exercise groups, with no significant difference between groups (0.5 (−0.4 to 1.3) vs 0.4 (−0.5 to 1.2) mg·L^{-1}, $P = 0.9$). Change in weight was correlated with change in CRP.

Conclusions.—Exercise training without weight loss is not associated with a reduction in CRP (Fig 4).

▶ C-reactive protein (CRP) is a marker of systemic inflammation and an independent predictor of cardiovascular disease in adults.[1] Achieving low levels of CRP appears to be of similar importance as achieving low levels of low-density lipoprotein cholesterol.[2] Statin medication lowers CRP, but increasing attention is being given to lifestyle strategies such as exercise and/or weight loss. Weight loss is an effective nonpharmacologic strategy for lowering CRP, with each 1 kg of weight loss translating to a mean 0.13 mg/L decrease in CRP.[3] The data from this exercise training study suggest no linkage between exercise training and change in CRP, in contrast to numerous cross-sectional studies that report an inverse relation between physical activity and CRP.[4] Cross-sectional studies typically use long-term physical activity patterns, and the contrast in activity and fitness is greater than can be achieved in training studies (in this study, just a 12% improvement in fitness). Nonetheless, a combination of weight loss and high physical activity should achieve CRP reduction in most adults, as shown in this study (see Fig 4).

D. C. Nieman, DrPH

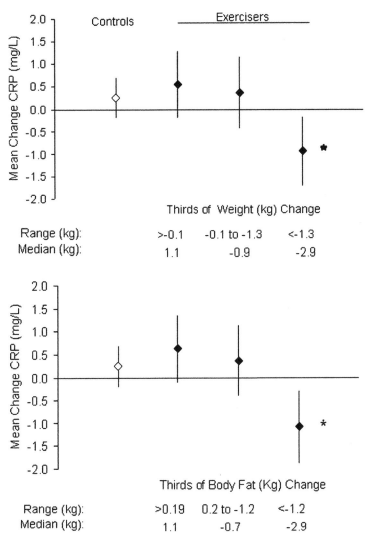

FIGURE 4.—Change in CRP for the control group (*open diamond*) and the exercise group with categorization by thirds of change weight and DEXA body fat (*closed diamonds*). Data represent the least squares means. *Error bars* indicate 95% CI. *P < 0.05 versus all other groups including the control group. (Reprinted from Church TS, Earnest CP, Thompson AM, et al. Exercise without weight loss does not reduce C-reactive protein: the INFLAME study. *Med Sci Sports Exerc.* 2010;42:708-716, with permission from the American College of Sports Medicine.)

References

1. Ridker PM. High-sensitivity C-reactive protein: potential adjunct for global risk assessment in the primary prevention of cardiovascular disease. *Circulation.* 2001;103:1813-1818.

2. Ridker PM. Inflammatory biomarkers and risks of myocardial infarction, stroke, diabetes, and total mortality: implications for longevity. *Nutr Rev.* 2007;65: S253-S259.
3. Selvin E, Paynter NP, Erlinger TP. The effect of weight loss on C-reactive protein: a systematic review. *Arch Intern Med.* 2007;167:31-39.
4. Beavers KM, Brinkley TE, Nicklas BJ. Effect of exercise training on chronic inflammation. *Clin Chim Acta.* 2010;411:785-793.

Aging, Persistent Viral Infections, and Immunosenescence: Can Exercise "Make Space"?

Simpson RJ (Univ of Houston, TX)
Exerc Sport Sci Rev 39:23-33, 2011

Background.—The biological aging and progressive deterioration in function of the immune system has been termed immunosenescence. Its characteristics include poor vaccine efficacy, reduced immune vigilance, and higher morbidity and mortality from infectious disease. Naïve antigen virgin T cells are important for providing immune responses to novel pathogens but are gradually replaced by clones of effector and effector-memory T cells. These less effective T cells take up space in the immune system, where numbers of T cells are tightly regulated, and crowd out naïve T-cell replacements. Persons who carry latent herpesvirus infections appear to be at higher risk for losing T-cell immunity because these reactivating viruses accumulate and shrink the naïve T-cell repertoire. Persistent infection with cytomegalovirus (CMV) infection may produce the most deleterious effects on T-cell immunity and immunosenescence. Methods to remove clones of terminally differentiated effector-memory T cells are costly, carry high risks, and produce potentially harmful side effects. It was hypothesized that regular physical exercise may offer an alternative, inexpensive, and safe strategy to manage the adverse effects of immunosenescence resulting from aging and reactivating viral infections. A theoretical framework was proposed to explain how acute exercise could remove excess clones of antigen-specific terminally differentiated T cells, expand naïve T-cell populations, and restore T cell-n-mediated immunity.

Development of Senescence.—T cells are developed within the thymus gland from bone marrow-n-derived progenitor cells. The thymus replenishes naïve T-cell numbers throughout life, but age-associated atrophy of the gland begins at birth, accelerates in puberty, and leaves just a small thymic mass by age 50 to 60 years. Then the thymus can no longer maintain effective naïve T-cell homeostasis and individuals are at higher risk for infection because of the diminished T-cell repertoire. In addition, senescent T cell numbers grow during normal immune responses to reactivating or invading pathogens. Theoretically, after a viral infection resolves, the excess clones of effector T cells will die by apoptosis, although a few survive as central memory cells that recirculate when the same infectious agent is encountered again. For some reactivating herpesviruses, many excess T-cell clones remain in the memory T-cell pool, reducing naïve T-cell repertoire.

Exercise Effects.—Moderate habitual exercise can aid in preventing functional declines in immune function in later life. Regular exercise may limit the opportunities for latent viral agents to reactivate, so the individual has fewer of these illnesses to handle. Exercise may help target apoptosis-resistant T cells by mobilizing them from peripheral tissues and sending them into apoptosis, making space for newly produced naïve T cells. For these possible roles to occur, three distinct phases must occur: (1) selective mobilization of senescent T cells from peripheral tissues to the blood compartment during exercise; (2) extravasation of senescent T cells from the circulation and their apoptosis in peripheral tissues during exercise recovery; and (3) generation of naïve T-cells to replace the lost senescent cells. Acute exercise preferentially mobilizes effector-memory and senescent T cells compared to naïve or lowly differentiated T cells. Exercise also evokes the mobilization of some T cells specific to CMV and Epstein-Barr viral antigens. Frequent shifts in T cells with acute exercise may produce cumulative long-term restorative effects on immunity. However, senescent cells are probably not localized to the peripheral blood component but are also found in other body tissues. Regardless, they are pulled out of the T-cell depository, so there are fewer peripheral T-cells. This should stimulate thymopoeisis through positive feedback and generate naïve antigen-virgin cells to replace the lost senescent T cells. Habitual exercise could induce lymphocytopenia and the apoptosis of terminally differentiated T cells in peripheral tissues, then increase thymic output to replace T-cell numbers with an expanded naïve T-cell repertoire.

Conclusions.—The proposed theoretical framework seeks to explain how exercise may make space in the immune storehouse by removing excess clones of antigen-specific T cells and then restoring the numbers of naïve T cells. Many future experimental studies are needed to support this hypothesis.

▶ There have been suggestions that regular moderate physical activity increases an individual's resistance to upper respiratory infections.[1] Masters athletes have noted that there is a critical weekly running distance. If they stay beneath this personal limit (commonly, about 50 km/wk), they remain healthier than their sedentary peers, but with further exertion, they show an increased liability to colds. Although there are several potential explanations for the adverse effects of excessive exercise, such as suppression of natural killer cell counts or a depression of secretary immunoglobulin function, reasons for the beneficial effects of moderate physical activity have been less clear. One possibility, particularly in older individuals, seems to be a slowing or a reversal of immunosenescence.[2,3] Simpson's review article offers an interesting if somewhat speculative explanation of one way in which this might come about. He suggests that as we age, the pool of T cells progressively develops memory function for various microorganisms, often those with no major pathological significance (such as the herpes simplex and Epstein-Barr viruses). Although the T-cell count still appears to be adequate, there remain relatively few circulating naive T cells that can respond to challenge from a novel micro-organism. Exercise could thus have a beneficial effect by bringing memory and senescent T cells into the circulation; the senescent cells would then escape into the tissues and their apoptosis would allow space for the thymus to generate new naive T cells (Fig 3 in the original article). There is some evidence to support this hypothesis, including positive effects of exercise on the naive/memory T-cell ratio and the T-cell response to mitogens.[3] The ever-increasing sophistication of surface marker identification should allow further exploration of Simpson's concept, with a potential to explore also interactions between regular moderate exercise and treatment with thymus-stimulating interleukins (ILs), such as IL-7.

R. J. Shephard, MD (Lond), PhD, DPE

References

1. Shephard RJ, Kavanagh T, Mertens DJ, Qureshi S, Clark M. Personal benefits of Masters athletic competition. *Br J Sports Med.* 1995;29:35-40.
2. Shinkai S, Konishi M, Shephard RJ. Aging and immune response to exercise. *Can J Physiol Pharmacol.* 1998;76:562-572.
3. Simpson RJ, Guy K. Coupling aging immunity with a sedentary lifestyle: has the damage already been done? — A mini-review. *Gerontology.* 2010;56:449-458.

The influence of prolonged cycling on monocyte Toll-like receptor 2 and 4 expression in healthy men

Oliveira M, Gleeson M (Loughborough Univ, UK)
Eur J Appl Physiol 109:251-257, 2010

Several studies have reported that some immune cell functions including monocyte Toll-like receptor (TLR) expression and antigen presentation are temporarily impaired following acute bouts of strenuous exercise, which could represent an 'open window' to upper respiratory tract infection (URTI). However, we do not know the time course of effects of acute exercise on human monocyte TLR expression. The purpose of the present study was to examine the effects of 1.5 h cycling at 75% VO_{2peak} on human monocyte TLR2 and TLR4 expression and how long it takes for TLR expression to return to pre-exercise values. Nine healthy endurance trained males (age 25 ± 5 years) had blood samples taken before and for up to 24 h after exercise and analysed using flow cytometry. Although there was an increase in the total monocyte cell count at 0, 1 and 4 h post-exercise ($P < 0.01$), exercise reduced monocyte TLR4 expression (geometric mean fluorescence intensity, corrected for non-specific binding; $P < 0.05$) by 32 and 45% at 0 and 1 h post-exercise, respectively, compared with pre-exercise values but had returned to baseline values by 4 h post-exercise. There were no statistically significant changes in TLR2 expression after exercise. In addition, a control resting study was conducted on six healthy endurance trained men (age 25 ± 2 years) to analyse any diurnal changes

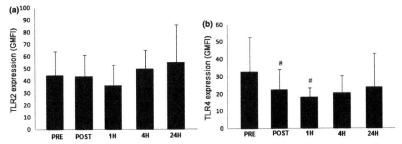

FIGURE 3.—CD14⁺ monocyte TLR2 (a) and TLR4 (b) expression (GMFI) after exercise. # Significantly different from PRE ($P < 0.05$). (Reprinted from Oliveira M, Gleeson M. The influence of prolonged cycling on monocyte Toll-like receptor 2 and 4 expression in healthy men. *Eur J Appl Physiol.* 2010;109:251-257. With kind permission of Springer Science+Business Media.)

on monocyte TLR2 and TLR4 expression but no changes were found across time ($P > 0.05$). This study showed that prolonged cycling at 75% VO_{2peak} temporarily reduces TLR4 expression, which may in part be responsible for post-exercise immunodepression (Fig 3).

▶ Exercise scientists have long attempted to offer a plausible explanation of the apparent increase in vulnerability to upper respiratory tract infections following participation in a marathon or ultramarathon event.[1] Suggestions to date, including a temporary decrease in the number and/or activity of circulating natural killer cells and decreased concentrations of mucosal immunoglobulins, have been less convincing. This article offers a new avenue of exploration of exercise-induced changes in the activity of toll-like receptors, transmembrane proteins located in the cell surface of antigen-presenting cells such as monocytes and macrophages. Toll-like receptors 2 and 4 (TLR2 and TLR4) are of particular interest because the respiratory syncytial virus induces inflammatory cytokines and chemokines through TLR2,[2] and TLR4 can recognize proteins from the outer envelope of the respiratory syncytial virus.[3] Indeed, TLR2 seems essential to the control of respiratory syncytial virus in vivo.[2] Furthermore, TLR activation leads to the activation of transcription factor kappa-B and interferon regulatory factors, with the release of interleukins 1, 6, and 12 and tumor necrosis factor-alpha.[4,5] Finally, the protein that is first recognized on the virus is degraded to immunogenic peptides that differentiate T-helper cells into their h1 and h2 subsets, with the production of interferon-gamma.[6] This report confirms earlier reports that prolonged vigorous exercise reduces the expression of TLRs on monocytes, documenting the time course of this response (Fig 3). The depression of TLR2 is relatively short-term, but TLR4 is still depressed at 24 hours. There remain several issues still to explore: How long does the reduced TLR4 expression continue beyond the 24-hour mark? Is an increase of body temperature a factor? What happens if exercise of similar intensity is prolonged to correspond to a marathon or an ultramarathon race? And how far is an exchange of monocytes between the blood stream and other body sites responsible for the observed response?

R. J. Shephard, MD (Lond), PhD, DPE

References

1. Nieman DC. Exercise, infection, and immunity. *Int J Sports Med.* 1994;15:S131-S141.
2. Murawski MR, Bowen GN, Cerny AM, et al. Respiratory syncytial virus activates innate immunity through Toll-like receptor 2. *J Virol.* 2009;83:1492-1500.
3. Kumar H, Kawai T, Akira S. Toll-like receptors and innate immunity. *Biochem Biophys Res Commun.* 2009;388:621-625.
4. Kaisho T, Akira S. Toll-like receptor function and signaling. *J Allergy Clin Immunol.* 2006;117:979-987.
5. Blander JM. Signalling and phagocytosis in the orchestration of host defence. *Cell Microbiol.* 2007;9:290-299.
6. Gleeson M, McFarlin B, Flynn M. Exercise and Toll-like receptors. *Exerc Immunol Rev.* 2006;12:34-53.

Pentraxin3 and high-sensitive C-reactive protein are independent inflammatory markers released during high-intensity exercise

Nakajima T, Kurano M, Hasegawa T, et al (The Univ of Tokyo, Bunkyo-ku, Japan; et al)
Eur J Appl Physiol 110:905-913, 2010

High-intensity exercise shares similarities with acute phase responses of inflammatory diseases. We investigated the influences of acute exercise on inflammatory markers, plasma pentraxin3 (PTX3) and serum high sensitive C-reactive protein (CRP) (hsCRP). Nine healthy male subjects (41 ± 3 years old) participated. Each subject performed three types of exercise; ergometer exercise at 70% workload of anaerobic threshold (AT) for 30 min (70% AT exercise), peak ergometer exercise (peak EX, 20 watt increase/min until fatigue) and resistance exercises of 70% 1 RM (70% RE) until exhaustion. We measured plasma PTX3, serum hsCRP, lactate, noradrenaline (NOR), white blood cells (WBC), interleukin-6 (IL-6) and myeloperoxidase (MPO), a marker of neutrophil degranulation. The effects of exercise on intracellular PTX3 and MPO in neutrophils were also investigated, by using flow cytometry analysis. Circulating PTX3 and hsCRP significantly increased immediately after 70% RE and peak EX, while they did not increase after 70% AT exercise. The exercise-induced fold increase in PTX3 and hsCRP relative to the resting level was positively correlated with the changes in WBC, NOR, lactate and MPO. The exercise-induced fold increase in IL-6 was positively correlated with that in NOR, but not with that in PTX3 and hsCRP. Neutrophils isolated immediately after 70% RE, but not 70% AT exercise, exhibited lower mean fluorescence for PTX3 and MPO than those from pre-exercise blood. These results provide the evidence that high-intensity exercises significantly increase circulatory PTX3 as well as hsCRP. The release from peripheral neutrophils is suggested to be involved in the exercise-induced plasma PTX3 increase (Fig 4).

▶ C-reactive protein (CRP) is one of a group of short pentraxins, and it is produced mainly in the liver in response to various sources of inflammation,

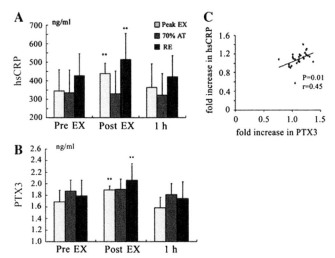

FIGURE 4.—Serum hsCRP (a) and plasma PTX3 (b) level before (Pre EX), immediately after (Post EX), and 1 h after EX. Peak EX, 70% AT exercise, and 70% RE. Values are means ± SE for nine subjects. **Significantly different from Pre EX, $p < 0.01$. c Correlations between the fold increase in hsCRP and that in PTX3 during exercises. (Reprinted from Nakajima T, Kurano M, Hasegawa T, et al. Pentraxin3 and high-sensitive C-reactive protein are independent inflammatory markers released during high-intensity exercise. *Eur J Appl Physiol.* 2010;110:905-913. With kind permission of Springer Science+Business Media.)

such as tissue injury. In contrast, the newly discovered long pentraxin molecule, pentraxin3 (PX3), is produced in various tissues, such as skeletal muscle and white cells, close to the site of injury.[1,2] Both CRP and PX3 levels were increased by all 3 patterns of exercise tested in this study, not only resistance exercise but also high-intensity anaerobic effort (Fig 4). Resting levels of CRP and PX3 were unrelated to each other, although the percentage increases in CRP and PX3 showed a moderate intercorrelation. The authors of this report suggest that PX3 is probably derived from neutrophils and that resting values may provide a better index of chronic inflammation than the measurement of resting CRP levels.

R. J. Shephard, MD (Lond), PhD, DPE

References

1. Presta M, Camozzi M, Salvatori G, Rusnati M. Role of the soluble pattern recognition receptor PTX3 in vascular biology. *J Cell Mol Med.* 2007;11:723-738.
2. Mantovani A, Garlanda C, Doni A, Bottazzi B. Pentraxins in innate immunity: from C-reactive protein to the long pentraxin PTX3. *J Clin Immunol.* 2008;28:1-13.

5 Metabolism and Obesity, Nutrition and Doping

Changes in the Salivary Biomarkers Induced by an Effort Test
de Oliveira VN, Bessa A, Lamounier RPMS, et al (Universidade Federal de Uberlândia, Brazil; et al)
Int J Sports Med 31:377-381, 2010

Physical exercise induces biochemical changes in the body that modify analytes in blood and saliva among other body fluids. This study analyzed the effect of an incremental effort test on the salivary protein profile to determine whether any specific protein is altered in response to such stress. We also measured thresholds of salivary alpha amylase, total salivary protein and blood lactate and searched for correlations among them. Twelve male cyclists underwent a progressive test in which blood and saliva samples were collected simultaneously at each stage. The salivary total protein profile revealed that physical exercise primarily affects the polypeptide corresponding to salivary alpha-amylase, the concentration of which increased markedly during the test. We observed thresholds of salivary alpha-amylase (sAAT), total salivary protein (PAT) and blood lactate (BLT) in 58%, 83% and 100% of our sample, respectively. Pearson's correlation indicates a strong and significant association between sAAT and BLT ($r = 0.84$, $p < 0.05$), sAAT and PAT ($r = 0.83$, $p < 0.05$) and BLT and PAT ($r = 0.90$, $p < 0.05$). The increased expression of the salivary alpha-amylase (sAA) polypeptide suggests that sAA is the main protein responsible for the increase in total protein concentration of whole saliva. Therefore, monitoring total protein concentration is an efficient tool and an alternative noninvasive biochemical method for determining exercise intensity (Fig 3).

▶ Exercise modifies saliva flow and thus the concentration of saliva constituents such as immunoglobulins, giving a spurious indication of changes in secretion. In an attempt to circumvent this problem, some biochemists have thus reported variables in relation to total grams of salivary protein. However, if the total protein content of saliva also changes in response to exercise (Fig 3), this may not provide a satisfactory point of reference. This study is

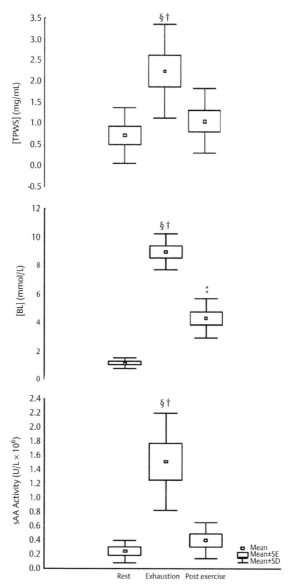

FIGURE 3.—Exercise intensity markers before the test, during exhaustion and after the test. Alterations in blood lactate (BL) concentrations, total protein concentration of whole saliva (TPWS) and salivary alpha-amylase (sAA) activity during rest, exhaustion and after the test. Plots display absolute values of the mean (± standard deviation) of blood lactate (BL) and salivary total protein (TPWS) concentrations as well as salivary alpha-amylase activity (sAA) at the moments of rest, exhaustion and 15 min after the last stage (post-exercise). (†) Indicates $p < 0.05$ vs. exhaustion and rest. (‡) Indicates $p < 0.05$ vs. 15' post-exercise and rest. (§) Indicates $p < 0.05$ vs. exhaustion and post-exercise. SD = Standard Deviation and SE = Standard Error. (Reprinted from de Oliveira VN, Bessa A, Lamounier RPMS, et al. Changes in the salivary biomarkers induced by an effort test. *Int J Sports Med.* 2010;31:377-381.)

based on a short progressive exercise test; the subjects were well hydrated and saliva production was stimulated by chewing gum, and in this situation there was a substantial increase in total salivary protein. Because there was an increase in some specific constituents, particularly salivary alpha-amylase, but not in others, it is difficult to attribute this to a reduction in salivary flow; it probably reflects an action of beta-adrenergic stimulation upon membrane-bound granules of the amylase. The authors suggest the interesting possibility that increases in salivary alpha-amylase could provide a noninvasive indication of the intensity of exercise. However, further research will be needed to ensure that the magnitude of this response is sufficiently consistent to be helpful in monitoring the intensity of effort.

R. J. Shephard, MD (Lond), PhD, DPE

Evaluation of three portable blood lactate analysers: Lactate Pro, Lactate Scout and Lactate Plus
Tanner RK, Fuller KL, Ross MLR (Australian Inst of Sport, Belconnen, Canberra, Australia)
Eur J Appl Physiol 109:551-559, 2010

Three portable blood lactate analysers, Lactate Pro (LP), Lactate Scout (LS) and Lactate Plus (L^+), were evaluated. Analyser reliability and accuracy was assessed. For reliability, intra- and inter-analyser comparisons demonstrated that the LP (intra-TE = 0.5 mM, inter-TE = 0.4 mM) and L^+ (intra-TE = 0.4, inter-TE = 0.4 mM) displayed greater overall reliability than the LS (intra- TE = 1.0, inter-TE = 0.8 mM). At BLa < 4.0 mM, the LP (intra-TE = 0.1 mM) demonstrated greater reliability than the LS (intra-TE = 0.5 mM) and L^+ (intra-TE = 0.4 mM). At BLa > 8.0 mM, the LP (intra-TE = 0.5 mM, inter-TE = 0.4 mM) and L^+ (intra- and inter-TE = 0.4 mM) displayed greater reliability than the LS (intra- TE = 1.1 mM, inter-TE = 0.9 mM). For accuracy, the L^+ (SEE = 0.6 mM) compared more favourably to the LP than the LS (SEE = 1.1 mM). At BLa ~ 1.0– 18.0 mM, the LS produced values that were up to 0.9 mM higher than the LP; the L^+ produced BLa that were within ± 0.1 mM. All portable analysers tended to under-read the ABL 700 analyser. The suitability of the LP and L^+ as accurate analysers is supported by strong correlations ($r = 0.91$ and $r = 0.94$) and limits of agreement ≤2.1 mM. This study showed that the LP and L^+, compared well to each other, displayed good reliability and accuracy when compared to a laboratory-based analyser. Although the LS also displayed relatively good reliability, it was not as reliable or accurate as the LP or L^+ (Table 6).

▶ The field measurement of blood lactate is important to regulate training for top athletes,[1] and the use of this approach has been greatly facilitated by the development of portable, battery-operated, hand-held analyzers that evaluate test strips. None of these devices work well in very humid environments (> 80%-90% relative humidity). All 3 models that were tested slightly

TABLE 6.—Accuracy Data for Lactate Pro, Lactate Scout and Lactate Plus Analysers Versus Radiometer ABL 700

	ABL Versus LP	ABL Versus LS	ABL Versus L*
Sample number	58	77	73
Mean ± SD	12.2 ± 2.5	12.5 ± 2.5	12.3 ± 2.3
Range (mM)	6.6–17.0	7.6–17.6	7.4–17.0
Mean bias, mM (±95% CI)	−0.7 (−1.0 to −0.4)	−0.4 (−0.7 to −0.1)	−0.8 (−1.1 to −0.6)
SEE, mM (±95% CI)	1.1 (0.9–1.3)	1.4 (1.2–1.6)	0.9 (0.7–1.0)
CV% (±95% CI)	8.9 (7.4–11.0)	11.9 (10.2–14.3)	7.4 (6.3–8.9)
Correlation r	0.913	0.837	0.936

underestimated lactate levels relative to laboratory measurements (Table 6), but they showed good intra- and interanalyzer reliabilities. The Lactate Scout appears to have a poorer reliability than the other 2 instruments, particularly at lactate concentrations < 8 mM/L, but it requires a much smaller blood sample (0.5 μL of blood), has a shorter analysis time, and has a substantial memory (250 readings) relative to the more commonly used Lactate Pro.

R. J. Shephard, MD (Lond), PhD, DPE

Reference

1 Jacobs I. Blood lactate: implications for training and sports performance, *Sports Med.* 1986;3:10-25.

Effect of glycogen availability on human skeletal muscle protein turnover during exercise and recovery
Howarth KR, Phillips SM, MacDonald MJ, et al (McMaster Univ, Hamilton, Ontario, Canada)
J Appl Physiol 109:431-438, 2010

We examined the effect of carbohydrate (CHO) availability on whole body and skeletal muscle protein utilization at rest, during exercise, and during recovery in humans. Six men cycled at ~75% peak O_2 uptake ($\dot{V}o_{2peak}$) to exhaustion to reduce body CHO stores and then consumed either a high-CHO (H-CHO; 71 ± 3% CHO) or low-CHO (L-CHO; 11 ± 1% CHO) diet for 2 days before the trial in random order. After each dietary intervention, subjects received a primed constant infusion of [1-^{13}C]leucine and L-[ring-^{2}H$_5$]phenylalanine for measurements of the whole body net protein balance and skeletal muscle protein turnover. Muscle, breath, and arterial and venous blood samples were obtained at rest, during 2 h of two-legged kicking exercise at ~45% of kicking ($\dot{V}o_{2peak}$), and during 1 h of recovery. Biopsy samples confirmed that the muscle glycogen concentration was lower in the L-CHO group versus the H-CHO group at rest, after exercise, and after recovery. The net leg protein balance was decreased in the L-CHO group compared with at rest and compared with the H-CHO condition, which was primarily due to an increase in protein degradation (area under the curve of the phenylalanine rate of appearance: 1,331 ± 162 μmol in the L-CHO group vs. 786 ± 51 μmol in the H-CHO group, $P < 0.05$) but also due to a decrease in protein synthesis late in exercise. There were no changes during exercise in the rate of appearance compared with rest in the H-CHO group. Whole body leucine oxidation increased above rest in the L-CHO group only and was higher than in the H-CHO group. The whole body net protein balance was reduced in the L-CHO group, largely due to a decrease in whole body protein synthesis. These data extend previous findings by others and demonstrate, using contemporary stable isotope methodology, that CHO availability influences the rates of skeletal muscle and whole body protein synthesis, degradation, and net balance during prolonged exercise in humans (Fig 5).

▶ When I have evaluated ultralong distance runners, I have often been impressed by the paucity of muscle tissue they show in regions of the body that do not contribute directly to their athletic performance. The logical conclusion seems that when body glycogen stores became depleted, the competitor drew upon muscle protein to maintain blood glucose through a process of

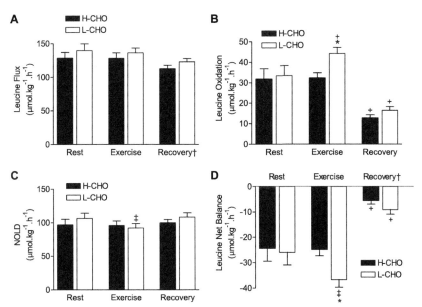

FIGURE 5.—Whole body leucine flux (*A*), leucine oxidation (*B*), nonoxidative leucine disposal (NOLD; *C*), and leucine net balance (*D*) at rest, during 2 h of two-leg knee extensor exercise, and during 1 h of recovery after a glycogen depletion protocol and subsequent H-CHO or L-CHO diet for ~48 h. Values are means ± SE; $n = 6$. *$P < 0.05$ vs. the H-CHO trial at the same time point; +$P < 0.05$ vs. rest in the same trial; ‡$P < 0.05$ vs. rest and recovery in the same trial; †main effect for diet ($P < 0.05$). (Reprinted from Howarth KR, Phillips SM, MacDonald MJ, et al. Effect of glycogen availability on human skeletal muscle protein turnover during exercise and recovery. *J Appl Physiol.* 2010;109:431-438, used with permission.)

gluconeogenesis. Previous studies have supported this view by showing that when glycogen levels were low, there was an increase of blood urea[1] and a net loss of muscle as assessed by measurements of arteriovenous nitrogen balance.[2,3] The present small-scale crossover study extends this information, using an infusion of stable amino acid isotopes; using such an approach, it is possible to distinguish between an increased breakdown of protein and a reduced protein synthesis, rather than simply reporting a net nitrogen balance. This study also differs from previous trials (in which 1 leg was glycogen depleted); here, both legs were depleted, and subjects then followed a high- or a low-carbohydrate diet for 2 days. Under the conditions of these experiments, the main adverse effect of the low-glycogen diet was upon protein synthesis nonoxidative leucine disposal rather than protein breakdown (flux) (Fig 5). However, it seems possible that this may have been influenced by the infusion of amino acids; moreover, protein intake was higher during the low-carbohydrate trial than during the high-carbohydrate phase. Further trials with a closer control of protein availability are thus desirable. The practical lesson from this study seems that the provision of carbohydrate to the endurance athlete is likely not only to enhance immediate performance but also to avert long-term loss of muscle protein.

R. J. Shephard, MD (Lond), PhD, DPE

References

1. Lemon PW, Mullin JP. Effect of initial muscle glycogen levels on protein catabolism during exercise. *J Appl Physiol*. 1980;48:624-629.
2. Van Hall G, Saltin B, Wagenmakers AJ. Muscle protein degradation and amino acid metabolism during prolonged knee-extensor exercise in humans. *Clin Sci (Lond)*. 1999;97:557-567.
3. Blomstrand E, Saltin B. Effect of muscle glycogen on glucose, lactate and amino acid metabolism during exercise and recovery in human subjects. *J Physiol*. 1999;514:293-302.

Physical Activity in U.S. Older Adults with Diabetes Mellitus: Prevalence and Correlates of Meeting Physical Activity Recommendations
Zhao G, Ford ES, Li C, et al (Natl Ctr for Chronic Disease Prevention and Health Promotion, Atlanta, GA)
J Am Geriatr Soc 59:132-137, 2011

Objectives.—To compare the prevalence and correlates of meeting current recommendations for physical activity in older adults with and without diabetes mellitus (DM) in the United States.

Design.—A cross-sectional, population-based sample.

Setting.—The 2007 Behavioral Risk Factor Surveillance Survey, which employs random-digit dialing to interview noninstitutionalized U.S. adults.

Participants.—Ninety-nine thousand one hundred seventy-two adults (18,370 with DM) aged 65 and older.

Measurements.—The age-adjusted prevalence and the odds ratios for physical activity patterns (defined on the basis of the physical activity guidelines from the American Diabetes Association (ADA 2007) and the Department of Health and Human Services (DHHS 2008)) were obtained using multiple logistic regression analyses. The correlates of meeting physical activity recommendations were assessed using log-binomial regression analyses.

Results.—Overall, 25% and 42% of older adults with diabetes mellitus met recommendations for total physical activity based on the ADA 2007 and the DHHS 2008 guidelines, respectively. Adults with DM were 31% to 34% ($P < .001$) less likely to engage in physical activity at recommended levels and 13% to 19% ($P < .001$) less likely to be physically active at insufficient levels than those without DM. Analyses limited to participants who reported no disability yielded similar results. In adults with DM, older age (≥ 75); being female; being non-Hispanic black; and having obesity, coronary heart disease, and disability were associated with less likelihood, whereas advanced educational status was associated with greater likelihood of meeting physical activity recommendations.

Conclusion.—In the United States, efforts to boost physical activity participation in older adults with DM are needed.

▶ Much effort has been exerted by public health organizations to improve physical activity participation, especially in people with obesity or obesity-related conditions such as diabetes mellitus. Despite these efforts, the data from this large population-based study demonstrated that most older adults with diabetes mellitus did not exercise enough to meet physical activity recommendations, even after accounting for disabilities and limitations in performing physical activity.[1] Thus there is a great need for health care professionals to continue to educate their patients with diabetes mellitus about the benefits of physical activity and to continuously prescribe physical activity for them.

D. C. Nieman, DrPH

Reference

1. Zhao G, Ford ES, Li C, Mokdad AH. Compliance with physical activity recommendations in US adults with diabetes. *Diabet Med.* 2008;25:221-227.

Prognostic Effect of Exercise Capacity on Mortality in Older Adults with Diabetes Mellitus
Nylen ES, Kokkinos P, Myers J, et al (Veterans Affairs Med Ctr, Washington, DC)
J Am Geriatr Soc 58:1850-1854, 2010

Objectives.—To investigate the prognostic effect of exercise capacity in older individuals with diabetes mellitus.

Design.—Retrospective data review in a clinic-based cohort.

Setting.—Veterans Affairs Medical Centers in Washington, District of Columbia, and Palo Alto, California.

Participants.—Two thousand eight hundred sixty-seven men aged 50 to 87 with type 2 diabetes mellitus.

Measurements.—Exercise tolerance testing with fitness categories based on peak metabolic equivalents of task (METs) achieved adjusted for age. All-cause mortality in age groups 50 to 65 (Group 1; n = 1,658) and older than 65 (Group 2; n = 1,209) was analyzed using adjusted Cox proportional hazards models.

Results.—After a mean ± standard deviation follow-up period of 7.8 ± 5.1 years, there were 324 deaths in Group 1 (20%) and 464 in Group 2 (38%). For each 1-MET increase in exercise capacity, mortality was 18% lower for the entire cohort (hazard ratio (HR) = 0.82, 95% confidence interval (CI) = 0.79−0.86), 23% lower for Group 1 (HR = 0.77, 95% CI = 0.73−0.82), and 16% lower for Group 2 (HR = 0.84, 95% CI = 0.8−0.89). When fitness categories were considered, the mortality risk was 30% to 80% lower for those who achieved more than 4 METs in both age groups.

Conclusion.—Augmented exercise capacity is associated with lower risk of mortality in people with type 2 diabetes mellitus aged 50 to 65 as well as in those older than 65. Thus, physical fitness, as represented by exercise capacity, lowers mortality risk in people with diabetes mellitus irrespective of age. These findings suggest that healthcare providers should be cognizant of the level of exercise capacity in individual patients and encourage a physically active lifestyle regardless of age (Fig 1).

▶ The findings of this study support an inverse association between exercise capacity and all-cause mortality in older individuals with type 2 diabetes mellitus (Fig 1). When fitness level was considered, a significant reduction of approximately 30% in mortality risk was noted at the relatively modest exercise

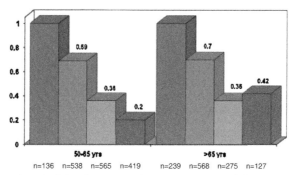

FIGURE 1.—Adjusted risk for all-cause mortality in two age groups of older men with diabetes mellitus according to exercise capacity. The graphs (read from left to right for both groups) depict the referant group (i.e., far left graph) ≤4 METs; next group is 4.1−6.0 METs; next group is 6.1−8.0 METs; and final group is > 8 METs. (Reprinted from Nylen ES, Kokkinos P, Myers J, et al. Prognostic effect of exercise capacity on mortality in older adults with diabetes mellitus. *J Am Geriatr Soc.* 2010;58:1850-1854. Reprinted with permission from 2010, Copyright the Authors. 2010, The American Geriatrics Society, John Wiley and Sons.)

capacity of 4.1 to 6.0 metabolic equivalents of task (METs) and 60% to 80% lower for the next fitness category (6.1 to 8.0 METs). This is consistent with the mortality reductions observed in populations without diabetes mellitus. The authors urge that "it is imperative that healthcare providers encourage a physically active lifestyle regardless of age. In addition, a compelling argument can be made that exercise capacity should be used to stratify mortality risk of the individual."

D. C. Nieman, DrPH

Brown fat as a therapy for obesity and diabetes
Cypess AM, Kahn CR (Harvard Med School, Boston, MA)
Curr Opin Endocrinol Diabetes Obes 17:143-149, 2010

Purpose of Review.—Human fat consists of white and brown adipose tissue (WAT and BAT). Though most fat is energy-storing WAT, the thermogenic capacity of even small amounts of BAT makes it an attractive therapeutic target for inducing weight loss through energy expenditure. This review evaluates the recent discoveries regarding the identification of functional BAT in adult humans and its potential as a therapy for obesity and diabetes.

Recent Findings.—Over the past year, several independent research teams used a combination of positronemission tomography and computed tomography (PET/CT) imaging, immunohistochemistry, and gene and protein expression assays to prove conclusively that adult humans have functional BAT. This has occurred against a backdrop of basic studies defining the origins of BAT, new components of its transcriptional regulation, and the role of hormones in stimulation of BAT growth and differentiation.

Summary.—Adult humans have functional BAT, a new target for antiobesity and antidiabetes therapies focusing on increasing energy expenditure. Future studies will refine the methodologies used to measure BAT mass and activity, expand our knowledge of critical-control points in BAT regulation, and focus on testing pharmacological agents that increase BAT thermogenesis and help achieve long-lasting weight loss and an improved metabolic profile.

▶ Brown fat is an interesting tissue in that small quantities can consume large amounts of energy, perhaps as much as 2 MJ/d. Futile metabolic cycles in this form of fat generate heat rather than serving normal metabolic functions. As the article of Cypess and Kahn indicates, there has been growing interest in exploiting this tissue in the fight against obesity and type II diabetes mellitus. Brown fat has long been recognized to play a significant role in the thermal homeostasis of infants, but the persistence of such tissue into adulthood has been a controversial issue. Recently, positron emission tomography has confirmed earlier suggestions from surface thermography, identifying substantial deposits in the interscapular region of adults and distinguishing such deposits from tumors[1,2] (Fig 1 in the original article). The brown adipose tissue contains

β_3-adrenergic agonist receptors, but attempts to stimulate its metabolism by the infusion of β_3-adrenergic drugs[3,4] have generally been unsuccessful. On the contrary, cold exposure appears to be an effective stimulus to brown fat metabolism, although possibly less so in obese than in normal-weight individuals.[5] This underlines the importance of some early observations from our laboratory.[6-9] We observed that there was an increased loss of body fat when subjects exercised in cold rather than comfortable thermal environments. Part of the difference seemed attributable to the wearing of heavier clothing, but we suspected at the time—and recent observations confirm this suspicion—that part of the benefit came from an activation of brown fat in the cold. This seems a strong argument to include winter endurance sports such as cross-country skiing as a valuable component of any campaign to normalize a patient's body mass index; there may even be a revival of our suggestions from the early 1980s, the provision of exercise rooms held at near freezing temperatures.

R. J. Shephard, MD (Lond), PhD, DPE

References

1. Hany TF, Gharehpapagh E, Kamel EM, Buck A, Himms-Hagen J, von Schulthess GK. Brown adipose tissue: a factor to consider in symmetrical tracer uptake in the neck and upper chest region. *Eur J Nucl Med Mol Imaging.* 2002;29:1393-1398.
2. Cohade C, Osman M, Pannu HK, Wahl RL. Uptake in supraclavicular area fat ("USA-Fat"): description on18F-FDGPET/CT. *J Nucl Med.* 2003;44:170-176.
3. Weyer C, Tataranni PA, Snitker S, Danforth E Jr, Ravussin E. Increase in insulin action and fat oxidation after treatment with CL 316,243, a highly selective beta3-adrenoceptor agonist in humans. *Diabetes.* 1998;47:1555-1561.
4. Larsen TM, Toubro S, van Baak MA, et al. Effect of a 28-d treatment with L-796568, a novel beta(3)-adrenergic receptor agonist, on energy expenditure and body composition in obese men. *Am J Clin Nutr.* 2002;76:780-788.
5. van Marken Lichtenbelt WD, Vanhommerig JW, Smulders NM, et al. Cold-activated brown adipose tissue in healthy men. *N Engl J Med.* 2009;360:1500-1508.
6. O'Hara WJ, Allen C, Shephard RJ, Allen G. Fat loss in the cold—a controlled study. *J Appl Physiol.* 1979;46:872-877.
7. O'Hara WJ, Allen C, Shephard RJ. Loss of body fat during an arctic winter expedition. *Can J Physiol Pharmacol.* 1977;55:1235-1241.
8. O'Hara WJ, Allen C, Shephard RJ. Loss of body weight and fat during exercise in a cold chamber. *Eur J Appl Physiol Occup Physiol.* 1977;37:205-218.
9. O'Hara WJ, Allen C, Shephard RJ. Treatment of obesity by exercise in the cold. *Can Med Assoc J.* 1977;117:773-778.

Sedentary behavior, physical activity, and concentrations of insulin among US adults
Ford ES, Li C, Zhao G, et al (Ctrs for Disease Control and Prevention, Atlanta, GA; et al)
Metabolism 59:1268-1275, 2010

Time spent watching television has been linked to obesity, metabolic syndrome, and diabetes, all conditions characterized to some degree by hyperinsulinemia and insulin resistance. However, limited evidence relates screen time (watching television or using a computer) directly to concentrations of insulin. We examined the cross-sectional associations between time spent watching television or using a computer, physical activity, and serum concentrations of insulin using data from 2800 participants aged at least 20 years of the 2003-2006 National Health and Nutrition Examination Survey. The amount of time spent watching television and using a computer as well as physical activity was self-reported. The unadjusted geometric mean concentration of insulin increased from 6.2 μU/mL among participants who did not watch television to 10.0 μU/mL among those who watched television for 5 or more hours per day ($P = .001$). After adjustment for age, sex, race or ethnicity, educational status, concentration of cotinine, alcohol intake, physical activity, waist circumference, and body mass index using multiple linear regression analysis, the log-transformed concentrations of insulin were significantly and positively associated with time spent watching television ($P = <.001$). Reported time spent using a computer was significantly associated with log-transformed concentrations of insulin before but not after accounting for waist circumference and body mass index. Leisure-time physical activity but not transportation or household physical activity was significantly and inversely associated with log-transformed concentrations of insulin. Sedentary behavior, particularly the amount of time spent watching

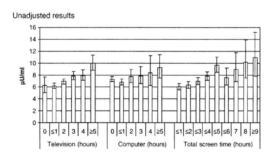

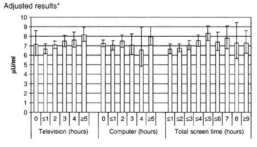

*Adjusted for age, gender, race or ethnicity, educational status, concentration of cotinine, alcohol intake, waist circumference, body mass index, and leisure-time physical activity.

FIGURE 1.—Unadjusted and adjusted geometric mean concentrations of insulin by hours of time spent watching television, using computers, and total screen time among 2800 US adults aged at least 20 years, National Health and Nutrition Examination Survey 2003-2006. (Reprinted from Ford ES, Li C, Zhao G, et al. Sedentary behavior, physical activity, and concentrations of insulin among US adults. *Metabolism.* 2010;59:1268-1275, with permission from Elsevier Inc.)

television, may be an important modifiable determinant of concentrations of insulin (Fig 1).

▶ As summarized in Fig 1, the amount of time spent watching television proved to be positively associated with serum insulin levels in US adults. Serum insulin is moderately associated with criterion-standard measures of insulin resistance and elevated risk of cardiovascular disease and diabetes. Spending time watching television is turning out to be quite hazardous to the health, with other studies showing links to obesity, metabolic syndrome, and diabetes.[1,2] Americans watch about 150 hours of television each month, promoting sedentary behavior and increased energy intake through snacking of energy-dense foods.[3]

D. C. Nieman, DrPH

References

1. Ford ES, Kohl HW III, Mokdad AH, Ajani UA. Sedentary behavior, physical activity, and the metabolic syndrome among U.S. adults. *Obes Res.* 2005;13:608-614.
2. Hu FB. Sedentary lifestyle and risk of obesity and type 2 diabetes. *Lipids.* 2003;38: 103-108.
3. Cleland VJ, Schmidt MD, Dwyer T, Venn AJ. Television viewing and abdominal obesity in young adults: is the association mediated by food and beverage consumption during viewing time or reduced leisure-time physical activity? *Am J Clin Nutr.* 2008;87:1148-1155.

Exercise and Type 2 Diabetes: American College of Sports Medicine and the American Diabetes Association: Joint Position Statement
American College of Sports Medicine; American Diabetes Association ()
Med Sci Sports Exerc 42:2282-2303, 2010

Although physical activity (PA) is a key element in the prevention and management of type 2 diabetes mellitus (T2DM), many with this chronic disease do not become or remain regularly active. High-quality studies establishing the importance of exercise and fitness in diabetes were lacking until recently, but it is now well established that participation in regular PA improves blood glucose control and can prevent or delay T2DM, along with positively affecting lipids, blood pressure, cardiovascular events, mortality, and quality of life. Structured interventions combining PA and modest weight loss have been shown to lower T2DM risk by up to 58% in high-risk populations. Most benefits of PA on diabetes management are realized through acute and chronic improvements in insulin action, accomplished with both aerobic and resistance training. The benefits of physical training are discussed, along with recommendations for varying activities, PA-associated blood glucose management, diabetes prevention, gestational diabetes, and safe and effective practices for PA with diabetes-related complications.

▶ This joint position statement on exercise and type II diabetes was coauthored by a writing team of 6 knowledgeable professionals from the American College of Sports Medicine (ACSM) and 3 from the American Diabetes Association. Having previously been a member of the Board of Directors and a vice president of ACSM, I am personally cognizant of the degree of scientific rigor with which these position statements are crafted and the intense scrutiny with which they are reviewed by the Pronouncements Committee. For this article, 295 separate articles were reviewed and referenced. For each research, clinical, or practice question, an evidence statement was produced and graded according to the evidence categories of each of the organizations.

Section headings include the acute effects of exercise, chronic effects of exercise training, physical activity (PA) in the prevention and control of type 2 diabetes as well as gestational diabetes, preexercise evaluation, recommended PA participation, exercise with nonoptimal blood glucose control, medication effects on exercise responses, exercise with complications of diabetes, and finally, adoption and maintenance of exercise by persons with diabetes. In short, this is a single source reference to consult about any question related to PA and type 2 diabetes. The writing group is to be congratulated and commended for their thorough coverage of this important topic.

C. Lebrun, MD

Body-Mass Index and Mortality among 1.46 Million White Adults
Berrington de Gonzalez A, Hartge P, Cerhan JR, et al (Natl Cancer Inst, Bethesda, MD; Mayo Clinic, Rochester, MN; et al)
N Engl J Med 363:2211-2219, 2010

Background.—A high body-mass index (BMI, the weight in kilograms divided by the square of the height in meters) is associated with increased mortality from cardiovascular disease and certain cancers, but the precise relationship between BMI and all-cause mortality remains uncertain.

Methods.—We used Cox regression to estimate hazard ratios and 95% confidence intervals for an association between BMI and all-cause mortality, adjusting for age, study, physical activity, alcohol consumption, education, and marital status in pooled data from 19 prospective studies encompassing 1.46 million white adults, 19 to 84 years of age (median, 58).

Results.—The median baseline BMI was 26.2. During a median follow-up period of 10 years (range, 5 to 28), 160,087 deaths were identified. Among healthy participants who never smoked, there was a J-shaped relationship between BMI and all-cause mortality. With a BMI of 22.5 to 24.9 as the reference category, hazard ratios among women were 1.47 (95 percent confidence interval [CI], 1.33 to 1.62) for a BMI of 15.0 to 18.4; 1.14 (95% CI, 1.07 to 1.22) for a BMI of 18.5 to 19.9; 1.00 (95% CI, 0.96 to 1.04) for a BMI of 20.0 to 22.4; 1.13 (95% CI, 1.09 to 1.17) for a BMI of 25.0 to 29.9; 1.44 (95% CI, 1.38 to 1.50) for a BMI of 30.0 to 34.9; 1.88 (95% CI, 1.77 to 2.00) for a BMI of 35.0 to 39.9; and 2.51 (95% CI, 2.30 to 2.73) for a BMI of 40.0 to 49.9. In general, the hazard ratios for the men were similar. Hazard ratios for a BMI below 20.0 were attenuated with longer-term follow-up.

Conclusions.—In white adults, overweight and obesity (and possibly underweight) are associated with increased all-cause mortality. All-cause mortality is generally lowest with a BMI of 20.0 to 24.9.

▶ The concept of a U-shaped relationship between body mass and health (Fig 1 in the original article) has been well documented since the studies of Andres.[1,2] It has provided the main basis for the current categorization of people as overweight and obese. Two important criticisms of these studies were that the population was biased (those purchasing life insurance in the United States and Canada) and that most of the height and weight data were self-reported, with a resultant risk of the underreporting of actual body mass. Controversy has remained on the extent to which health is compromised by a body mass index (BMI) in the range 25 to 29.9 kg/m^2,[3-8] possibly because of small sample size and differences in age or follow-up period. A recent analysis examined prospective data from some 900 000 subjects enrolled in studies looking at cardiovascular risk factors,[3] concluding that the optimal BMI was 22.5 to 25.0 kg/m^2, with health risk from being either overweight or obese; critics of this analysis noted that the inclusion of smokers and individuals with preexisting cancers could have underestimated the importance of BMI to health. de Gonzalez and associates have now conducted an analysis based on a very large sample of Americans enrolled in prospective studies of cancer. The initial median age was 58 years, and participants were drawn from 19 major prospective studies. Over a follow up averaging 10 years, there were a large number of deaths (160 087), and this allowed statistical adjustment of prognosis for age, study, smoking habits, physical activity, alcohol consumption, education, and marital status. As in the original studies of Andres, height and body mass were obtained by questionnaire and in many cases were probably self-reports. Participants also had some bias, particularly restriction to white Americans. The data for subjects initially free of cancer or cardiovascular disease show clearly distortion of the relationship by smoking although leaving the optimal BMI range suggested by Andres (20-25 kg/m^2). One new feature of the de Gonzalez analysis is the inclusion of some information on physical activity; apparently, this had little effect on the shape of the relationship, except that the adverse significance of a low BMI tended to be less for active individuals. This effect was also reduced in studies where the follow-up was for more than 15 years, suggesting that a part of the left-hand side of the curve reflects preexisting morbidity.

R. J. Shephard, MD (Lond), PhD, DPE

References

1. Society of Actuaries. *Build Study, 1979.* Chicago, IL: Society of Actuaries; 1979.
2. Andres R. Discussion: assessment of health status. In: Bouchard C, Shephard RJ, Stephens T, et al., eds. *Exercise, Fitness and Health.* Champaign, IL: Human Kinetics; 1990:133-136.
3. Flegal KM, Graubard BI, Williamson DF, Gail MH. Cause-specific excess deaths associated with underweight, overweight, and obesity. *JAMA.* 2007;298:2028-2037.
4. Orpana HM, Berthelot JM, Kaplan MS, Feeny DH, McFarland B, Ross NA. BMI and mortality: results from a national longitudinal study of Canadian adults. *Obesity (Silver Spring).* 2010;18:214-218.

5. Calle EE, Rodriguez C, Walker-Thurmond K, Thun MJ. Overweight, obesity, and mortality from cancer in a prospectively studied cohort of U.S. adults. *N Engl J Med*. 2003;348:1625-1638.

6. Adams KF, Schatzkin A, Harris TB, et al. Overweight, obesity, and mortality in a large prospective cohort of persons 50 to 71 years old. *N Engl J Med*. 2006; 355:763-778.

7. Pischon T, Boeing H, Hoffmann K, et al. General and abdominal adiposity and risk of death in Europe. *N Engl J Med*. 2008;359:2105-2120.

8. Prospective Studies Collaboration. Body-mass index and cause-specific mortality in 900 000 adults: collaborative analyses of 57 prospective studies. *Lancet*. 2009;373: 1083-1096.

Physical Activity Attenuates the Genetic Predisposition to Obesity in 20,000 Men and Women from EPIC-Norfolk Prospective Population Study
Li S, Zhao JH, Luan J, et al (Inst of Metabolic Science, Cambridge, UK; et al)
PLoS Med 7:e1000332, 2010

Background.—We have previously shown that multiple genetic loci identified by genome-wide association studies (GWAS) increase the susceptibility to obesity in a cumulative manner. It is, however, not known whether and to what extent this genetic susceptibility may be attenuated by a physically active lifestyle. We aimed to assess the influence of a physically active lifestyle on the genetic predisposition to obesity in a large population-based study.

Methods and Findings.—We genotyped 12 SNPs in obesity-susceptibility loci in a population-based sample of 20,430 individuals (aged 39–79 y) from the European Prospective Investigation of Cancer (EPIC)-Norfolk cohort with an average follow-up period of 3.6 y. A genetic predisposition score was calculated for each individual by adding the body mass index (BMI)-increasing alleles across the 12 SNPs. Physical activity was assessed using a self-administered questionnaire. Linear and logistic regression models were used to examine main effects of the genetic predisposition score and its interaction with physical activity on BMI/obesity risk and BMI change over time, assuming an additive effect for each additional BMI-increasing allele carried. Each additional BMI-increasing allele was associated with 0.154 (standard error [SE] 0.012) kg/m^2 ($p = 6.73 \times 10^{-37}$) increase in BMI (equivalent to 445 g in body weight for a person 1.70 m tall). This association was significantly ($p_{interaction} = 0.005$) more pronounced in inactive people (0.205 [SE 0.024] kg/m^2 [$p = 3.62 \times 10^{-18}$; 592 g in weight]) than in active people (0.131 [SE 0.014] kg/m^2 [$p = 7.97 \times 10^{-21}$; 379 g in weight]). Similarly, each additional BMI-increasing allele increased the risk of obesity 1.116-fold (95% confidence interval [CI] 1.093–1.139, $p = 3.37 \times 10^{-26}$) in the whole population, but significantly ($p_{interaction} = 0.015$) more in inactive individuals (odds ratio [OR] = 1.158 [95% CI 1.118–1.199; $p = 1.93 \times 10^{-16}$]) than in active individuals (OR = 1.095 (95% CI 1.068–1.123; $p = 1.15 \times 10^{-12}$]). Consistent with the cross-sectional observations, physical activity modified the association between the genetic predisposition score and change in BMI during follow-up ($p_{interaction} = 0.028$).

Conclusions.—Our study shows that living a physically active lifestyle is associated with a 40% reduction in the genetic predisposition to common obesity, as estimated by the number of risk alleles carried for any of the 12 recently GWAS-identified loci (Fig 1).

▶ "I can't do anything about my weight, Doctor. It's in my genes." This is a frequent excuse advanced by the overweight patient. The article by Li and associates reports on a massive study of 20 430 adults, looking at 12 genetic loci consistently associated with obesity[1-5] in relation to a questionnaire assessment of their physical activity. There is certainly a strong influence of genotype. Among active individuals, the body mass index (BMI) increases from around 25.5 kg per m² as the burden of unfavorable genes is increased. However, there is also a striking (gene × environment) interaction. Thus, those who are

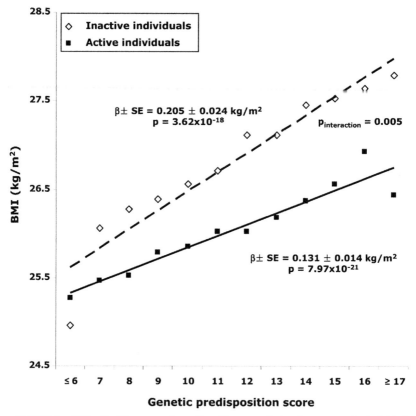

FIGURE 1.—BMI with different genetic predisposition scores in inactive versus active individuals. (Reprinted from Li S, Zhao JH, Luan J, et al. Physical activity attenuates the genetic predisposition to obesity in 20,000 men and women from EPIC-Norfolk prospective population study. *PLoS Med.* 2010;7:e1000332, with permission from Li et al.)

physically active have a much lower BMI at all levels of genetic susceptibility (Fig 1). Perhaps even more importantly, the slope of genetic effect is much weaker (379 g per allele then 592 g per allele) in those who are active. Taking a genetic predisposition score of 11 as the divider between low and high genetic susceptibility, in active subjects, genetic susceptibility adds only 0.4 kg per m^2 to the average BMI. The benefit of exercise is greatest in those who are most active, but some attenuation of genetic predisposition occurs even with quite low levels of physical activity. The figure seems worth showing to patients who claim that overweight runs in the family! The impact of an increase of physical activity upon the burden of obesity is probably even greater than these BMI data indicate; those who exercise regularly are likely to have heavier muscles and bones than those who are sedentary, and a smaller proportion of their BMI is attributable to fat.

R. J. Shephard, MD (Lond), PhD, DPE

References

1. Frayling TM, Timpson NJ, Weedon MN, et al. A common variant in the FTO gene is associated with body mass index and predisposes to childhood and adult obesity. *Science*. 2007;316:889-894.
2. Scuteri A, Sanna S, Chen WM, et al. Genome-wide association scan shows genetic variants in the FTO gene are associated with obesity-related traits. *PLoS Genet*. 2007;3:e115.
3. Loos RJ, Lindgren CM, Li S, et al. Common variants near MC4R are associated with fat mass, weight and risk of obesity. *Nat Genet*. 2008;40:768-775.
4. Willer CJ, Speliotes EK, Loos RJ, et al. Six new loci associated with body mass index highlight a neuronal influence on body weight regulation. *Nat Genet*. 2009;41:25-34.
5. Thorleifsson G, Walters GB, Gudbjartsson DF, et al. Genome-wide association yields new sequence variants at seven loci that associate with measures of obesity. *Nat Genet*. 2009;41:18-24.

The Effects of Exercise-Induced Weight Loss on Appetite-Related Peptides and Motivation to Eat
Martins C, Kulseng B, King NA, et al (Norwegian Univ of Science and Technology; Queensland Univ of Technology, Brisbane, Australia; et al)
J Clin Endocrinol Metab 95:1609-1616, 2010

Context.—The magnitude of exercise-induced weight loss depends on the extent of compensatory responses. An increase in energy intake is likely to result from changes in the appetite control system toward an orexigenic environment; however, few studies have measured how exercise impacts on both orexigenic and anorexigenic peptides.

Objective.—The aim of the study was to investigate the effects of medium-term exercise on fasting/postprandial levels of appetite-related hormones and subjective appetite sensations in overweight/obese individuals.

Design and Setting.—We conducted a longitudinal study in a university research center.

Participants and Intervention.—Twenty-two sedentary overweight/obese individuals (age, 36.9 ± 8.3 yr; body mass index, 31.3 ± 3.3 kg/m^2) took part in a 12-wk supervised exercise programme (five times per week, 75% maximal heart rate) and were requested not to change their food intake during the study.

Main Outcome Measures.—We measured changes in body weight and fasting/postprandial plasma levels of glucose, insulin, total ghrelin, acylated ghrelin (AG), peptide YY, and glucagon-like peptide-1 and feelings of appetite.

Results.—Exercise resulted in a significant reduction in body weight and fasting insulin and an increase in AG plasma levels and fasting hunger sensations. A significant reduction in postprandial insulin plasma levels and a tendency toward an increase in the delayed release of glucagon-like peptide-1 (90–180 min) were also observed after exercise, as well as a significant increase (127%) in the suppression of AG postprandially.

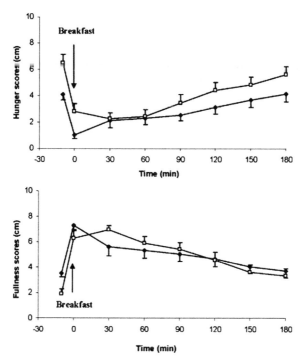

FIGURE 4.—Subjective feelings of hunger (*top*) and fullness (*bottom*) (cm) over time after breakfast, before (◆) and after a 12-wk exercise intervention (□). Values represent means ± SEM for 15 subjects. Repeated measures ANOVA showed a significant effect of time ($P < 0.0001$) and exercise ($P < 0.01$), but no interactions for hunger and a significant effect of time ($P < 0.0001$), and a time*exercise interaction ($P < 0.01$) for fullness feelings. (Reprinted from Martins C, Kulseng B, King NA, et al. The effects of exercise-induced weight loss on appetite-related peptides and motivation to eat. *J Clin Endocrinol Metab.* 2010;95:1609-1616, with permission from The Endocrine Society.)

Conclusions.—Exercise-induced weight loss is associated with physiological and biopsychological changes toward an increased drive to eat in the fasting state. However, this seems to be balanced by an improved satiety response to a meal and improved sensitivity of the appetite control system (Fig 4).

▶ Many interested in obesity have objected that exercise is an ineffective treatment for those who are overweight because it stimulates appetite through an upregulation of orexigenic hormones; the resulting increase in the ingestion of food counters even a substantial investment in physical activity.[1] This study, although relatively small in subject numbers, offers some objective information on this issue. The exercise program was quite vigorous (5 days/week for 12 weeks, at 75% of maximal heart rate, and requiring a net energy expenditure of some 2 megajoules per session). The levels of orexigenic hormones (total ghrelin and acyl ghrelin) and anorexigenic (glucagon-like peptide-1 and polypeptide YY) peptides were measured, and subjective assessments of appetite were made using a visual analog scale. Although hunger in the fasting state was increased following the 12 weeks of exercise (Fig 4), the sense of satiety following a standard meal was also enhanced. The plasma ghrelin levels matched these findings; although increased when fasting, levels were decreased following a standard meal. This is a different type of response from the compensatory upregulation of appetite seen with dieting alone, and it provides 1 more reason to advocate an appropriate exercise program for those who are obese.

R. J. Shephard, MD (Lond), PhD, DPE

Reference

1. Epstein LH, Wing RR. Aerobic exercise and weight. *Addict Behav.* 1980;5: 371-388.

Combined effects of weight loss and physical activity on all-cause mortality of overweight men and women
Østergaard JN, Grønbæk M, Schnohr P, et al (Univ of Southern Denmark, Copenhagen; Bispebjerg Univ Hosp, Copenhagen, Denmark; et al)
Int J Obes 34:760-769, 2010

Objective.—To estimate the excess deaths associated with weight loss in combination with leisure time physical activity among overweight or obese people.

Design.—Prospective cohort study.

Subjects.—In two consecutive examinations in 1976–1978 and 1981–1983, 11 135 people participated in the Copenhagen City Heart Study. Of these, 3078 overweight or obese participants lost weight or remained weight stable from 1976–1978 to 1981–1983, and were without pre-existing diagnosis of diabetes, stroke, ischaemic heart disease or cancer in 1981–1983. They were followed up until 2007 in the Danish Civil Registration System, with a <0.2% loss to follow-up only.

Measurements.—The following measurements were taken: body mass index (BMI) and physical activity in 1976–1978 and 1981–1983 and hazard ratio (HR) of mortality during 53 976 person-years of follow-up.

Results.—Of the initially overweight or obese subjects who either lost weight or remained weight stable, 2060 died. Overall, weight loss was associated with excess mortality when compared with weight stability. Weight loss was associated with a higher mortality among those who became physically *inactive*, compared with those who remained active while losing weight (men: HR 2.25, 95% confidence interval 1.31–3.84; women: 1.43, 1.07–1.91). However, losing weight while remaining physically active was still associated with excess mortality when compared with those who were weight stable and initially active (men: 1.72, 1.27–2.34; women: 1.57, 1.06–2.31). Among those who remained physically *inactive*, weight loss seemed associated with excess mortality when compared with weight loss among those who became active, although not statistically significant (men: 2.00, 0.94–4.29; women: 1.40, 0.82–2.39). Finally, weight loss among those who became physically active was not associated with excess mortality when compared with those who were weight stable and initially *inactive* (men: 1.12, 0.61–2.07; women: 1.19, 0.58–2.43).

Conclusion.—Weight loss among the overweight or obese seemed hazardous to survival. However, weight loss seemed less hazardous to survival among those who remained physically active or those who became active (Table 3).

▶ There is general agreement that obesity should be prevented whenever possible, and most physicians would also seek to correct cases of established obesity. Such treatment leads to favorable changes in a number of cardiovascular and metabolic risk factors.[1,2] However, it is less clearly established that the reduction in these risk factors leads to a corresponding improvement in prognosis, and some studies have suggested that weight loss may increase all-cause mortality rates for those who are initially obese.[3-6] In epidemiological studies, it is of course difficult to control for confounding variables such as pre-existing disease conditions that may precipitate weight loss.[7] Nevertheless, studies such as this report, with careful control of other variables, continue to show a substantial increase of all-cause mortality in those who lose weight relative to those whose weight remains stable (Table 3). Part of the problem may arise from the fact that a negative energy balance induces a concomitant loss of muscle tissue,[8,9] and this would offer one explanation why the adverse effect of losing weight is much less apparent (and indeed no longer statistically significant) in those who were initially inactive but become active during the weight-loss process (Table 3). It is also possible that adding exercise to a weight-loss regimen encourages a preferential loss of the more harmful visceral fat. This study does not necessarily argue against recommending weight loss in the obese, but it does underline the importance of accomplishing

TABLE 3.—Hazard Ratio and 95% Confidence Intervals of All-Cause Mortality Associated with Weight Loss and Change in Physical Activity Among 1692 Overweight and Obese Men and 1386 Overweight and Obese Women in the Copenhagen City Heart Study (1976–1978 to 1981–1983)

Groups in Focus	Reference Group	HR[a]	95% CI	P-Value[b]	HR, 10 Years After[a,c]	95% CI	P-Value[b]
Men							
WL	WS	1.84	(1.41–2.39)	<0.01	1.20	(1.05–1.38)	<0.01
Change in physical activity	Initial physical activity						
PAPA-WL	PAxx-WS	1.72	(1.27–2.34)	<0.01	1.18	(1.01–1.38)	0.04
PAPI-WL	PAxx-WS	3.87	(2.32–6.46)	<0.01	1.84	(1.36–2.49)	<0.01
PIPI-WL	PIxx-WS	1.96	(0.93–4.11)	0.08	0.91	(0.73–1.13)	0.77
PIPA-WL	PIxx-WS	1.12	(0.61–2.07)	0.72	0.99	(0.71–1.38)	0.97
Women							
WL	WS	1.73	(1.24–2.41)	<0.01	1.28	(1.08–1.51)	<0.01
Change in physical activity	Initial physical activity						
PAPA-WL	PAxx-WS	1.57	(1.06–2.31)	0.02	1.22	(1.00–1.49)	0.05
PAPI-WL	PAxx-WS	2.17	(1.21–3.91)	0.01	1.73	(1.28–2.33)	<0.01
PIPI-WL	PIxx-WS	3.06	(1.40–6.71)	<0.01	1.49	(0.98–2.26)	0.06
PIPA-WL	PIxx-WS	1.19	(0.58–2.43)	0.63	0.95	(0.64–1.40)	0.80

Abbreviations: CI, confidence interval; HR, hazard ratio; PAPA, physically active in both 1976–1978 and 1981–1983; PAPI, physically active in 1976–1978, but *inactive* in 1981–1983; PAxx, initially physically active; PIPA, physically *inactive* in 1976–1978, but active in 1981–1983; PIPI, physically *inactive* in both 1976–1978 and 1981–1983; PIxx, initially physically *inactive*; WL, weight loss (decline in BMI > 1 kg m^{-2} (BMI = weight(kg) height(m)$^{-2}$)); WS, weight stable (BMI within ± 1 kg m^{-2}).

[a]Adjusted for age, time between the two examinations, time since the second examination in 1981–1983, change in daily smoking habits, initial body mass index, height, education and marital status.

[b]P-value for the difference between the group in focus and the reference group.

[c]The hazard ratio 10 years after the second examination in 1981–1983.

this by a combination of dieting and a substantial level of physical activity, rather than by dieting alone.

R. J. Shephard, MD (Lond), PhD, DPE

References

1. Bacon SL, Sherwood A, Hinderliter A, Blumenthal JA. Effects of exercise, diet and weight loss on high blood pressure. *Sports Med.* 2004;34:307-316.
2. Poobalan A, Aucott L, Smith WCS, et al. Effects of weight loss in overweight/obese individuals and long-term lipid outcomes: a systematic review. *Obes Rev.* 2004;5: 43-50.
3. Lee IM, Paffenbarger RS. Is weight loss hazardous? *Nutr Rev.* 1996;54:S116-S124.
4. Higgins M, D'Agostino R, Kannel W, Cobb J, Pinsky J. Benefits and adverse effects of weight loss. Observations from the Framingham Study. *Ann Intern Med.* 1993; 119:758-763.
5. Mikkelsen KL, Heitmann BL, Keiding N, Sørensen TI. Independent effects of stable and changing body weight on total mortality. *Epidemiology.* 1999;10:671-678.
6. Nilsson PM, Nilsson JA, Hedblad B, Berglund G, Lindgärde F. The enigma of increased non-cancer mortality after weight loss in healthy men who are overweight or obese. *J Intern Med.* 2002;252:70-78.

7. Berentzen T, Sørensen TI. Effects of intended weight loss on morbidity and mortality: possible explanations of controversial results. *Nutr Rev.* 2006;64: 502-507.

8. Allison DB, Zannolli R, Faith MS, et al. Weight loss increases and fat loss decreases all-cause mortality rate: results from two independent cohort studies. *Int J Obes Relat Metab Disord.* 1999;23:603-611.

9. Heitmann BL, Erikson H, Ellsinger BM, Mikkelsen KL, Larsson B. Mortality associated with body fat, fat-free mass and body mass index among 60-years-old Swedish men-a 22-years follow-up. The study of men born in 1913. *Int J Obes Relat Metab Disord.* 2000;24:33-37.

Maintaining a High Physical Activity Level Over 20 Years and Weight Gain

Hankinson AL, Daviglus ML, Bouchard C, et al (Northwestern Univ, Chicago, IL; Pennington Biomedical Res Ctr, Baton Rouge, LA; et al)

JAMA 304:2603-2610, 2010

Context.—Data supporting physical activity guidelines to prevent long-term weight gain are sparse, particularly during the period when the highest risk of weight gain occurs.

Objective.—To evaluate the relationship between habitual activity levels and changes in body mass index (BMI) and waist circumference over 20 years.

Design, Setting, and Participants.—The Coronary Artery Risk Development in Young Adults (CARDIA) study is a prospective longitudinal study with 20 years of follow-up, 1985-1986 to 2005-2006. Habitual activity was defined as maintaining high, moderate, and low activity levels based on sex-specific tertiles of activity scores at baseline. Participants comprised a population-based multicenter cohort (Chicago, Illinois; Birmingham, Alabama; Minneapolis, Minnesota; and Oakland, California) of 3554 men and women aged 18 to 30 years at baseline.

Main Outcome Measures.—Average annual changes in BMI and waist circumference.

Results.—Over 20 years, maintaining high levels of activity was associated with smaller gains in BMI and waist circumference compared with low activity levels after adjustment for race, baseline BMI, age, education, cigarette smoking status, alcohol use, and energy intake. Menmaintaining high activity gained 2.6 fewer kilograms per year (+0.15 BMI units; 95% confidence interval [CI], 0.11-0.18 vs +0.20 in the lower activity group; 95% CI, 0.17-0.23), and women maintaining higher activity gained 6.1 fewer kilograms per year (+0.17 BMI units; 95% CI, 0.12-0.21 vs +0.30 in the lower activity group; 95% CI, 0.25-0.34). Men maintaining high activity gained 3.1 fewer centimeters in waist circumference per year (+0.52 cm; 95% CI, 0.43-0.61 cm vs 0.67 cm in the lower activity group; 95% CI, 0.60-0.75 cm) and women maintaining higher activity gained 3.8 fewer centimeters per year (+0.49 cm; 95% CI, 0.39-0.58 cm vs 0.67 cm in the lower activity group; 95% CI, 0.60-0.75 cm).

Conclusion.—Maintaining high activity levels through young adulthood may lessen weight gain as young adults transition to middle age, particularly in women.

▶ Canadian recommendations for minimum population levels of physical activity have traditionally been substantially higher than those proposed for the United States. One reason for advocating a greater weekly volume of activity was the fear that US recommendations were insufficient to tackle the growing epidemic of obesity in North America.[1-4] However, this year, Health Canada finally yielded to fears that the levels of activity demanded by the existing Canadian recommendations were unlikely to be achieved by a large segment of the population, and it thus drastically reduced the recommended minima of weekly activity. The 20-year longitudinal study of initially young adults conducted by Hankinson and associates provides further fuel for this debate. Absolute values for daily energy expenditures were obtained by questionnaire, and are thus somewhat suspect. Nevertheless, when subjects were grouped by physical activity tertiles, there was a substantially smaller weight gain in the most active third of the population, amounting over 20 years of adult life to an average difference of 2.6 kg in the men and 6.1 kg in the women (Fig in the original article). Even the top third of the sample were not highly active, although they did meet current US physical activity recommendations. The difference in estimated daily energy expenditures between the most active and the least active tertiles was some 3.3 MJ for the men and 0.8 MJ for the women. Based on these intergroup differences in weight gain, Hankinson and associates concluded that the current US recommendations were adequate. However, it is worth underlining that although weight gains were smaller in the most active tertiles, they also showed substantial accumulations of body fat over the 20-year study. Outcomes would indeed be better if the former Canadian standards were to be achieved.

R. J. Shephard, MD (Lond), PhD, DPE

References

1. Lee IM, Djoussé L, Sesso HD, Wang L, Buring JE. Physical activity and weight gain prevention. *JAMA.* 2010;303:1173-1179.
2. Saris WH, Blair SN, van Baak MA, et al. How much physical activity is enough to prevent unhealthy weight gain? Outcome of the IASO 1st Stock Conference and consensus statement. *Obes Rev.* 2003;4:101-114.
3. Erlichman J, Kerbey AL, James WP. Physical activity and its impact on health outcomes. Paper 2: Prevention of unhealthy weight gain and obesity by physical activity: an analysis of the evidence. *Obes Rev.* 2002;3:273-287.
4. Di Pietro L, Dziura J, Blair SN. Estimated change in physical activity level (PAL) and prediction of 5-year weight change in men: the Aerobics Center Longitudinal Study. *Int J Obes Relat Metab Disord.* 2004;28:1541-1547.

Maintaining a High Physical Activity Level Over 20 Years and Weight Gain

Hankinson AL, Daviglus ML, Bouchard C, et al (Northwestern Univ, Chicago, IL; Pennington Biomed Res Ctr, Baton Rouge, LA; et al)
JAMA 304:2603-2610, 2010

Context.—Data supporting physical activity guidelines to prevent long-term weight gain are sparse, particularly during the period when the highest risk of weight gain occurs.

Objective.—To evaluate the relationship between habitual activity levels and changes in body mass index (BMI) and waist circumference over 20 years.

Design, Setting, and Participants.—The Coronary Artery Risk Development in Young Adults (CARDIA) study is a prospective longitudinal study with 20 years of follow-up, 1985-1986 to 2005-2006. Habitual activity was defined as maintaining high, moderate, and low activity levels based on sex-specific tertiles of activity scores at baseline. Participants comprised a population-based multicenter cohort (Chicago, Illinois; Birmingham, Alabama; Minneapolis, Minnesota; and Oakland, California) of 3554 men and women aged 18 to 30 years at baseline.

Main Outcome Measures.—Average annual changes in BMI and waist circumference.

Results.—Over 20 years, maintaining high levels of activity was associated with smaller gains in BMI and waist circumference compared with low activity levels after adjustment for race, baseline BMI, age, education, cigarette smoking status, alcohol use, and energy intake. Men maintaining high activity gained 2.6 fewer kilograms per year (+0.15 BMI units; 95% confidence interval [CI], 0.11-0.18 vs +0.20 in the lower activity group; 95% CI, 0.17-0.23), and women maintaining higher activity gained 6.1 fewer kilograms per year (+0.17 BMI units; 95% CI, 0.12-0.21 vs +0.30 in the lower activity group; 95% CI, 0.25-0.34). Men maintaining high activity gained 3.1 fewer centimeters in waist circumference per year (+0.52 cm; 95% CI, 0.43-0.61 cm vs 0.67 cm in the lower activity group; 95% CI, 0.60-0.75 cm) and women maintaining higher activity gained 3.8 fewer centimeters per year (+0.49 cm; 95% CI, 0.39-0.58 cm vs 0.67 cm in the lower activity group; 95% CI, 0.60-0.75 cm).

Conclusion.—Maintaining high activity levels through young adulthood may lessen weight gain as young adults transition to middle age, particularly in women.

▶ In this 20-year study, only 1 in 8 subjects managed to maintain high levels of physical activity. Their reward was gaining less weight as they transitioned from young adulthood into middle age. High physical activity levels, however, were not sufficient to entirely prevent age-related weight gain. At all activity levels, men and women experienced gains in weight (Fig 1 in the original article). The authors caution that "some age-related weight gain may be unavoidable in our society" and that even vigorously active runners gain weight through middle age.[1] This study also determined that 30 minutes or more of daily physical activity was needed to slow down age-related weight gain. Although not calculated, keeping the body mass index below 25 as one gets older may require 60 minutes or more of daily physical activity with a tight rein on energy intake and uncommon motivation.[2]

D. C. Nieman, DrPH

References

1. Williams PT, Wood PD. The effects of changing exercise levels on weight and age-related weight gain. *Int J Obes (Lond)*. 2006;30:543-551.
2. Di Pietro L, Dziura J, Blair SN. Estimated change in physical activity level (PAL) and prediction of 5-year weight change in men: the Aerobics Center Longitudinal Study. *Int J Obes Relat Metab Disord*. 2004;28:1541-1547.

Effects of mechanical massage, manual lymphatic drainage and connective tissue manipulation techniques on fat mass in women with cellulite
Bayrakci Tunay V, Akbayrak T, Bakar Y, et al (Hacettepe Univ, Ankara, Turkey; Abant Izzet Baysal Univ, Bolu, Turkey)
J Eur Acad Dermatol Venereol 24:138-142, 2010

Objective.—To evaluate and compare the effectiveness of three different noninvasive treatment techniques on fat mass and regional fat thickness of the patients with cellulites.

Methods.—Sixty subjects were randomized into three groups. Group 1 ($n = 20$) treated with mechanical massage (MM), group 2 ($n = 20$) treated with manual lymphatic drainage (MLD) and group 3 ($n = 20$) treated with connective tissue manipulation (CTM) techniques. Subjects were evaluated by using standardized photographs, body composition analyzer (TBF 300) (body weight (BW), body mass index (BMI), fat %, fat mass (FM), fat free mass (FFM), total body water (TBW)), circumference measurement from thigh, waist-hip ratio (WHR), fat thickness measurements from abdomen, suprailium and thigh regions with skin fold caliper.

Results.—All groups had an improvement in thinning of the subcutaneous fat after the treatment ($P < 0.05$). Thigh circumference decreased by an average of 0.5 cm in all groups and thigh fat thickness decreased 1.66 mm in Group 1, 2.21 mm in Group 2 and 3.03 mm in Group 3. Abdomen and suprailium fat thicknesses decreased 2.4 and 2.58 mm in Group 1, 1.78 and 2 mm in Group 2 and 1.23 and 0.64 mm in Group 3, respectively. The mean difference in waist-hip ratio was 0.1 cm in all groups.

Conclusion.—All the treatment techniques are effective in decreasing the regional fat values of the patients with cellulites.

▶ This randomized clinical trial compared 3 noninvasive treatment techniques to reduce cellulite in women. The 3 techniques are described as manual massage, which used electric stimulation and manual massage (3 sessions per week for 5 weeks), manual lymphatic drainage and wearing of pressured varicose vein stockings between sessions (4 times a week for 5 weeks), and connective tissue manipulation (4 times a week for 5 weeks). All groups had reduction of subcutaneous fat after treatment. There are several important limitations to this study. There are multiple measures used in the study, and multiple testing may be a problem. Also, it is unclear whether the evaluators were blinded as to patient group. Also, there was no control group. Finally, there is no discussion of clinical significance because reduction in fat thickness is quite small. However, besides objective measures of fat thickness, the authors also asked the patients to assess any change in body contour based on before and after photographs. The results indicated that 25% to 30% of body contour improved. Thus, although there are clear limitations to this study, the authors do include a measure of patient self-assessment of improvement, which may be the most appropriate measure in this case because it relates to body image.

D. E. Feldman, PT, PhD

Short-Term Recovery from Prolonged Exercise: Exploring the Potential for Protein Ingestion to Accentuate the Benefits of Carbohydrate Supplements
Betts JA, Williams C (Univ of Bath, UK; Loughborough Univ, Leicestershire, UK)
Sports Med 40:941-959, 2010

This review considers aspects of the optimal nutritional strategy for recovery from prolonged moderate to high intensity exercise. Dietary carbohydrate represents a central component of post-exercise nutrition. Therefore, carbohydrate should be ingested as early as possible in the post-exercise period and at frequent (i.e. 15- to 30-minute) intervals throughout recovery to maximize the rate of muscle glycogen resynthesis. Solid and liquid carbohydrate supplements or whole foods can achieve this aim with equal effect but should be of high glycaemic index and ingested following the feeding schedule described above at a rate of at least 1 g/kg/h in order to rapidly and sufficiently increase both blood glucose and insulin concentrations throughout recovery. Adding ≥ 0.3 g/kg/h of protein to a carbohydrate supplement results in a synergistic increase in insulin secretion that can, in some circumstances, accelerate muscle glycogen resynthesis. Specifically, if carbohydrate has not been ingested in quantities sufficient to maximize the rate of muscle glycogen resynthesis, the inclusion of protein may at least partially compensate for the limited availability of ingested carbohydrate. Some studies have reported improved physical performance with ingestion of carbohydrate-protein mixtures, both during exercise and during recovery prior to a subsequent exercise test. While not all of the evidence supports these ergogenic benefits, there is clearly the potential for improved performance under certain conditions, e.g. if the additional protein increases the energy content of a supplement and or the carbohydrate fraction is ingested at below the recommended rate. The underlying mechanism for such effects may be partly

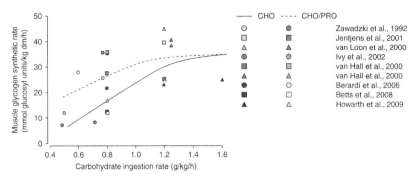

FIGURE 2.—Reported rates of muscle glycogen resynthesis across nine studies that have measured muscle glycogen concentrations over >2−6 hours post-exercise with varied carbohydrate (CHO) ingestion rates either with or without protein (PRO).[8,9,17,20,33-35,39,75] Any published studies that have not matched for either carbohydrate or available energy or did not measure absolute glycogen concentrations have been excluded.[71,83,84] The apparent difference between treatments in the study by Jentjens et al.[20] is a product of large inter-individual variation during the exercise-induced component of glycogen resynthesis and is not statistically significant. **dm** = dry mass. *Editor's Note:* Please refer to original journal article for full references. (Reprinted from Betts JA, Williams C. Short-term recovery from prolonged exercise: exploring the potential for protein ingestion to accentuate the benefits of carbohydrate supplements. *Sports Med.* 2010;40:941-959.)

due to increased muscle glycogen resynthesis during recovery, although there is varied support for other factors such as an increased central drive to exercise, a blunting of exercise-induced muscle damage, altered metabolism during exercise subsequent to recovery, or a combination of these mechanisms (Fig 2).

▶ The rapid restoration of intramuscular and hepatic glycogen stores is plainly important to many classes of athletes. The concept of speeding the recovery process and thus enhancing performance[1] by adding protein to ingested carbohydrate thus has some interest (although one suspects that outside the laboratory, the competitor will eat a diet containing protein and carbohydrate). Perhaps more important is which components of protein are likely to enhance an insulinotropic response and thus favor glycogen storage. This review article cites 18 articles that report increased insulin levels with ingestion of 0.3 to 0.5 g/kg of protein each hour; it also underlines the work of van Loon and associates,[2] indicating that the primary amino acids involved in this process are leucine, phenylalanine, and tyrosine. Hydrolyzed whey may be an even more effective stimulus to glycogen resynthesis.[3] Unfortunately, for those who may be seeking a new dietary breakthrough, it seems that the benefits of added protein or amino acids are most obvious when the individual is taking less than the optimum amount of carbohydrate during the recovery period (Fig 2).

R. J. Shephard, MD (Lond), PhD, DPE

References

1. Williams MB, Raven PB, Fogt DL, Ivy JL. Effects of recovery beverages on glycogen restoration and endurance exercise performance. *J Strength Cond Res.* 2003;17:12-19.

2. van Loon LJ, Saris WH, Verhagen H, Wagenmakers AJ. Plasma insulin responses after ingestion of different amino acid or protein mixtures with carbohydrate. *Am J Clin Nutr.* 2000;72:96-105.

3. Morifuji M, Kanda A, Koga J, et al. Post-exercise carbohydrate plus whey protein hydrolysates supplementation increases skeletal muscle glycogen level in rats. *Amino Acids.* 2010;38:1109-1115.

Caffeinated chewing gum increases repeated sprint performance and augments increases in testosterone in competitive cyclists

Paton CD, Lowe T, Irvine A (Eastern Inst of Technology, Napier, New Zealand; Bay of Plenty Polytechnic, Tauranga, New Zealand; Waikato Inst of Technology, Hamilton, New Zealand)

Eur J Appl Physiol 110:1243-1250, 2010

This investigation reports the effects of caffeinated chewing gum on fatigue and hormone response during repeated sprint performance with competitive cyclists. Nine male cyclists (mean ± SD, age 24 ± 7 years, VO_{2max} 62.5 ± 5.4 mL kg^{-1} min^{-1}) completed four high-intensity experimental sessions, consisting of four sets of 30 s sprints (5 sprints each set). Caffeine (240 mg) or placebo was administered via chewing gum following the second set of each experimental session. Testosterone and cortisol concentrations were assayed in saliva samples collected at rest and after each set of sprints. Mean power output in the first 10 sprints relative to the last 10 sprints declined by 5.8 ± 4.0% in the placebo and 0.4 ± 7.7% in the caffeine trials, respectively. The reduced fatigue in the caffeine trials equated to a 5.4% (90% confidence limit ± 3.6%, effect size 0.25; ±0.16) performance enhancement in favour of caffeine. Salivary testosterone increased rapidly from rest (~53%) and prior to treatments in all trials. Following caffeine treatment, testosterone increased by a further 12 ± 14% (ES 0.50; ± 0.56) relative to the placebo condition. In contrast, cortisol concentrations were not elevated until after the third exercise set; following the caffeine treatment cortisol was reduced by 21 ± 31% (ES −0.30; ± 0.34) relative to placebo. The acute ingestion of caffeine via chewing gum attenuated fatigue during repeated, high-intensity sprint exercise in competitive cyclists. Furthermore, the delayed fatigue was associated with substantially elevated testosterone concentrations and decreased cortisol in the caffeine trials.

▶ Caffeine is one of the few ergogenic aids that is both effective and legally permitted, and it is widely used by competitive cyclists. One of the advantages claimed for ingestion by chewing gum rather than standard beverages is that the rate of absorption is increased, although bioavailability does not seem to be altered. Absorption is in the blood stream directly, bypassing hepatic metabolism and avoiding possible gastric distress.[1] In this small study, caffeinated gum (dose of 240 mg) was compared with a placebo (but unfortunately not with a caffeinated beverage). The caffeine was effective in reducing fatigue;

peak power output increased by 5.5% (Fig 2 in the original article), enough to influence competitive success[2]; testosterone levels were higher; and there was a smaller decrease in cortisol concentrations. The biochemical basis of the enhanced performance in short sprints remains to be clarified[3,4]; possible factors include greater arousal and increased central drive, and the higher levels of testosterone may also help muscle anabolism.

R. J. Shephard, MD (Lond), PhD, DPE

References

1. Kamimori GH, Karyekar CS, Otterstetter R, et al. The rate of absorption and relative bioavailability of caffeine administered in chewing gum versus capsules to normal healthy volunteers. *Int J Pharm.* 2002;234:159-167.
2. Paton CD, Hopkins WG. Variation in performance of elite cyclists from race to race. *Eur J Sport Sci.* 2006;6:25-31.
3. Graham TE. Caffeine and exercise: metabolism, endurance and performance. *Sports Med.* 2001;31:785-807.
4. Davis JK, Green JM. Caffeine and anaerobic performance: ergogenic value and mechanisms of action. *Sports Med.* 2009;39:813-832.

Ginger (*Zingiber officinale*) Reduces Muscle Pain Caused by Eccentric Exercise

Black CD, Herring MP, Hurley DJ, et al (Georgia College and State Univ, Milledgeville; Univ of Georgia, Athens)
J Pain 11:894-903, 2010

Ginger has been shown to exert anti-inflammatory effects in rodents, but its effect on human muscle pain is uncertain. Heat treatment of ginger has been suggested to enhance its hypoalgesic effects. The purpose of this study was to examine the effects of 11 days of raw (study 1) and heat-treated (study 2) ginger supplementation on muscle pain. Study 1 and 2 were identical double-blind, placebo controlled, randomized experiments with 34 and 40 volunteers, respectively. Participants consumed 2 grams of either raw (study 1) or heated (study 2) ginger or placebo for 11 consecutive days. Participants performed 18 eccentric actions of the elbow flexors to induce pain and inflammation. Pain intensity, perceived effort, plasma prostaglandin E_2, arm volume, range-of-motion and isometric strength were assessed prior to and for 3 days after exercise. Results Raw (25%, $-.78$ SD, $P = .041$) and heat-treated (23%, $-.57$ SD, $P = .049$) ginger resulted in similar pain reductions 24 hours after eccentric exercise compared to placebo. Smaller effects were noted between both types of ginger and placebo on other measures. Daily supplementation with ginger reduced muscle pain caused by eccentric exercise, and this effect was not enhanced by heat treating the ginger.

Perspective.—This study demonstrates that daily consumption of raw and heat-treated ginger resulted in moderate-to-large reductions in muscle pain following exercise-induced muscle injury. Our findings agree with those showing hypoalgesic effects of ginger in osteoarthritis patients and further demonstrate ginger's effectiveness as a pain reliever (Fig 2).

▶ Unlike many forms of alternative medicine, there seems to be some theoretical basis for the use of ginger in the treatment of muscle pain, although most of the relevant articles have appeared in other-than-mainstream scientific journals. Reports have noted an ability of ginger preparations to block the activity of cyclooxygenases[1-3] and to inhibit the production of proinflammatory cytokines.[4,5] Tests in rats have also suggested a reduction in paw edema and a decrease in behavior suggestive of pain.[6,7] At first inspection, this study seems well designed, with a randomized double-blinded protocol. Treatment with either raw or cooked ginger (2 g/day for 11 days) led to a substantial reduction in reported symptoms following eccentric exercise of the elbow flexor

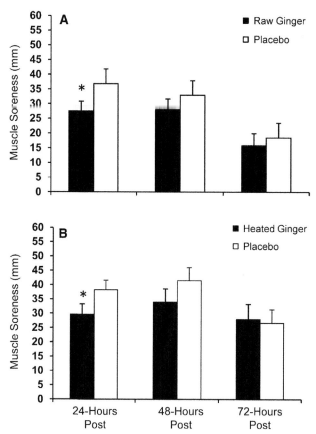

FIGURE 2.—Ratings of arm muscle pain intensity 24, 48, and 72 hours after eccentric exercise. Preexercise muscle pain was "0" on a 0 to 100 VAS scale and is therefore not included. *Indicates a significant ($P < .05$) difference from placebo. Values are mean ± SE. (Reprinted from Black CD, Herring MP, Hurley DJ, et al. Ginger (*Zingiber officinale*) reduces muscle pain caused by eccentric exercise. *J Pain.* 2010;11:894-903.)

muscles (Fig 2). However, this result must be accepted with caution because objective data such as limb swelling, range of motion, and prostaglandin E2 concentrations were unaffected by treatment. Moreover, although specific precautions were taken to maintain blinding as to treatment, this is difficult to achieve with a strongly flavored and easily recognized substance such as ginger. In fact, debriefing revealed that most subjects were aware whether they had been in the experimental group (an important point to check in any supposedly double-blinded trial). It may be worth repeating the experiment with even more stringent blinding precautions, but at present, it seems likely that the difference in reported symptoms was a placebo response.

R. J. Shephard, MD (Lond), PhD, DPE

References

1. Lantz RC, Chen GJ, Sarihan M, Solyom AM, Jolad SD, Timmermann BN. The effect of extracts from ginger rhizome on inflammatory mediator production. *Phytomedicine.* 2007;14:123-128.
2. Nurtjahja-Tjendraputra E, Ammit AJ, Roufogalis BD, Tran VH, Duke CC. Effective anti-platelet and COX-1 enzyme inhibitors from pungent constituents of ginger. *Thromb Res.* 2003;111:259-265.
3. Tjendraputra E, Tran VH, Liu-Brennan D, Roufogalis BD, Duke CC. Effect of ginger constituents and synthetic analogues on cyclooxygenase-2 enzyme in intact cells. *Bioorg Chem.* 2001;29:156-163.
4. Tripathi S, Bruch D, Kittur DS. Ginger extract inhibits LPS induced macrophage activation and function. *BMC Complement Altern Med.* 2008;8:1.
5. Grzanna R, Phan P, Polotsky A, Lindmark L, Frondoza CG. Ginger extract inhibits beta-amyloid peptide-induced cytokine and chemokine expression in cultured THP-1 monocytes. *J Altern Complement Med.* 2004;10:1009-1013.
6. Ojewole JA. Analgesic, antiinflammatory and hypoglycaemic effects of ethanol extract of Zingiber officinale (Roscoe) rhizomes (Zingiberaceae) in mice and rats. *Phytother Res.* 2006;20:764-772.
7. Young HY, Luo YL, Cheng HY, Hsieh WC, Liao JC, Peng WH. Analgesic and anti-inflammatory activities of [6]-gingerol. *J Ethnopharmacol.* 2005;96:207-210.

High Prevalence of Vitamin D Insufficiency in Athletes and Dancers
Constantini NW, Arieli R, Chodick G, et al (Hadassah-Hebrew Univ Med Ctr, Jerusalem, Israel; Tel Aviv Univ, Israel; et al)
Clin J Sport Med 20:368-371, 2010

Objective.—Vitamin D insufficiency is prevalent in various populations worldwide but with scarce data on physically active individuals. Vitamin D is important to athletes, affecting bone mass, immunity, and physical performance. This study evaluated the prevalence of vitamin D insufficiency and deficiency among young athletes and dancers.

Design.—Cross-sectional study.

Setting.—Sport medicine clinic.

Patients.—Data on 98 athletes and dancers (age, 14.7 ± 3.0 years; range, 10-30 years; 53% men), who had undergone screening medical evaluations, were extracted from medical records.

Independent Variable.—Serum 25(OH)D concentrations.

Main Outcome Measures.—Serum 25(OH)D concentrations, age, sex, sport discipline, month of blood test, and serum ferritin. Vitamin D insufficiency was defined as serum 25(OH)D concentration <30 ng/mL.

Results.—Mean serum 25(OH)D concentration was 25.3 ± 8.3 ng/mL. Seventy-three percent of participants were vitamin D insufficient. Prevalence of vitamin D insufficiency was higher among dancers (94%), basketball players (94%), and Tae Kwon Do fighters (67%) and among athletes from indoor versus outdoor sports (80% vs 48%; $P = 0.002$). 25(OH)D levels adjusted for age and sex correlated with serum ferritin and season.

Conclusions.—In this study, conducted among young athletes and dancers from various disciplines in a sunny country, a high prevalence of vitamin D insufficiency was identified. A higher rate of vitamin D insufficiency was found among participants who practice indoors, during the winter months, and in the presence of iron depletion. Given the importance of vitamin D to athletes for several reasons, we suggest that athletes and dancers be screened for vitamin D insufficiency and treated as needed (Table 1).

▶ It is possible to construct athletic facilities with good natural lighting. I have pleasant memories of a leisurely prebreakfast swim at the Swiss National Athletic Center in Mägglingen, with my spirits lifted by a glorious view over the distant snow-capped Alps. But too often, like the athletic building that I inherited at the University of Toronto, the structure dedicated to the enhancement of physical health seems totally devoid of windows. It is thus not surprising that athletes who spend much of their time training within such desirable facilities show serum vitamin D levels that fall far below the commonly accepted desirable level of 30 ng per mL (Table 1). This deficit carries adverse consequences for many aspects of health, increasing the risks of osteoporosis, cancer, heart disease, autoimmune disorders, and premature all-cause mortality.[1-4] It is also associated with some impairment of athletic performance[5,6] and an increased risk of upper respiratory infections. Particularly in northern climates, the situation during the winter months is compounded by relatively short hours of daylight.[7] The study of Constantini and associates was conducted in Israel, where sunshine is plentiful through most of the year; nevertheless, there remained

TABLE 1.—Clinical Data and Iron Status in Athletes Across Serum 25(OH)D Groups

	<15 ng/mL	15-19.9 ng/mL	20-29.9 ng/mL	≥30 ng/mL	P
		Vitamin D Group			
n	6	19	47	26	
Males, n (%)	3 (50)	8 (42)	24 (51)	17 (65)	0.47
Age, y	15.9 ± 7.1	14.6 ± 2.7	14.6 ± 2.8	14.6 ± 2.3	0.785
Sample taken in winter, n (%)*	5 (83)	15 (79)	26 (55)	7 (27)	0.002
Ferritin, ng/mL	16.5 ± 3.7	21.4 ± 10.9	25.4 ± 17.5	35.1 ± 19.0	0.014
Iron depletion, n (%)	5 (83)	10 (53)	18 (42)	4 (16)	0.006

Values are n (%) or mean ± SD as appropriate.
*November to April.

a statistically significant seasonal difference in vitamin D levels (Table 1). The subjects were a mixed population of young adults; about half of the participants in outdoor sports had less than desirable levels of vitamin D, but the problem was much more prevalent among those who exercised indoors, becoming almost universal in gymnasts and basketball players. A poor overall diet may have contributed to the vitamin deficiency seen in the gymnasts. Unfortunately, their data are not presented separately, and the number of gymnasts is not specified. However, there is a clear association between a low vitamin D level and a low serum ferritin (Table 1). Deliberate restriction of food intake seems a less likely factor contributing to the prevalence of vitamin D deficiency among the basketball players. The practical lessons for the sports physician are 2-fold: first, both exercise and training should be undertaken outdoors where possible and second, if competitors must spend long hours training indoors, then their vitamin D levels should be checked and vitamin supplements provided as required.

R. J. Shephard, MD (Lond), PhD, DPE

References

1. Hintzpeter B, Mensink GB, Thiefelder W, Müller MJ, Scheidt-Nave C. Vitamin D status and health correlates among German adults. *Eur J Clin Nutr.* 2008;62: 1079-1089.
2. Holick MF, Chen TC. Vitamin D deficiency: a worldwide problem with health consequences. *Am J Clin Nutr.* 2008;87:1080S-1086S.
3. Lee JH, O'Keefe JH, Bell D, Hensrud DD, Holick MF. Vitamin D deficiency an important, common, and easily treatable cardiovascular risk factor? *J Am Coll Cardiol.* 2008;52:1949-1956.
4. Melamed ML, Michos ED, Post W, Astor B. 25-hydroxyvitamin D levels and the risk of mortality in the general population. *Arch Intern Med.* 2008;168: 1629-1637.
5. Ward KA, Das G, Berry JL, et al. Vitamin D status and muscle function in post-menarchal adolescent girls. *J Clin Endocrinol Metab.* 2009;94:559-563.
6. Cannell JJ, Hollis BW, Sorenson MB, Taft TN, Anderson JJ. Athletic performance and Vitamin D. *Med Sci Sports Exerc.* 2009;41:1102-1110.
7. Holick MF. Vitamin D deficiency. *N Engl J Med.* 2007;357:266-281.

Dietary and Physical Activity Patterns in Children with Obstructive Sleep Apnea
Spruyt K, Capdevila OS, Serpero LD, et al (Univ of Louisville, KY)
J Pediatr 156:724-730, 2010

Objective.—To assess dietary and physical activity patterns and morning circulating blood levels of the orexigenic hormones ghrelin and visfatin in children with either obesity, obstructive sleep apnea (OSA), or both conditions.

Study Design.—In this cross-sectional design, 5- to 9-year-old participants (n = 245) from the community were identified. After overnight polysomnography, caregivers filled out a food and physical activity questionnaire, and the child underwent a fasting blood draw for ghrelin and visfatin plasma levels.

TABLE 1.—Demographic Characteristics in 245 Children and their Parents

	OSA(−)		OSA(+)		Test Statistic	P Value	Scheffé Post Hoc
	OSA(−)OB(−) (1)	OSA(−)OB(+) (2)	OSA(+)OB(−) (3)	OSA(+)OB(+) (4)			
Sex (%,female:male)	34.4/ 38.0		4.1/ 6.1	7.3/ 10.2	$\chi^2(2) = 0.803$	.669	
Ethnicity* (%)	46.1/ 22.0/ 4.1		4.9/ 4.1/ 1.2	11.4/ 5.3/ 0.8	$\chi^2(4) = 3.219$	.552	
Age (years)	6.9 ± 0.6 (6.8-7.0)		6.7 ± 0.6 (6.4-7.0)	6.9 ± 0.66 (6.7-7.1)	F(2, 242) = 1.1	.327	
BMI	15.9 ± 1.23 (15.2-16.5)	19.9 ± 3.6 (19.4-20.6)	15.5 ± 0.8 (15.2-15.9)	21.6 ± 5.1 (20.1-23.2)	F(3, 241) = 52.4	.000	(1) vs (2); (1) vs (4); (2) vs (4): $P = .04$; (2) vs (3); (3) vs (4)
Parental characteristics (%)							
Father's schooling†	5.5/ 36.3/ 25.4/ 9		0.5/ 3.5/ 2/ 2.5	1.5/ 7.5/ 3.5/ 3	$\chi^2(6) = 5.6$	.466	
Mother's schooling†	2.7/ 39/ 23.3/ 9		0/ 4.9/ 2.7/ 1.3	0.9/ 9/ 5.4/ 1.8	$\chi^2(6) = 1.3$	.974	
Father smoking (yes)	28.8		3.4	3.4	$\chi^2(2) = 4.0$	.135	
Mother smoking (yes)	24.3		1.4	4.1	$\chi^2(2) = 3.1$	.208	
Father snore (yes)	62.4		6.9	13.9	$\chi^2(2) = 1.1$	.486	
Mother snore (yes)	38.7		2.8	10.1	$\chi^2(2) = 4.4$	.113	

Data are shown as mean ± SD with (95% CI).
*White non-Hispanic/ African-American/ Other.
†Junior high school/ high school/ college/ graduate.

Results.—Compared with control subjects, obese children with OSA ate 2.2-times more fast food, ate less healthy food such as fruits and vege-tables, and were 4.2-times less frequently involved in organized sports. OSA was positively correlated with plasma ghrelin levels (R^2, 0.73; $P < .0001$), but not visfatin levels, particularly when obesity was present.

Conclusion.—OSA and obesity in children may adversely impact dietary preferences and may be particularly detrimental to daily physical activity patterns. Furthermore, increased ghrelin levels support the presence of increased appetite and caloric intake in obese patients with OSA, which in turn may further promote the severity of the underlying conditions (Table 1).

▶ The abstract to this cross-sectional study appears to infer causation, which is not appropriate. Moreover, it is not necessarily the combination of obesity and sleep apnea that causes problems, since the level of obesity in itself is much greater in those children with sleep apnea (Table 1).[1,2] Nevertheless, any com-pounding of the effects of obesity by obstructive sleep apnea is an issue that merits further study. Logical bases for such an association might include the eating of fast foods as a reaction to stress and disturbed sleep.[3,4] The very low physical activity levels observed in this particular population are a continuing challenge to sports physicians.

R. J. Shephard, MD (Lond), PhD, DPE

References

1. Lutter M, Sakata I, Osborne-Lawrence S, et al. The orexigenic hormone ghrelin defends against depressive symptoms of chronic stress. *Nat Neurosci.* 2008;11: 752-753.
2. Nguyen-Rodriguez STCC, Chou CP, Unger JB, Spruijt-Metz D. BMI as a moderator of perceived stress and emotional eating in adolescents. *Eat Behav.* 2008;9:238-246.
3. Zheng H, Berthoud HR. Neural systems controlling the drive to eat: mind versus metabolism. *Physiology (Bethesda).* 2008;23:75-83.
4. Gozal D. Sleep-disordered breathing and school performance in children. *Pediatrics.* 1998;102:616-620.

Exercise and Glycemic Imbalances: A Situation-Specific Estimate of Glucose Supplement

Francescato MP, Geat M, Accardo A, et al (Univ of Udine, Italy; Univ of Trieste, Italy; et al)
Med Sci Sports Exerc 43:2-11, 2011

Purpose.—The purposes of this study were to describe a newly devel-oped algorithm that estimates the glucose supplement on a patient- and situation-specific basis and to test whether these amounts would be appro-priate for maintaining blood glucose levels within the recommended range in exercising type 1 diabetic patients.

Methods.—The algorithm first estimates the overall amount of glucose oxidized during exercise on the basis of the patient's physical fitness, exer-cise intensity, and duration. The amount of supplemental CHO to be consumed before or during the effort represents a fraction of the burned quantity depending on the patient's usual therapy and insulin sensitivity and on the time of day the exercise is performed. The algorithm was tested in 27 patients by comparing the estimated amounts of supplemental CHO with the actual amounts required to complete 1-h constant-intensity walks. Each patient performed three trials, each of which started at different time intervals after insulin injection (81 walks were performed overall). Glycemia was tested every 15 min.

Results.—In 70.4% of the walks, independent of the time of day, the amount of CHO estimated by the algorithm would be adequate to allow the patients to complete the exercise with a glucose level within the selected thresholds (i.e., 3.9–10 mmol·L^{-1}).

Conclusions.—The algorithm provided a satisfactory estimate of the CHO needed to complete the exercises. Although the performance of the algorithm still requires testing for different exercise intensities, durations, and modalities, the results indicate its potential usefulness as a tool for preventing immediate exercise-induced glycemic imbalances (i.e., during exercise) in type 1 diabetic patients, in particular for spontaneous physical activities not planned in advance, thus allowing all insulin-dependent patients to safely enjoy the benefits of exercise.

▶ Exercise is strongly recommended for patients with type I diabetes mellitus, in part because of their high risk of cardiovascular disease[1-3] and in part because of the positive effects of exercise on self-esteem and overall quality of life.[4] However, it remains a challenge for diabetic patients to maintain normoglycemia in the face of the increased uptake of blood glucose seen during exercise and particularly during the recovery period, and such problems can have a strong negative effect on motivation to exercise for some patients with type I diabetes.[5] The study of Francescato et al represents an attempt to develop an individualized algorithm (Fig 1 in the original article) that will help to adjust carbohydrate intake to keep the blood sugar level within a broadly acceptable range (3.9-10.0 mmol/L) during and following exercise. Their approach was evaluated on 27 middle-aged adults (aged an average of 44 years), who had been diagnosed with diabetes an average of 22 years previously. Only one form of exercise was evaluated (60 minutes of treadmill walking at 65% of maximal heart rate, commencing 90-270 minutes after lunch). However, even with this standardization of effort, the algorithm failed to keep patients within the desired range in 30% of instances. Plainly, there remains a need for further research, including comparisons with other approaches to the avoidance of hypoglycemia. At the present time, patients who are receiving guidance from this algorithm must continue to watch for hypoglycemia following a bout of exercise.

R. J. Shephard, MD (Lond), PhD, DPE

References

1. Haider DG, Pleiner J, Francesconi M, Wiesinger GF, Müller M, Wolzt M. Exercise training lowers plasma visfatin concentrations in patients with type 1 diabetes. *J Clin Endocrinol Metab.* 2006;91:4702-4704.

2. Laaksonen DE, Atalay M, Niskanen LK, et al. Aerobic exercise and the lipid profile in type 1 diabetic men: a randomized controlled trial. *Med Sci Sports Exerc.* 2000;32:1541-1548.
3. Lehmann R, Kaplan V, Bingisser R, Bloch K, Spinas G. Impact of physical activity on cardiovascular risk factors in IDDM. *Diabetes Care.* 1997;20:1603-1611.
4. Steppel JH, Horton ES. Exercise in the management of type 1 diabetes mellitus. *Rev Endocr Metab Disord.* 2003;4:355-360.
5. Brazeau AS, Rabasa-Lhoret R, Strychar I, Mircescu H. Barriers to physical activity among patients with type 1 diabetes. *Diabetes Care.* 2008;31:2108-2109.

Effect of n-3 Fatty Acids and Antioxidants on Oxidative Stress after Exercise

McAnulty SR, Nieman DC, Fox-Rabinovich M, et al (Appalachian State Univ, Boone, NC)
Med Sci Sports Exerc 42:1704-1711, 2010

Purpose.—n-3 fatty acids are known to exert multiple beneficial effects including anti-inflammatory actions that may diminish oxidative stress. Supplementation with antioxidant vitamins has been proposed to counteract oxidative stress and improve antioxidant status. Therefore, this project investigated the effects of daily supplementation in 48 trained cyclists over 6 wk and during 3 d of continuous exercise on F_2-isoprostanes (oxidative stress), plasma n-3 fatty acids, and antioxidant status (oxygen radical absorption capacity and ferric-reducing antioxidant potential).

Methods.—Cyclists were randomized into n-3 fatty acids (N3) ($n = 11$) (2000 mg of eicosapentaenoic acid and 400 mg of docosahexaenoic acid), a vitamin—mineral (VM) complex ($n = 12$) emphasizing vitamins C (2000 mg), E (800 IU), A (3000 IU), and selenium (200 μg), a VM and n-3 fatty acid combination (VN3) ($n = 13$), or placebo (P) ($n = 12$). Blood was collected at baseline and preexercise and postexercise. A 4×3 repeated-measures ANOVA was performed to test main effects.

Results.—After exercise, F_2-isoprostanes were higher in N3 (treatment effect $P = 0.014$). Eicosapentaenoic acid and docosahexaenoic acid plasma values were higher after supplementation (interaction effect $P = 0.001$ and 0.006, respectively) in both n-3 supplemented groups. Oxygen radical absorption capacity declined similarly among all groups after exercise. Ferric-reducing antioxidant potential exhibited significant interaction ($P = 0.045$) and significantly increased after exercise in VN3 and VM ($P < 0.01$).

Conclusions.—This study indicates that supplementation with n-3 fatty acids alone significantly increases F_2-isoprostanes after exhaustive exercise. Lastly, antioxidant supplementation augments plasma antioxidant status and modestly attenuates but does not prevent the significant n-3 fatty acid associated increase in F_2-isoprostanes postexercise (Fig 3).

▶ The optimum diet is probably based on the ingestion of reasonable and well-balanced amount of the natural foods to which humankind has adapted over

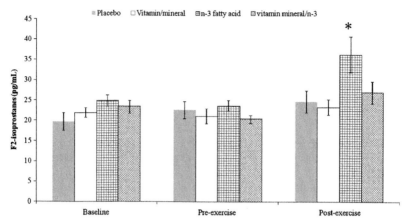

FIGURE 3.—F_2-isoprostane values over time among four treatments. Treatment effect ($P = 0.014$), time effect ($P = 0.002$), and treatment × time interaction ($P = 0.224$). *$P \leq 0.0125$ after Bonferroni correction versus placebo value at baseline ($n = 12$). Values are presented as mean ± SEM. (Reprinted from McAnulty SR, Nieman DC, Fox-Rabinovich M, et al. Effect of n-3 fatty acids and antioxidants on oxidative stress after exercise. *Med Sci Sports Exerc.* 2010;42:1704-1711.)

many millennia. However, in recent years, people have ingested a wide range of supplements in the hope of either prolonging their longevity or enhancing their physical performance. Omega-3 fatty acids, a prominent component of the Inuit diet,[1] have become a popular purchase. In sedentary or moderately active individuals, it is argued that such supplements counter the excessive proportion of omega-6 fatty acids in the modern diet, with a reduction of inflammatory, arrhythmic, thrombotic, and hyperlipemic tendencies.[2] Against these postulated advantages, there have also been fears that the administration of omega-3 fatty acids may increase lipid peroxidation,[3] particularly during heavy exercise. This randomized controlled trial was conducted in young and well-trained cyclists (average training volume more than 200 km per week). The experimental group received a substantial dose of omega-3 fatty acids (2000 mg of eicosapentaenoic acid and 400 mg of docosahexaenoic acid) for a period of 6 weeks. They performed exhausting exercises, cycling for 3 hours on 3 successive days at 57% of their maximal power output. The data confirm that following exercise, the experimental group showed a substantial increase in the traditional marker of oxidative stress (F_2-isoprostanes) (Fig 3). Moreover, this adverse outcome was only partially reversed by the simultaneous ingestion of large doses of antioxidants. Plainly, caution is thus needed when recommending omega-3 supplements to those who are proposing to engage in very heavy exercise. Further studies are also needed in those members of the general population who are most likely to use omega-3 supplements (the elderly and those with atherosclerotic heart disease).

R. J. Shephard, MD (Lond), PhD, DPE

References

1. Shephard RJ, Rode A. *The Health Consequences of "Modernization": Evidence from Circumpolar Peoples.* London: Cambridge University Press; 1996.

2. Simopoulos AP. The importance of the ratio of omega-6/omega-3 essential fatty acids. *Biomed Pharmacother.* 2002;56:365-379.
3. Mori TA. Effect of fish and fish oil-derived omega-3 fatty acids on lipid oxidation. *Redox Rep.* 2004;9:193-197.

Effect of purple sweet potato leaves consumption on exercise-induced oxidative stress and IL-6 and HSP72 levels
Chang W-H, Hu S-P, Huang Y-F, et al (Taipei Med Univ, Taiwan)
J Appl Physiol 109:1710-1715, 2010

The aim of this study was to evaluate the effects of purple sweet potato leaves (PSPL) consumption on oxidative stress markers in a healthy, nontrained, young male population after completing a running exercise protocol. A crossover design was applied, with 15 subjects participating in a two-step dietary intervention period. Each subject was given a high-(PSPL group) or low-polyphenol (control group) diet for 7 days with a 14-day washout period. After each dietary intervention period, all subjects performed 1 h of treadmill running at a speed corresponding to 70% of each subject's individual maximal oxygen uptake ($\dot{V}_{O_{2max}}$). Blood samples were taken before exercise and at 0, 1, and 3 h after exercise. Compared with the control group, PSPL consumption significantly increased plasma total poly-phenols concentration and total antioxidant power (i.e., the ferric-reducing ability of plasma) in the PSPL group. The markers of oxidative damage, plasma TBARS and protein carbonyl, significantly decreased. Plasma IL-6 concentration also decreased. However, no significant difference was found in HSP72 levels between the two groups. These findings indicate that consuming a high-polyphenol diet for 7 days can modulate antioxidative status and decrease exercise-induced oxidative damage and pro-inflammatory cytokine secretion.

▶ Flavonoids provide many of the colors in fruits and vegetables, where they serve as defenders against microbes, radiation from the sun, and other insults. Whether flavonoids have beneficial influences in humans is a hot topic among scientists, but there is growing support for multiple health and fitness benefits. Flavonoid-rich plant extracts are being tested by an increasing number of investigative teams as performance aids and countermeasures to exercise-induced inflammation, delayed onset muscle soreness, and oxidative stress.[1] This study provides additional evidence that the consumption of flavonoid-rich foods, extracts, or products for 1 week or longer prior to intense exercise attenuates oxidative stress and inflammation in both trained and untrained individuals.[1] Some question the value of using nutritional supplements as countermeasures to exercise-induced oxidative stress and inflammation because these may interfere with important signaling mechanisms for training adaptations. Another viewpoint is that nutritional supplements attenuate but do not totally block exercise-induced oxidative stress and inflammation, analogous to the beneficial use of ice packs to reduce swelling following mild injuries.[2]

D. C. Nieman, DrPH

References

1. Nieman DC, Stear SJ, Castell LM, Burke LM. A-Z of nutritional supplements: dietary supplements, sports nutrition foods and ergogenic aids for health and performance: part 15. *Br J Sports Med*. 2010;44:1202-1205.
2. Yfanti C, Akerström T, Nielsen S, et al. Antioxidant supplementation does not alter endurance training adaptation. *Med Sci Sports Exerc*. 2010;42:1388-1395.

Transdermal Patch Drug Delivery Interactions with Exercise
Lenz TL, Gillespie N (Creighton Univ, Omaha, NE)
Sports Med 41:177-183, 2011

Transdermal drug delivery systems, such as the transdermal patch, continue to be a popular and convenient way to administer medications. There are currently several medications that use a transdermal patch drug delivery system. This article describes the potential untoward side effects of increased drug absorption through the use of a transdermal patch in individuals who exercise or participate in sporting events. Four studies have been reported that demonstrate a significant increase in the plasma concentration of nitroglycerin when individuals exercise compared with rest. Likewise, several case reports and two studies have been conducted that demonstrate nicotine toxicity and increased plasma nicotine while wearing a nicotine patch in individuals who exercise or participate in sporting events compared with rest. Healthcare providers, trainers and coaches should be aware of proper transdermal patch use, especially while exercising, in order to provide needed information to their respective patients and athletes to avoid potential untoward side effects. Particular caution should be given to individuals who participate in an extreme sporting event of long duration. Further research that includes more medications is needed in this area.

▶ The issue of an exercise-related increase in the absorption of insulin from intramuscular depots is well documented in this article, but it is important to recognize that when a person is exercising under warm conditions, the skin blood flow is also increased manyfold and there can be a similar type of increase in the rate of absorption of medications from dermal patches. The review article of Lenz and Gillespie brings together a number of studies and case reports documenting an increased absorption of both nitroglycerin and nicotine from dermal pads during and immediately following exercise. These are but 2 of many drugs approved for transdermal delivery, and there is a need to examine the potential toxicity of other drugs such as painkillers and hormones. The issue seems important because the instructions provided with the patches in general do not seem to discuss the effects of exercise. Case reports have described nausea, palpitations, severe fatigue, and tremor when nicotine patches were worn in conjunction with a squash game or a karate class; laboratory tests also described statistically significant increases in blood nicotine levels following 20 to 30 minutes of exercise, although under the conditions of the experiment the change was no more than 12%, not much more than the effect of smoking a single cigarette. The effect would probably be more serious following a marathon or ultramarathon event, and coaches should warn former smokers of this problem.

R. J. Shephard, MD (Lond), PhD, DPE

Effects of High Intensity Exercise on Isoelectric Profiles and SDS-PAGE Mobility of Erythropoietin
Voss S, Lüdke A, Romberg S, et al (German Sport Univ Cologne, Germany)
Int J Sports Med 31:367-371, 2010

Exercise induced proteinuria is a common phenomenon in high performance sports. Based on the appearance of so called "effort urines" in routine doping analysis the purpose of this study was to investigate the influence of exercise induced proteinuria on IEF profiles and SDS-PAGE relative mobility values (rMVs) of endogenous human erythropoietin (EPO). Twenty healthy subjects performed cycle-ergometer exercise until exhaustion. VO_2max, blood lactate, urinary proteins and urinary creatinine were analysed to evaluate the exercise performance and proteinuria. IEF and SDS-PAGE analyses were performed to test for differences in electrophoretic behaviour of the endogenous EPO before and after exercise. All subjects showed increased levels of protein/creatinine ratio after performance ($8.8 \pm 5.2-26.1 \pm 14.4$). IEF analysis demonstrated an elevation of the relative amount of basic band areas ($13.9 \pm 11.3-36.4 \pm 12.6$). Using SDS-PAGE analysis we observed a decrease in rMVs after exercise and no shift in direction of the recombinant human EPO (rhEPO) region ($0.543 \pm 0.013-0.535 \pm 0.012$). Following identification criteria of the World Anti Doping Agency (WADA) all samples were negative. The implementation of the SDS-PAGE method represents a good solution to distinguish between results influenced by so called effort urines and results of rhEPO abuse. Thus this method can be used to confirm adverse analytical findings (Fig 4).

▶ In addition to the evaluation of indirect measures such as hemoglobin concentration and reticulocyte percentages, observers can assess an athlete's abuse of recombinant human erythropoietin (rhEPO) based on the excretion of this substance in urine,[1] using isoelectric focusing (ISF) and double-blotting techniques. There is general agreement that such methodology provides an adequate basis for distinguishing endogenous erythropoietin from rhEPO, both in urine specimens collected at rest and in samples obtained following strenuous exercise. However, beginning in 2008, biosimilar erythropoietins such as epoetin delta made their appearance in pharmacies, and these compounds were much

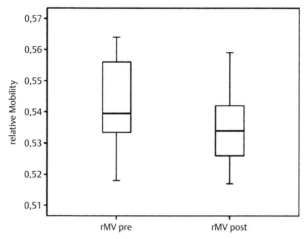

FIGURE 4.—Change in relative mobility values of EPO for all samples before and after high intensive exercise, using SDS-PAGE Analysis (p = 0.001). (Reprinted from Voss S, Lüdke A, Romberg S, et al. Effects of high intensity exercise on isoelectric profiles and SDS-PAGE mobility of erythropoietin. *Int J Sports Med.* 2010;31:367-371.)

less readily distinguished from endogenous erythropoietin, creating public suspicion that some abusers had escaped detection.[2] Sodium dodecyl sulfate polyacrylamide gel electrophoresis (SDS-PAGE) offers an alternative approach to the assay of erythropoietins. SDS causes a dissociation of oligomeric proteins and their binding as subunits to form complexes of constant charge/mass ratio; epoetin delta can be distinguished because it has a lower molecular weight and thus a faster electrophoretic migration rate than its endogenous counterpart.[3] This report demonstrates a narrowing of the distinction between normal and abnormal urine when ISF testing is applied to urine collected after vigorous exercise. With SDS-PAGE analyses, there is a small decrease in relative motility (rMV) in postexercise urine samples (Fig 4), and none of the 20 volunteers had values in excess of 0.558, the World Anti-Doping Agency 99.9% confidence limit for a suspicious sample. SDS-PAGE thus seems another useful tool in the armamentarium of an antidoping laboratory.

R. J. Shephard, MD (Lond), PhD, DPE

References

1. Lasne F, de Ceaurriz J. Recombinant erythropoietin in urine. *Nature.* 2000;8:635.
2. Damsgaard, R. Legalities 'lag behind doping work'. http://news.bbc.co.uk/2/hi/science/nature/7517332.stm. Accessed June 22, 2010.
3. Kohler M, Ayotte C, Desharnais P, et al. Discrimination of recombinant and endogenous urinary erythropoietin by calculating relative mobility values from SDS gels. *Int J Sports Med.* 2008;29:1-6.

Screening for recombinant human erythropoietin using [Hb], reticulocytes, the OFF$_{hr\ score}$, OFF$_{z\ score}$ and Hb$_{z\ score}$: status of the Blood Passport

Bornø A, Aachmann-Andersen NJ, Munch-Andersen T, et al (Copenhagen Muscle Res Centre, Denmark)

Eur J Appl Physiol 109:537-543, 2010

Haemoglobin concentration ([Hb]), reticulocyte percentage (retic%) and OFF$_{hr\ score}$ are well-implemented screening tools to determine potential recombinant human erythropoietin (rHuEpo) abuse in athletes. Recently, the International Cycling Union implemented the OFF$_{z\ score}$ and the Hb$_{z\ score}$ in their anti-doping testing programme. The aim of this study is to evaluate the sensitivity of these indirect screening methods. Twenty-four human subjects divided into three groups with eight subjects each (G1; G2 and G3) were injected with rHuEpo. G1 and G2 received rHuEpo for a 4-week period with 2 weeks of "boosting" followed by 2 weeks of "maintenance" and a wash-out period of 3 weeks. G3 received rHuEpo for a 10-week period (boost = 3 weeks; maintenance = 7 weeks; wash out = 1 week). Three, seven and eight of the 24 volunteers exceeded the cut-off limits for OFF$_{hr\ score}$, [Hb] and retic%, respectively. One subject from G1, nobody from G2, and seven subjects from G3 exceeded the cut-off limit for Hb$_{z\ score}$. In total, ten subjects exceeded the cut-off limit for the OFF$_{z\ score}$; two subjects from G1, two subjects from G2 and six subjects from G3. In total, indirect screening methods were able to indicate rHuEpo injections in 58% of subjects. However, 42% of our rHuEpo-injected subjects were not detected. It should be emphasised that the test frequency in real world anti-doping is far less than the present study, and hence the detection rate will be lower (Table 1).

▶ When screening for any type of doping, contest organizers face 2 opposing challenges: detecting as large a proportion of drug abusers as possible while simultaneously avoiding the embarrassment of excluding athletes through false-positive test results. In the case of blood doping, the regulations of the International Cycling Union (UCI, version 19.01.2009) allow laboratories to make 1 in 1000 false-positive diagnoses. Decisions are based on hemoglobin concentrations and reticulocyte percentages (R%). For the World Anti-Doping Agency, the cut-off limit of hemoglobin is 170 g/L; the UCI also assesses a cyclist to be suspicious of doping if R% is < 0.2% or > 2.4%. Male athletes are banned from competition if the OFF$_{hr\ score}$ ([Hb] (g/L) − 60 $\sqrt{R\%}$) exceeds 1.33. The corresponding z scores are:

$$\mathrm{OFF}_{z\ score} = (\mathrm{OFF}_{current} - \mathrm{OFF}_{mean})/\sqrt{(\sigma^2(1 + 1/n))}$$

$$\mathrm{Hb}_{z\ score} = (\mathrm{Hb}_{current} - \mathrm{Hb}_{mean})/\sqrt{(\sigma^2(1 + 1/n))}$$

where *n* is the number of blood samples used in establishing the athlete's passport and σ^2 is the within-subject variance.

TABLE 1.—Number of Subjects Exceeding Various Cut Offs for Haemoglobin Concentration (g/dl); Retic%, Percentage of Reticulocytes; $OFF_{hr\ score}$, $OFF_{z\ score}$ and $Hb_{z\ score}$ (Points)

Method/Group	Pre	Boost	Maint.	Wash Out	Total
[Hb] $\geq$ 17.0 g/dl					
G1	–	–	1 (6.3)	1 (4.8)	1/8 (2.4)
G2	1 (6.3)	–	1 (10.0)	3 (18.8)	3/8 (12.5)
G3	–	1 (1.8)	3 (21.6)	1 (20.0)[a]	3/8 (11.7)
Total	1 (1.6)	1 (0.8)	5 (16.2)	5 (15.6)	7/24 (9.9)
%retic. $\geq$ 2.4%					
G1	–	2 (8.7)	–	–	2/8 (4.8)
G2	–	2 (8.3)	1 (2.5%)	–	2/8 (2.3)
G3	1 (3.4)	4 (16.4)	–	–[a]	4/8 (8.2)
Total	1 (1.6)	8 (12.0)	1 (0.9)	–	8/24 (5.0)
%retic. $\leq$ 0.2%					
G1, G2, G3	–	–	–	–	–
$OFF_{hr} \geq 133$					
G1	–	–	–	–	–
G2	–	–	–	2 (6.3)	2/8 (3.1)
G3	–	–	–	1 (20.0)[a]	1/8 (0.9)
Total	–	–	–	3 (5.6)	3/24 (1.6)
$OFF_{z\ score} \geq 3.09$					
G1	–	–	2 (12.5)	2 (14.3)	2/8 (6.0)
G2	–	–	–	2 (6.3)	2/8 (3.1)
G3	–	–	–5 (16%)	3 (60%)[a]	6/8 (10)
Total	–	–	7 (9.4)	7 (11.1)	10/24 (6.2)
$Hb_{z\ score} \geq 3.09$					
G1	1 (2.2)	1 (6.3)	1 (4.8)	1/8 (3.6)	
G2	–	–	–	–	
G3	1 (1.8)	7 (26.0)	2 (40.0%)[a]	7/8 (14.5)	
Total	2 (0.8)	8 (12.3)	3 (2.2)	8/24 (5.0)	

The numbers in parentheses denotes the sensitivity (percentage of samples within the pre, boost, maintenance or wash-out period exceeding the various cut offs).

Total denotes the number of subjects in each group exceeding the cut off and the numbers in parentheses denotes the sensitivity post the first rHuEpo injection.

[a]Samples missing for three subjects.

An athlete with a z value of > 3.09 will be subject to a 14-day suspension. These cut-off points are all compatible with the 1 in 1000 false-positive limit. Moreover, when using these criteria, Sharpe et al[1] were able to detect all 39 athletes who had received thrice weekly 18 to 20 IU/kg maintenance doses of recombinant human erythropoietin (rHuEpo). Bornø and associates tested the ability of the 5 potential standards to detect an alternative treatment plan, a single weekly maintenance dose of 60 to 65 IU/kg (Table 1). Despite the use of what is acknowledged to be an effective maintenance dose of rHuEpo,[2] similar in total amount to that used by Sharpe et al,[1] the passport of more than a half of the trial participants remained within permitted limits; further, some of the subjects who were detected exceeded the allowable ceiling only on 1 or 2 occasions, and with the less frequent blood sampling likely in the real world of athletics, overall detection rates would likely have been even lower than 42%. Plainly, success in detecting rHuEpo abuse depends greatly on details of the treatment schedule, and the standards currently imposed by the UCI do not guarantee the absence of blood doping during competition.

R. J. Shephard, MD (Lond), PhD, DPE

References

1. Sharpe K, Ashenden MJ, Schumacher YO. A third generation approach to detect erythropoietin abuse in athletes. *Haematologica.* 2006;91:356-363.
2. Lundby C, Achman-Andersen NJ, Thomsen JJ, Norgaard AM, Robach P. Testing for recombinant human erythropoietin in urine: problems associated with current anti-doping testing. *J Appl Physiol.* 2008;105:417-419.

Stability of Hemoglobin Mass During a 6-Day UCI ProTour Cycling Race
Garvican LA, Eastwood A, Martin DT, et al (Australian Inst of Sport, Canberra; Flinders Univ, Adelaide, Australia; et al)
Clin J Sport Med 20:200-204, 2010

Objective.—Blood doping in endurance sport is a growing problem. The purpose of this study was to determine the reliability of total hemoglobin mass (Hb_{mass}) measurement in the field and to establish the variability of Hb_{mass} during a cycling race, to assess its viability as an additional anti-doping detection parameter.

Design.—Control-matched longitudinal study.

Setting.—International Cycling Union's (UCI) ProTour stage race.

Participants.—Six professional cyclists and 5 recreationally active controls.

Interventions.—Seventy-two Hb_{mass} tests using the optimized carbon monoxide rebreathing method were performed over 7 consecutive days, before and throughout the tour. Fasted venous blood was obtained for measurement of hematocrit (Hct) and hemoglobin concentration [Hb] in the morning before stages 1, 3, and 6 (D_1, D_3, and D_6).

Main Outcome Measures.—Reliability of Hb_{mass} measurement was established using typical error calculated from 2 baseline measures. Individual change scores and coefficients of variation were used to assess stability during racing.

Results.—Typical error for Hb_{mass} was 1.3% [95% confidence limits (CL): 0.9%, 2.5%]. Calculated 95% and 99.99% CL for percent change in Hb_{mass} were ±3.6% and ±7.2%, respectively. Mean Hb_{mass} remained within ±1.9% of baseline in cyclists and ±0.5% in controls. In all cases, individual change scores for both cyclists and controls fell within the 95% CL. There was a decrease in Hct (8.1% ± 2.8%) and [Hb] (9.7% ± 3.2%) throughout the tour in cyclists but not in controls.

Conclusions.—We demonstrate that Hb_{mass} can be measured reliably via CO-rebreathing during a cycling tour. Unlike [Hb] and Hct, Hb_{mass} remains stable over 6 days of racing in professional cyclists and may have potential in an antidoping context (Fig 1).

▶ The detection of blood doping remains a challenge, and the more evidence that can be brought to bear on this question, the greater the likelihood of detecting cheaters.[1] A biological passport[2] is one promising approach. Items noted on the passport have included hemoglobin concentration, hematocrit,

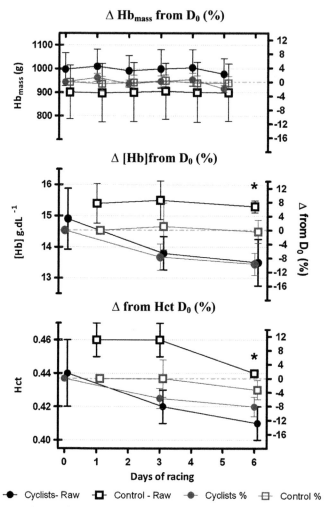

FIGURE 1.—Hb_{mass}, [Hb], and Hct (mean ± SD) before and throughout a 6-day cycling race in 6 professional cyclists (circles) and 5 recreationally active controls (squares). Raw units are shown on the left x axis (black symbols), and change (%) from baseline (D_0) shown on the right y axis (gray symbols). *Denotes a substantial difference between the groups in the change scores from D_0 ($P < 0.05$). (Reprinted from Garvican LA, Eastwood A, Martin DT, et al. Stability of hemoglobin mass during a 6-day UCI Pro-Tour cycling race. *Clin J Sport Med.* 2010;20:200-204, with permission from Lippincott Williams & Wilkins.)

and reticulocyte count, but these measures are all susceptible to effects from changes in hydration status and thus plasma volume. The article by Garvican and associates suggests that this information should be supplemented with a measure of total hemoglobin, a statistic that would be relatively independent of any changes in plasma volume. The technique of measuring hemoglobin mass is now relatively simple; it involves the rebreathing of 1.2 mL/kg of carbon monoxide and subsequent determination of the percentage of carboxy hemoglobin in 200 μL of capillary blood.[3] The entire test can be completed in 15 minutes or less, and the resulting values for hemoglobin mass are stable within ±3% over both a 6-day race (Fig 1) and a year in which training loads may vary. This compares with the 6% change in hemoglobin mass associated with the removal and subsequent reinfusion of 1 unit of blood.[4]

R. J. Shephard, MD (Lond), PhD, DPE

References

1. Borrione P, Mastrone A, Salvo RA, Spaccamiglio A, Grasso L, Angeli A. Oxygen delivery enhancers: past, present, and future. *J Endocrinol Invest*. 2008;31: 185-192.
2. Ashenden MJ. A strategy to deter blood doping in sport. *Haematologica*. 2002;87: 225-232.
3. Prommer N, Schmidt W. Loss of CO from the intravascular bed and its impact on the optimised CO-rebreathing method. *Eur J Appl Physiol*. 2007;100:383-391.
4. Pottgiesser T, Umhau M, Ahlgrim C, Ruthardt S, Roecker K, Schumacher YO. Hb mass measurement suitable to screen for illicit autologous blood transfusions. *Med Sci Sports Exerc*. 2007;39:1748-1756.

The Impact of Acute Gastroenteritis on Haematological Markers Used for the Athletes Biological Passport – Report of 5 Cases

Schumacher YO, Pottgiesser T (Medizinische Universitätsklinik Freiburg, Germany)

Int J Sports Med 32:147-150, 2011

The haematological module of the "Athletes Biological Passport" (ABP) is used to detect blood doping through the longitudinal variation of blood variables, such as haemoglobin concentration (Hb). Sporting federations have opened disciplinary procedures against athletes based on ABP results. Suspicious athletes try to explain the variations in their blood values with dehydration caused by gastrointestinal (GI) problems. The aim of the present report is to describe haemoglobin concentration, a key variable of the ABP, during acute gastroenteritis in athletes. 5 athletes with severe gastroenteritis were studied in retrospective. Blood test results (Hb, white blood cell count (WBC) and differential, CRP) obtained on hospital admission for GI problems were compared to data obtained from the same athletes in states of good health on previous occasions. During GI problems, athletes displayed marked inflammatory constellations with increased CRP and typical WBC shifts. Hb was not affected and remained mostly unchanged. This is in line with basic physiologic fluid regulation, where plasma volume is kept constant, even under conditions of severe dehydration. It is therefore unlikely that fluid loss associated with gastroenteritis will cause athletes blood data to reach levels of abnormality that will be suspicious of blood doping (Fig 1).

▶ Athletes who are accused of blood doping because of wide swings in their hematological profile relative to their biological passport[1] have sometimes

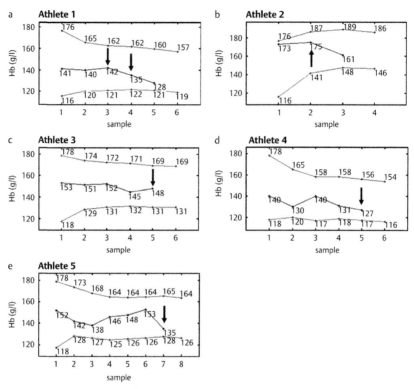

FIGURE 1.—Athlete 1–5: Individual profiles for haemoglobin concentration (g/l) calculated for each athlete using the ABP software. The red lines define the upper and lower individual limit (99.9%) for haemoglobin concentration. The samples obtained during gastroenteritis are indicated by an arrow. (Reprinted from Schumacher YO, Pottgiesser T. The impact of acute gastroenteritis on haematological markers used for the athletes biological passport — report of 5 cases. *Int J Sports Med.* 2011;32:147-150, with permission from Georg Thieme Verlag KG Stuttgart.)

pleaded that gastrointestinal problems (which can lead to several liters of fluid loss) have caused dehydration, a decrease in plasma volume, and thus a high hemoglobin concentration. The authors evaluated the validity of this excuse, examining longitudinal data on 5 athletes (2 soccer players and 3 cyclists) who had developed severe gastroenteritis (at least 3 episodes of vomiting and diarrhea within the previous 12 hours). Despite these symptoms, their hemoglobin levels all remained well within the permitted range (Fig 1). Other markers of true pathology were an increase in white cell count and C-reactive protein. In addition to any treatment that may be received, the plasma fluid volume tends to show little change because most of the fluid loss during gastroenteritis is from the intracellular and interstitial water.[2,3] This small case study suggests that gastroenteritis cannot be accepted as an alibi for unusual hemoglobin concentrations.

R. J. Shephard, MD (Lond), PhD, DPE

References

1. Sottas PE, Robinson N, Saugy M. The athlete's biological passport and indirect measures of blood doping. *Handb Exp Pharmacol*. 2010:305-326.
2. Costill DL, Cote R, Fink W. Muscle water and electrolytes following varied levels of dehydration in man. *J Appl Physiol*. 1976;40:6-11.
3. Dill DB, Costill DL. Calculation of percentage changes in volumes of blood, plasma, and red cells in dehydration. *J Appl Physiol*. 1974;37:247-248.

6 Cardiorespiratory Disorders

Syncope is unrelated to supine and postural hypotension following prolonged exercise

Murrell CJ, Cotter JD, George K, et al (Univ of Otago, Dunedin, New Zealand; Liverpool John Moores Univ, UK; et al)
Eur J Appl Physiol 111:469-476, 2011

Syncope is widely reported following prolonged exercise. It is often assumed that the magnitude of exercise-induced hypotension (post-exercise hypotension; PEH), and the hypotensive response to postural change (initial orthostatic hypotension; IOH) are predictors of syncope post-exercise. The aim of this study was to determine the relationship between PEH, IOH, the residual IOH and syncope following prolonged exercise. Blood pressure (BP; Finometer) was measured continuously in 19 athletes (47 ± 20 years; BMI: 23.2 ± 2.2 $kg\,m^2$; $\dot{V}O_2$ max: 51.3 ± 10.8 $mL\,kg^{-1}\,min^{-1}$) whilst supine and during head-up tilt (HUT) to 60° for 15 min (or to syncope), prior to and following 4 h of running at 70–80% maximal heart rate. Syncope developed in 15 of 19 athletes post-exercise [HUT-time completed, Pre: 14:39 (min:s) ± 0:55; Post: 5:59 ± 4:53; $P < 0.01$]. PEH was apparent (−7 ± 7 mmHg; −8 ± 8%), but was unrelated to HUT-time completed ($r^2 = 0.09$; $P > 0.05$). Although the magnitude of IOH was similar to post-exercise [−28 ± 12 vs. −20 ± 14% (pre-exercise); $P > 0.05$], the BP recovery following IOH was incomplete [−9 ± 9 vs. −1 ± 11 (pre-exercise); $P < 0.05$]; however, neither showed a relation to HUT-time completed ($r^2 = 0.18$, $r^2 = 0.01$; $P > 0.05$, respectively). Although an inability to maintain BP is a common feature of syncope post-exercise, the magnitude of PEH, IOH and residual IOH do not predict time to syncope. Practically, endurance athletes who present with greater hypotension are not necessarily at a greater risk of syncope than those who present with lesser reductions in BP.

▶ Syncope is a common occurrence at the end of an athletic event[1-3]; the study of Murrell et al is based on trained runners with an average age of 47 years, and 15 of their 19 subjects developed syncope following a run of 38 km during a period of 4 hours. There are many potential causes of postrace collapse, including arrhythmias, hypoglycemia, and hyponatremia, but probably the commonest reason is a sudden drop in systemic blood pressure, as blood pools in the widely dilated veins of the legs and abdomen[4]; this pooling acts in combination with increased circulating concentrations of vasodilator substances and a rapid decrease in sympathetic tone. In contrast to previous reports,[5] this study found no relationship between the tolerance of a head-up tilt (timed to impairment of consciousness) and either postexercise hypotension or immediate orthostatic hypotension. Thus, it seems that athletes who demonstrate the greatest hypotension following an event are not necessarily the individuals who are at the greatest risk of collapse.

R. J. Shephard, MD (Lond), PhD, DPE

References

1. Gratze G, Mayer H, Skrabal F. Sympathetic reserve, serum potassium, and orthostatic intolerance after endurance exercise and implications for neurocardiogenic syncope. *Eur Heart J.* 2008;29:1531-1541.
2. Holtzhausen LM, Noakes TD. The prevalence and significance of post-exercise (postural) hypotension in ultramarathon runners. *Med Sci Sports Exerc.* 1995; 27:1595-1601.
3. Holtzhausen LM, Noakes TD. Collapsed ultraendurance athlete: proposed mechanisms and an approach to management. *Clin J Sport Med.* 1997;7:292-301.
4. Smith JJ, Porth CM, Erickson M. Hemodynamic response to the upright posture. *J Clin Pharmacol.* 1994;34:375-386.
5. Halliwill JR. Mechanisms and clinical implications of post-exercise hypotension in humans. *Exerc Sport Sci Rev.* 2001;29:65-70.

An independent and external validation of QRISK2 cardiovascular disease risk score: a prospective open cohort study
Collins GS, Altman DG (Univ of Oxford, UK)
BMJ 340:c2442, 2010

Objective.—To evaluate the performance of the QRISK2 score for predicting 10-year cardiovascular disease in an independent UK cohort of patients from general practice records and to compare it with the NICE version of the Framingham equation and QRISK1.

Design.—Prospective cohort study to validate a cardiovascular risk score.

Setting.—365 practices from United Kingdom contributing to The Health Improvement Network (THIN) database.

Participants.—1.58 million patients registered with a general practice between 1 January 1993 and 20 June 2008, aged 35-74 years (9.4 million person years) with 71 465 cardiovascular events.

Main Outcome Measures.—First diagnosis of cardiovascular disease (myocardial infarction, angina, coronary heart disease, stroke, and transient ischaemic stroke) recorded in general practice records.

Results.—QRISK2 offered improved prediction of a patient's 10-year risk of cardiovascular disease over the NICE version of the Framingham equation. Discrimination and calibration statistics were better with QRISK2. QRISK2 explained 33% of the variation in men and 40% for women, compared with 29% and 34% respectively for the NICE Framingham and 32% and 38% respectively for QRISK1. The incidence rate of cardiovascular events (per 1000 person years) among men in the high risk group was 27.8 (95% CI 27.4 to 28.2) with QRISK2, 21.9 (21.6 to 22.2) with NICE Framingham, and 24.8 (22.8 to 26.9) with QRISK1. Similarly, the incidence rate of cardiovascular events (per 1000 person years) among women in the high risk group was 24.3 (23.8 to 24.9) with QRISK2, 20.6 (20.1 to 21.0) with NICE Framingham, and 21.8 (18.9 to 24.6) with QRISK1.

Conclusions.—QRISK2 is more accurate in identifying a high risk population for cardiovascular disease in the United Kingdom than the NICE version of the Framingham equation. Differences in performance between QRISK2 and QRISK1 were marginal (Table 3).

▶ Although the danger of a cardiac catastrophe while exercising is relatively low, sports physicians have long sought a simple procedure that would be of help to them both in identifying vulnerable individuals and in encouraging such people to take preventive measures, including an appropriate increase in their habitual physical activity. For many years, the most reliable tool for this purpose has seemed to be the Framingham Risk Factor Score.[1] However, critics have argued that the score is derived from a middle-class US population, using what 30 years ago were perceived as the main risk factors for cardiovascular disease (age, sex, systolic blood pressure, smoking status, and blood lipid data). In 2008, Hippisley-Cox and colleagues in the United Kingdom[2] introduced a new risk score (the QRISK2); this adds to the traditional Framingham risk factors the important items of body mass index, family history of cardiovascular disease, social deprivation, self-assigned ethnicity, and chronic conditions associated with cardiovascular risk (type 2 diabetes mellitus, treated hypertension, rheumatoid arthritis, renal disease, and atrial fibrillation). The 10-year risk of cardiovascular disease can be ascertained by entering these variables into

TABLE 3.—Discrimination and Model Performance Statistics for QRISK2, QRISK1, and NICE Framingham (Version of the Framingham Equation Recommended by NICE) in Estimating 10-year Risk of a Cardiovascular Event in the THIN Cohort

	QRISK2	QRISK1	NICE Framingham
Women			
AUROC statistic	0.801	0.799	0.774
D statistic (95% CI)	1.66 (1.56 to 1.76)	1.61 (1.50 to 1.71)	1.47 (1.29 to 1.64)
R^2 statistic (95% CI)	39.5 (36.6 to 42.4)	38.2 (35.1 to 41.3)	33.8 (28.5 to 39.2)
Brier score* (95% CI)	0.052 (0.050 to 0.054)	0.052 (0.050 to 0.054)	0.054 (0.051 to 0.057)
Men			
AUROC statistic	0.773	0.771	0.750
D statistic (95% CI)	1.45 (1.31 to 1.59)	1.42 (1.28 to 1.55)	1.30 (1.12 to 1.48)
R^2 statistic (95% CI)	33.3 (28.9 to 37.8)	32.3 (28.3 to 36.4)	28.7 (23.1 to 34.3)
Brier score* (95% CI)	0.076 (0.074 to 0.078)	0.076 (0.074 to 0.079)	0.082 (0.079 to 0.085)

AUROC = area under the receiver operating characteristics curve.
*Lower score indicates better accuracy of risk estimates.

appropriate software. This study by Collins and Altman reports the testing of the new formula in a prospective study of 1.6 million adults aged 35 to 74 years, although unfortunately the authors excluded patients who were already receiving statins, blood lipid values were not available for many of the samples, and cardiovascular outcomes (first diagnosis of myocardial infarction, angina, coronary heart disease, stroke, or transient ischemic stroke) were based on primary practice records, which have questionable accuracy. Despite these several important limitations, the QRISK2 appeared to give a better prediction of cardiovascular events than the Framingham formula (Table 3), and about a half of those patients who would have been classed as high risk by their Framingham score were downgraded to low risk. Nevertheless, there remains scope for better predictions; in terms of predicting cardiovascular events over the next 10 years, even the new QRISK2 score explains only 33% of the variation in men and 40% in women (Table 3).

R. J. Shephard, MD (Lond), PhD, DPE

References

1. Anderson KM, Odell PM, Wilson PW, Kannel WB. Cardiovascular disease risk profiles. *Am Heart J.* 1991;121:293-298.
2. Hippisley-Cox J, Coupland C, Vinogradova Y, et al. Predicting cardiovascular risk in England and Wales: prospective derivation and validation of QRISK2. *BMJ.* 2008;336:1475-1482.

Association among basal serum BDNF, cardiorespiratory fitness and cardiovascular disease risk factors in untrained healthy Korean men
Jung SH, Kim J, Davis JM, et al (Univ of South Carolina, Columbia; et al)
Eur J Appl Physiol 111:303-311, 2011

Evidence suggests that serum brain-derived neurotrophic factor (serum BDNF) can be affected by cardiorespiratory fitness (CRF), but this relationship is far from clear. Recent reports show an inverse relationship between serum BDNF and CRF in healthy individuals, and other studies suggest a possible association between serum BDNF and cardiovascular disease. However, the possible interaction between serum BDNF, CRF, and cardiovascular disease risk has not been studied. The purpose of this study was to examine the association among serum BDNF, CRF, and cardiovascular disease risk factors in healthy men. The investigation involved a large sample of men ($n = 995$, age range: 20–76 years) who live in the central area of South Korea and were recruited into the Preventive Health Study. Our study showed a significant inverse relationship between serum BDNF and relative VO_2max ($r = -0.412$, $p < 0.0001$) and heart rate reserve ($r = -0.194$, $p < 0.0001$). Serum BDNF was positively correlated with body mass index ($r = 0.80$, $p < 0.0001$), total cholesterol ($r = 0.185$, $p < 0.0001$), and triglyceride ($r = 0.320$, $p < 0.0001$). Our data suggest that serum BDNF may be associated with effects of increased CRF on cardiovascular disease. However, more research is clearly needed before a determination of whether, and to what extent, serum BDNF may be responsible for some of the health benefits associated with CRF (Fig 1).

▶ Perhaps because of the growing availability of measurement techniques, several journals have recently published articles drawing attention to associations between physical fitness, cardiovascular disease, and the concentration of novel circulating peptides, for example, soluble CD40 ligand.[1] The article of Jung and associates looks to confirm reported associations between regular physical activity, blood levels of brain-derived neurotrophic factor (BDNF), and cardiovascular disease,[2-4] using a much larger sample (men, 14-76 years) than in previous investigations. Whole circulating amounts of BDNF were measured because much of the circulating BDNF is stored in the platelets. BDNF concentrations were inversely related to cardiorespiratory fitness (mL O_2/[kg.min], as assessed by both Bruce treadmill test and heart rate reserve, Fig 1); however, β coefficients dropped progressively from −0.13 to −0.09 as covariate adjustment was made for other cardiac risk factors (body mass index, age, triglyceride, and high-density lipoprotein cholesterol concentrations). At first inspection, the findings seem to run counter to suggestions that regular exercise enhances brain BDNF concentrations, with an increase of neural plasticity and a reduction of various neural problems, including Alzheimer disease.[5-7] Jung et al offer several possible explanations for their findings. Possibly increased levels of body fat may cause BDNF to be liberated from platelets into the plasma, or

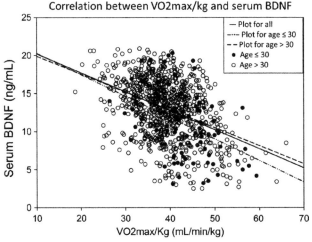

FIGURE 1.—Results of correlation between basal serum BDNF and maximal oxygen consumption. a Correlation (*a solid line*) between serum BDNF and VO_2max ml/kg/min ($N = 955$, $r = -0.412$, $r^2 = 0.169$, $p < 0.0001$) with a linear regression results in the equation: serum BDNF = 22.685 − $(0.249 \times VO_2$max ml/kg/min), SEE = 0.715. b Correlation (*a dash-dot-dot line*) between serum BDNF and VO_2max ml/kg/min ($N = 90$, r = −0.430, $r^2 = 0.185$, $p < 0.0001$) with a linear regression results in the equation: serum BDNF = 23.096 − $(0.282 \times VO_2$max ml/kg/min), SEE = 2.764. c Correlation (*a dash-dash line*) between serum BDNF and VO_2max ml/kg/min ($N = 865$, $r = -03.89$, $r^2 = 0.152$, $p < 0.0001$) with a linear regression results in the equation: serum BDNF = 22.235 − $(0.235 \times VO_2$max ml/kg/min), SEE = 0.749. (Reprinted from Jung SH, Kim J, Davis JM, et al. Association among basal serum BDNF, cardiorespiratory fitness and cardiovascular disease risk factors in untrained healthy Korean men. *Eur J Appl Physiol*. 2011;111:303-311. With kind permission of Springer Science+Business Media.)

a low level of fitness may in some way counter the transfer of BDNF from the blood stream into the brain. Given the growing prevalence of Alzheimer disease in an aging population, the effects of exercise on circulating and cerebral BDNF seem important areas for further study.

R. J. Shephard, MD (Lond), PhD, DPE

References

1. Geertsma L, Lucas SJ, Cotter JD, Hock B, McKenzie J, Fernyhough LJ. The cardiovascular risk factor soluble CD40 ligand (CD 154), but not soluble CD40 is lowered by ultra-endurance exercise in athletes. *Br J Sports Med*. 2011;45: 42-45.
2. Chan KL, Tong KY, Yip SP. Relationship of serum brain-derived neurotrophic factor (BDNF) and health-related lifestyle in healthy human subjects. *Neurosci Lett*. 2008;447:124-128.
3. Currie J, Ramsbottom R, Ludlow H, Nevill A, Gilder M. Cardio-respiratory fitness, habitual physical activity and serum brain derived neurotrophic factor (BDNF) in men and women. *Neurosci Lett*. 2009;451:152-155.
4. Nofuji Y, Suwa M, Moriyama Y, et al. Decreased serum brain-derived neurotrophic factor in trained men. *Neurosci Lett*. 2008;437:29-32.
5. Barnes DE, Whitmer RA, Yaffe K. Physical activity and dementia: the need for prevention trials. *Exerc Sport Sci Rev*. 2007;35:24-29.
6. Komulainen P, Pedersen M, Hänninen T, et al. BDNF is a novel marker of cognitive function in ageing women: the DR's EXTRA Study. *Neurobiol Learn Mem*. 2008;90:596-603.
7. Yaffe K, Barnes D, Nevitt M, Lui LY, Covinsky K. A prospective study of physical activity and cognitive decline in elderly women: women who walk. *Arch Intern Med*. 2001;161:1703-1708.

Combined Impact of Lifestyle-Related Factors on Total and Cause-Specific Mortality among Chinese Women: Prospective Cohort Study

Nechuta SJ, Shu X-O, Li H-L, et al (Vanderbilt Univ School of Medicine, Nashville, TN; Shanghai Cancer Inst, China; et al)

PLoS Med 7:e1000339, 2010

Background.—Although cigarette smoking, excessive alcohol drinking, obesity, and several other well-studied unhealthy lifestyle-related factors each have been linked to the risk of multiple chronic diseases and premature death, little is known about the combined impact on mortality outcomes, in particular among Chinese and other non-Western populations. The objective of this study was to quantify the overall impact of lifestyle-related factors beyond that of active cigarette smoking and alcohol consumption on all-cause and cause-specific mortality in Chinese women.

Methods and Findings.—We used data from the Shanghai Women's Health Study, an ongoing population-based prospective cohort study in China. Participants included 71,243 women aged 40 to 70 years enrolled during 1996–2000 who never smoked or drank alcohol regularly. A healthy lifestyle score was created on the basis of five lifestyle-related factors shown to be independently associated with mortality outcomes

TABLE 3.—Adjusted HRs for Lifestyle-Related Factors and Risk of All-Cause, Cardiovascular, and Cancer Mortality Among Nonsmoking and Nondrinking Women Aged 40–70 y at Baseline (n = 71,243), Shanghai Women's Health Study, 1996–2007

Lifestyle Factor	All-Cause (n = 2,860 deaths)			CVD (n = 775)			Cancer (n = 1,351)		
	n Deaths/Cohort	Age and SES-Adjusted[a] HR (95% CI)	Further Adjusted[b] HR (95% CI)	n Deaths	Age and SES-Adjusted[a] HR (95% CI)	Further Adjusted[b] HR (95% CI)	n Deaths	Age and SES-Adjusted[a] HR (95% CI)	Further Adjusted[b] HR (95% CI)
BMI (kg/m^2)									
≥30 (obese)	257/3,560	1.00 (Reference)	1.00 (Reference)	104	1.00 (Reference)	1.00 (Reference)	99	1.00 (Reference)	1.00 (Reference)
<18.5 (underweight)	149/2,402	1.52 (1.24–1.86)	1.83 (1.48–2.26)	42	1.18 (0.82–1.69)	1.61 (1.10–2.35)	60	1.43 (1.03–1.97)	1.64 (1.18–2.30)
25.0–29.99 (overweight)	1,027/21,328	0.83 (0.72–0.95)	0.85 (0.74–0.98)	299	0.62 (0.50–0.77)	0.64 (0.51–0.80)	483	0.97 (0.78–1.21)	0.99 (0.80–1.23)
18.5–24.99 (normal)	1,427/43,953	0.82 (0.72–0.94)	0.91 (0.80–1.05)	330	0.53 (0.43–0.66)	0.61 (0.48–0.77)	709	0.95 (0.77–1.17)	1.02 (0.82–1.27)
WHR									
≥0.830	1,477/23,766	1.00 (Reference)	1.00 (Reference)	447	1.00 (Reference)	1.00 (Reference)	631	1.00 (Reference)	1.00 (Reference)
0.786 to <0.830	811/23,730	0.81 (0.74–0.88)	0.80 (0.73–0.87)	219	0.79 (0.67–0.93)	0.82 (0.69–0.96)	407	0.88 (0.78–1.00)	0.87 (0.76–0.99)
<0.786	572/23,747	0.74 (0.67–0.82)	0.68 (0.61–0.76)	109	0.56 (0.45–0.69)	0.52 (0.42–0.66)	313	0.84 (0.73–0.97)	0.80 (0.69–0.93)
Exercise participation (MET, h/d)									
None	1,579/46,093	1.00 (Reference)	1.00 (Reference)	417	1.00 (Reference)	1.00 (Reference)	729	1.00 (Reference)	1.00 (Reference)
>0–1.99	812/17,284	0.91 (0.83–0.99)	0.92 (0.85–1.00)	232	0.90 (0.76–1.06)	0.92 (0.78–1.08)	406	1.04 (0.92–1.18)	1.04 (0.92–1.18)
≥2.0	469/7,866	0.86 (0.77–0.96)	0.89 (0.80–0.99)	126	0.76 (0.62–0.94)	0.79 (0.65–0.97)	216	0.96 (0.82–1.12)	0.96 (0.82–1.12)
Spouse smoke[c]									
Ever	1,315/38,994	1.00 (Reference)	1.00 (Reference)	352	1.00 (Reference)	1.00 (Reference)	634	1.00 (Reference)	1.00 (Reference)
Never	987/24,797	0.92 (0.84–1.00)	0.92 (0.85–1.00)	253	0.84 (0.72–0.99)	0.86 (0.73–1.01)	479	0.93 (0.83–1.05)	0.94 (0.83–1.06)
Fruit and vegetable intake (g/d)									
<404.3	1,313/23,742	1.00 (Reference)	1.00 (Reference)	384	1.00 (Reference)	1.00 (Reference)	522	1.00 (Reference)	1.00 (Reference)
404.3 to <626.5	823/23,752	0.83 (0.76–0.91)	0.85 (0.78–0.93)	207	0.78 (0.66–0.92)	0.81 (0.68–0.96)	437	1.03 (0.91–1.18)	1.05 (0.92–1.19)
≥626.5	724/23,749	0.82 (0.75–0.90)	0.85 (0.77–0.93)	184	0.81 (0.68–0.97)	0.84 (0.70–1.00)	392	1.01 (0.89–1.16)	1.03 (0.90–1.18)

[a] HRs are estimated from Cox proportional hazards regression models using age as the time-scale and adjusted for education, occupation, and income.
[b] Additionally adjusted for other lifestyle factors in the table.
[c] Excludes women without information on exposure to spousal smoking (n = 7,452).

(normal weight, lower waist-hip ratio, daily exercise, never exposed to spouse's smoking, higher daily fruit and vegetable intake). The score ranged from zero (least healthy) to five (most healthy) points. During an average follow-up of 9 years, 2,860 deaths occurred, including 775 from cardiovascular disease (CVD) and 1,351 from cancer. Adjusted hazard ratios for mortality decreased progressively with an increasing number of healthy lifestyle factors. Compared to women with a score of zero, hazard ratios (95% confidence intervals) for women with four to five factors were 0.57 (0.44–0.74) for total mortality, 0.29 (0.16–0.54) for CVD mortality, and 0.76 (0.54–1.06) for cancer mortality. The inverse association between the healthy lifestyle score and mortality was seen consistently regardless of chronic disease status at baseline. The population attributable risks for not having 4–5 healthy lifestyle factors were 33% for total deaths, 59% for CVD deaths, and 19% for cancer deaths.

Conclusions.—In this first study, to our knowledge, to quantify the combined impact of lifestyle-related factors on mortality outcomes in Chinese women, a healthier lifestyle pattern—including being of normal weight, lower central adiposity, participation in physical activity, nonexposure to spousal smoking, and higher fruit and vegetable intake—was associated with reductions in total and cause-specific mortality among lifetime nonsmoking and nondrinking women, supporting the importance of overall lifestyle modification in disease prevention (Table 3).

▶ Many studies on the effects of physical activity and other aspects of lifestyle upon mortality are confounded by the very strong effects of 2 variables that are difficult for investigators to assess accurately: smoking and drinking habits. This very large prospective cohort study comes from Shanghai, China, where in contrast to the men, very few women appear either to smoke or to drink. The study is based upon nonsmokers and nondrinkers, with a 5-point scale awarded for lifestyle characteristics (daily exercise, a healthy diet, a normal body mass, a normal waist to hip ratio, and avoidance of exposure to second-hand smoke). It shows that even in a population that avoids smoking and drinking, there is a substantial improvement of prognosis with the adoption of other components of a favorable lifestyle (relative risks over 9 years for those initially aged 40-70 years and having an unweighted good score on 4 of the 5 items studied: overall mortality 0.57, cardiovascular disease 0.29, and cancer 0.76). Possible reverse causation of health problems modifying physical activity or body mass was excluded by omitting data from the first 3 years of the follow-up period. A questionnaire assessed the type, intensity, duration, and frequency of exercise, which was summarized in terms of the individual's average number of metabolic equivalent (MET)-hours per day, 1 MET-hour being equivalent to about 15 minutes of moderate exercise in this age group. Multiple regression hazard analysis demonstrated independent benefits of physical activity, as thus assessed, in terms of overall mortality and cardiovascular disease but not cancer (Table 3). The benefits of a normal body mass and a normal waist to hip ratio were also statistically independent of each other. The data from this study underline the potential for a substantial lifestyle-induced improvement in health prospects even among those individuals who neither smoke nor drink alcohol.

R. J. Shephard, MD (Lond), PhD, DPE

Beyond sudden death in the athlete: how to identify family members at risk
Quarta G, Lambiase P, Elliott P (Univ College London, UK)
Br J Sports Med 45:189-192, 2011

Sudden death in young athletes is always a catastrophic event which focuses medical and public attention on the prevention of similar tragedies in other sporting participants. In this review article, we discuss the importance of evaluation of family members, who, by virtue of the familial nature of many of the diseases that cause sudden cardiac death, are potentially at risk of a similar outcome. We show that a systematic approach to the clinical evaluation of relatives of sudden death victims has a high yield in the identification of other affected family members and may prevent further catastrophic events in the same family.

▶ Although sudden death during exercise is a rare event (the probable incidence in young adults is about 0.5/100 000 competitors per year), it would be nice if one could discover a reliable method of distinguishing vulnerable individuals during routine preparticipation examinations. Italian investigators continue to argue strongly for the value of a resting electrocardiogram (ECG),[1] based mainly on a decrease of sudden deaths in Italy some 15 to 20 years after introducing mandatory ECG screening of athletes. However, 2 major problems remain: the physician is seeking to identify a very rare event and published standards of ECG normality devised for the general population are generally not appropriate for endurance athletes.[2,3] The classic World Health Organization criteria of a successful screening test[4] are not satisfied: the prevalence of sudden death within the athletic community is low, the ECG lacks both sensitivity and specificity, and application of mandatory testing to the entire population leads to many false-positive results, with unnecessary anxiety, expense, and exclusions from sport. One important aspect of clinical examination, sometimes overlooked by proponents of the ECG, is a careful family history looking for reports of sudden death before the age of 45 years in the next of kin. Many of the conditions causing sudden cardiac death (for instance, hypertrophic cardiomyopathy, long QT syndrome, and Brugada syndrome) have a strong genetic component. Quarta and associates follow previous authors[5,6] in suggesting that it may be particularly useful to carry out careful laboratory testing of someone who has a relative who died at an early age; their protocol includes ECG testing, echocardiography, Holter monitoring, and pharmacological challenges (sodium channel blockers for Brugada syndrome and epinephrine challenge to reveal catecholamine polymorphic ventricular tachycardia). Certainly, by concentrating on families that have a history of sudden death, they have taken a first step toward increasing prevalence, one of the prerequisites for successful screening.

R. J. Shephard, MD (Lond), PhD, DPE

References

1. Pelliccia A, Corrado D. Can ECG screening prevent sudden death in athletes? Yes. *BMJ*. 2010;341:c4923.
2. Shephard RJ. Preparticipation screening of young athletes: An effective investment? In: Shephard RJ, Alexander MJL, Cantu RC, et al., eds. *Year Book of Sports Medicine, 2005*. Philadelphia, PA: Elsevier/Mosby; 2005. xix–xvi.
3. Shephard RJ. Is the ECG screening of North American athletes now warranted? *Clin J Sports Med*. In Press.
4. Andermann A, Blancquaert I, Beauchamp S, Déryc V. Revisiting Wilson and Jungner in the genomic age: a review of screening criteria over the past 40 years. *Bull World Health Organ*. 2008;86:317-319.
5. Behr ER, Dalageorgou C, Christiansen M, et al. Sudden arrhythmic death syndrome: familial evaluation identifies inheritable heart disease in the majority of families. *Eur Heart J*. 2008;29:1670-1680.
6. Tan HL, Hofman N, van Langen IM, van der Wal AC, Wilde AA. Sudden unexplained death: heritability and diagnostic yield of cardiological and genetic examination in surviving relatives. *Circulation*. 2005;112:207-213.

Rapid loss of appendicular skeletal muscle mass is associated with higher all-cause mortality in older men: the prospective MINOS study

Szulc P, Munoz F, Marchand F, et al (Univ of Lyon, France; Société de Secours Minière de Bourgogne, Montceau les Mines, France)

Am J Clin Nutr 91:1227-1236, 2010

Background.—Changes in body composition underlying the association between weight loss and higher mortality are not clear.

Objective.—The objective was to investigate the association between changes in body composition of the appendicular (4 limbs) and central (trunk) compartments and all-cause mortality in men.

Design.—In men aged ≥50 y, body composition was assessed every 18 mo for 7.5 y with a whole-body dual-energy X-ray absorptiometry scan. Mortality was assessed for 10 y. Data were analyzed by logistic regression and Cox model and adjusted for age, body mass index (BMI), educational level, lifestyle, physical performance, comorbidities, body composition, and serum concentrations of 17β-estradiol and 25-hydroxycholecalciferol.

Results.—Of 715 men who were followed up, 137 (19.2%) died. Mortality was higher in men with the fastest weight loss [lowest compared with middle tertile odds ratio (OR): 2.31; 99% CI: 1.05, 5.09]. Faster loss of appendicular skeletal muscle mass (ASMM) was predictive of mortality (lowest compared with middle tertile OR: 3.60; 99% CI: 1.64, 7.89). Faster loss in ASMM remained a strong predictor of mortality after adjustment for weight loss (OR: 3.41; 99% CI: 1.51, 7.71). Faster loss in ASMM was the strongest predictor of death in the stepwise procedures when it was analyzed jointly with changes in the mass of other compartments. Loss in ASMM calculated over 36 mo was also a stronger predictor of death than were changes in the mass of other compartments (hazard ratio: 1.33 per 1-SD decrease; 95% CI: 1.06, 1.66).

Conclusion.—The accelerated loss of ASMM is predictive of all-cause mortality in older men regardless of age, BMI, lifestyle, physical performance, health status, body composition, and serum 17β-estradiol and 25-hydroxycholecalciferol (Table 4).

▶ Is the well-recognized association between mortality and loss of body mass[1-3] (Table 4) more than an expression of the link between a deterioration in skeletal muscle and loss of bone tissue and inadequate physical activity and thus premature death? Certainly, loss of muscle strength has previously been linked to increased mortality.[4,5] In this prospective study of older men, the association with loss of appendicular skeletal muscle remained after statistical adjustment of data for a large number of baseline variables, including age, body mass index, lifestyle (smoking and alcohol consumption together with estimates

TABLE 4.—Multivariate Analysis of the Association Between Prospectively Assessed Changes in Body Composition and Mortality in 715 Men[1]

Variable	Lower Tertile	Middle Tertile	Upper Tertile
Logistic regression[2]			
Weight	2.31 (1.05, 5.09)[3]	1.00	1.62 (0.72, 3.67)
Lean body mass	3.92 (1.70, 9.06)[4]	1.00	3.19 (1.38, 7.40)[5]
ASMM	3.60 (1.64, 7.89)[4]	1.00	1.08 (0.46, 2.54)
Central lean mass	2.21 (0.98, 5.01)	1.00	2.87 (1.28, 6.41)[3]
Visceral lean mass	1.94 (0.85, 4.45)	1.00	3.50 (1.55, 7.91)[4]
Fat body mass	2.02 (0.94, 4.36)	1.00	1.36 (0.62, 2.98)
Appendicular fat mass	1.24 (0.57, 2.70)	1.00	1.44 (0.68, 3.05)
Central fat mass	1.68 (0.79, 3.56)	1.00	1.31 (0.61, 2.81)
Cox's model: survival calculated since baseline, ie, first measurement in 1995–1996[6]			
Weight	1.96 (1.01, 3.82)[3]	1.00	1.49 (0.74, 3.01)
Lean body mass	2.78 (1.38, 5.57)[4]	1.00	2.70 (1.34, 5.44)[4]
ASMM	2.40 (1.29, 4.46)[4]	1.00	0.96 (0.47, 1.98)
Central lean mass	1.92 (0.95, 3.90)	1.00	2.50 (1.25, 4.97)[4]
Visceral lean mass	1.73 (0.85, 3.52)	1.00	2.69 (1.36, 5.32)[4]
Fat body mass	1.65 (0.87, 3.12)	1.00	1.22 (0.62, 2.38)
Appendicular fat mass	1.10 (0.57, 2.11)	1.00	1.28 (0.68, 2.39)
Central fat mass	1.67 (0.90, 3.09)	1.00	1.25 (0.66, 2.36)
Cox's model: survival calculated since the last DXA measurement[6]			
Weight	1.54 (0.78, 3.05)	1.00	0.90 (0.43, 1.90)
Lean body mass	2.73 (1.33, 5.60)[4]	1.00	2.26 (1.09, 4.68)[5]
ASMM	2.16 (1.15, 4.09)[5]	1.00	0.95 (0.45, 2.02)
Central lean mass	1.64 (0.81, 3.22)	1.00	1.55 (0.77, 3.13)
Visceral lean mass	1.73 (0.85, 3.51)	1.00	1.75 (0.87, 3.52)
Fat body mass	1.37 (0.72, 2.62)	1.00	0.79 (0.39, 1.59)
Appendicular fat mass	0.81 (0.42, 1.59)	1.00	0.83 (0.43, 1.61)
Central fat mass	1.32 (0.71, 2.47)	1.00	0.74 (0.38, 1.45)

[1]ASMM, appendicular skeletal muscle mass; DXA, dual-energy X-ray absorptiometry.
[2]All values are odds ratios; 99% CIs in parentheses.
[3]$P < 0.01$.
[4]$P < 0.001$.
[5]$P < 0.005$.
[6]All values are hazard ratios; 99% CIs in parentheses.

of leisure and occupational physical activity), health status (ischemic heart disease, hypertension, stroke, diabetes mellitus, Parkinson disease, and respiratory disease), body composition, and serum 17 beta-estradiol and 25-hydroxycholecalciferol levels. This report confirms the findings of an association between loss of muscle and mortality noted in a smaller previous study from Framingham,[6] but nevertheless cannot exclude the possibility that poor nutrition secondary to depression or diseases developing over the course of the 10 years of observation were responsible for loss of weight and mortality. It is unfortunate that the study did not distinguish between intentional and nonintentional weight loss, which would have separated out most of those developing disease during follow-up. The initial questionnaire analysis may also have lacked the sensitivity to make an accurate classification of habitual physical activity levels. Given the cross-sectional nature of the analysis, if there were an association with physical activity, it would remain difficult to determine whether muscle loss restricted physical activity and increased the cardiovascular strain imposed by a given bout of exercise or whether low levels of physical activity had preceded muscle loss. Despite these issues, the article shows that a loss of limb muscle may provide a useful empirical gauge of a patient's prognosis.

R. J. Shephard, MD (Lond), PhD, DPE

References

1. Iribarren C, Sharp DS, Burchfiel CM, Petrovitch H. Association of weight loss and weight fluctuation with mortality among Japanese American men. *N Engl J Med.* 1995;333:686-692.
2. Wannamethee SG, Shaper AG, Walker M. Weight change, weight fluctuation, and mortality. *Arch Intern Med.* 2002;162:2575-2580.
3. Nguyen ND, Center JR, Eisman JA, Nguyen TV. Bone loss, weight loss, and weight fluctuation predict mortality risk in elderly men and women. *J Bone Miner Res.* 2007;22:1147-1154.
4. Buchman AS, Wilson RS, Boyle PA, Bienias JL, Bennett DA. Change in motor function and risk of mortality in older persons. *J Am Geriatr Soc.* 2007;55:11-19.
5. Metter EJ, Talbot LA, Schragger M, Conwit RA. Arm-cranking muscle power and arm isometric muscle strength are independent predictors of all-cause mortality in men. *J Appl Physiol.* 2004;96:814-821.
6. Roubenoff R, Parise H, Payette HA, et al. Cytokines, insulin-like growth factor 1, sarcopenia, and mortality in very old community-dwelling men and women: the Framingham Heart Study. *Am J Med.* 2003;115:429-435.

Cardiovascular Screening in College Athletes With and Without Electrocardiography: A Cross-sectional Study
Baggish AL, Hutter AM Jr, Wang F, et al (Massachusetts General Hosp, Boston; Harvard Univ, Cambridge, MA)
Ann Intern Med 152:269-275, 2010

Background.—Although cardiovascular screening is recommended for athletes before participating in sports, the role of 12-lead electrocardiography (ECG) remains uncertain. To date, no prospective data that compare screening with and without ECG have been available.

Objective.—To compare the performance of preparticipation screening limited to medical history and physical examination with a strategy that integrates these with ECG.

Design.—Cross-sectional comparison of screening strategies.

Setting.—University Health Services, Harvard University, Cambridge, Massachusetts.

Participants.—510 collegiate athletes who received cardiovascular screening before athletic participation.

Measurements.—Each participant had routine history and examination–limited screening and ECG. They received transthoracic echocardiography (TTE) to detect or exclude cardiac findings with relevance to sports participation. The performance of screening with history and examination only was compared with that of screening that integrated history, examination, and ECG.

Results.—Cardiac abnormalities with relevance to sports participation risk were observed on TTE in 11 of 510 participants (prevalence, 2.2%). Screening with history and examination alone detected abnormalities in 5 of these 11 athletes (sensitivity, 45.5% [95% CI, 16.8% to 76.2%]; specificity, 94.4% [CI, 92.0% to 96.2%]). Electrocardiography detected 5 additional participants with cardiac abnormalities (for a total of 10 of 11 participants), thereby improving the overall sensitivity of screening to 90.9% (CI, 58.7% to 99.8%). However, including ECG reduced the specificity of screening to 82.7% (CI, 79.1% to 86.0%) and was associated with a false-positive rate of 16.9% (vs. 5.5% for screening with history and examination only).

Limitation.—Definitive conclusions regarding the effect of ECG inclusion on sudden death rates cannot be made.

Conclusion.—Adding ECG to medical history and physical examination improves the overall sensitivity of preparticipation cardiovascular screening in athletes. However, this strategy is associated with an increased rate of false-positive results when current ECG interpretation criteria are used.

▶ The merit of preparticipation electrocardiography (ECG) screening of athletes as a means of preventing exercise-related sudden death has long been controversial.[1-4] Pelliccia and Corrado[5] have recently advanced the study of Baggish and associates as new evidence supporting their claim of the value of ECG screening in saving the lives of athletes in a cost-effective manner. It is thus important to make a critical analysis of the evidence that Baggish et al have presented. Their study is based on a relatively small sample (510 college athletes). It compares history and physical examination alone against a combination of such information with the findings from a 12-lead resting ECG. Much depends, of course, on the skills devoted to these respective evaluations. The clinical examination was conducted by a noncardiologist and was of 8 minutes duration. The ECG evaluation also unfortunately failed to use athlete-specific criteria of normality! Thus, the initial comparison must be judged as relatively weak. The gold standard for a correct diagnosis was not cardiac death as seen in a prospective trial but rather a cross-sectional comparison with observations of suggestive or diagnostic abnormalities noted during limited echocardiographic imaging. The claim was made that ECG testing detected 11 abnormal individuals, as against 5 from history and physical examination alone. However, it is hard to believe that 11 of the 510 college athletes were at imminent risk of sudden death; most estimates of the annual risk of death while exercising are closer to 1 incident per 100 000 athletes. It seems significant that only 3 rather than 11 patients were ultimately asked to restrict their sport participation; further, we are not told whether these 3 were uniquely identified by ECG, nor do we have any information to tell us whether this advice lengthened or shortened their life span! Pelliccia and Corrado[5] created further confusion by suggesting that both the American Heart Association (AHA) and the European Society of Cardiology called for cardiovascular screening, without pointing out that the American recommendation was firmly against ECG screening.[6] Among the many problems associated with ECG screening, the AHA underlined low test specificity, a high false-positive rate, and the costs and logistics of accurate interpretation. As Bahr[7] recently underlined, the concept of preparticipation ECG evaluation ignores many of the 10 classical Wilson-Jungner criteria for the usefulness of a screening test,[8] particularly the need for a substantial disease prevalence and an appropriate level of sensitivity and specificity in the test procedure. Certainly, the article of Baggish et al is not sufficient to reverse the stand of North American cardiologists against preparticipation ECG screening.

R. J. Shephard, MD (Lond), PhD, DPE

References

1. Shephard RJ. Preparticipation screening of young athletes: an effective investment?. In: Shephard RJ, Alexander MJL, Cantu RC, et al., eds. *Year Book of Sports Medicine, 2005.* Philadelphia, PA: Elsevier/Mosby; 2005:xix-xxv.
2. Shephard RJ. Mass ECG screening of young athletes. *Br J Sports Med.* 2008;42: 707-708.
3. Chaitman R. An electrocardiogram should not be included in routine preparticipation screening of young athletes. *Circulation.* 2007;116:2610-2615.
4. Myerburg RJ, Vetter VL. Electrocardiograms should be included in preparticipation screening of athletes. *Circulation.* 2007;116:2616-2626.
5. Pelliccia A, Corrado D. Can electrocardiographic screening prevent sudden death in athletes? Yes. *BMJ.* 2010;341:c4923.
6. Maron BJ, Thompson PD, Ackerman MJ, et al. Recommendations and considerations related to preparticipation screening for cardiovascular abnormalities in competitive athletes: 2007 update: a scientific statement from the American Heart Association Council on Nutrition, Physical Activity, and Metabolism: endorsed by the American College of Cardiology Foundation. *Circulation.* 2007; 115:1643-1655.
7. Bahr R. Can electrocardiographic screening prevent sudden death in athletes? No. *BMJ.* 2010;341:c4914.
8. Andermann A, Blancquaert I, Beauchamp S, Déry V. Revisiting Wilson and Jungner in the genomic age: a review of screening criteria over the past 40 years. *Bull World Health Organ.* 2008;86:317-319.

Vagal Threshold Determination. Effect of Age and Gender
Botek M, Stejskal P, Krejci J, et al (Palacky Univ Olomouc, Czech Republic)
Int J Sports Med 31:768-772, 2010

Progressive increases in exercise intensity cause significant decreases in vagal activity (VA) until a critical point called the vagal threshold (T_{VA}) is reached. This is where further increases in exercise intensity cause negligible change in VA. This study was designed to develop the algorithm for the T_{VA} determination and to assess the effects of age and gender on its level. The sample consisted of 40 subjects who were divided according to age and gender into 4 groups with 10 subjects each: G_1-Men age 25—31, G_2-Men age 40—57, G_3-Women age 24—28, and G_4-Women age 43—56. The vagal responses were assessed by spectral analysis of the heart rate variability method while walking on a treadmill in a steady-state at intensities of 20—70 % of the maximal heart rate reserve (MHRR). The mean intensity of 45 % MHRR was suggested as the T_{VA} level which is related neither to age nor gender. Heart rate related to T_{VA} ($T_{VA\text{-}HR}$) was affected by gender. High frequency power at T_{VA} was influenced by age. The $T_{VA\text{-}HR}$ was considered to be a promising tool for the prescription of a safe level of physical activity for subjects with higher risks of health complications involving elevated sympathoadrenal activity during exercise (Fig 3).

▶ In patients subject to abnormalities of heart rhythm, the common practice among exercise prescribers is to conduct a medically supervised graded stress test, noting the heart rate and/or the intensity of effort when such abnormalities first appear. In general, this provides a satisfactory method of determining a safe intensity of effort for training and/or rehabilitation. However, it is arguable that

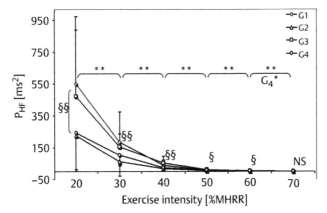

FIGURE 3.—Effect of incremental exercise intensity on high frequency power in tested groups (Results). (Reprinted from Botek M, Stejskal P, Krejci J, et al. Vagal threshold determination. Effect of age and gender. *Int J Sports Med.* 2010;31:768-772, with permission from Georg Thieme Verlag KG Stuttgart.)

anxiety during a formal medically supervised stress test may cause an increased release of catecholamines, with the onset of arrhythmias at a lower heart rate than would be the case when exercising in a more relaxed setting. Botek and associates here propose a somewhat more complicated method of determining a safe intensity of effort, arguing that the danger point comes when increases of heart rate are mediated by augmented sympathetic activity rather than vagal withdrawal. The transition point seems to be at/or around 50% of maximal heart rate (Fig 3). Since this threshold also seems to be independent of age and sex, a standard 50% of maximal heart rate might provide an appropriate guide to exercise prescription, rather than needing to carry out a spectral analysis of heart rate on every patient. There is some evidence supporting the new technique,[1,2] but further study (particularly of interindividual variability in this threshold) seems needed before the new approach can be recommended to replace a traditional graded stress test.

R. J. Shephard, MD (Lond), PhD, DPE

References

1. Billman GE. Cardiac autonomic neural remodeling and susceptibility to sudden cardiac death: effect of endurance exercise training. *Am J Physiol Heart Circ Physiol.* 2009;297:H1171-H1193.
2. Vanoli E, Adamson PB, Hull SS Jr, Foreman RD, Schwartz PJ. Prediction of unexpected sudden death among healthy dogs by a novel marker of autonomic neural activity. *Heart Rhythm.* 2008;5:300-305.

Prevalence and Prognostic Significance of Exercise-Induced Right Bundle Branch Block
Stein R, Nguyen P, Abella J, et al (Hospital de Clinicas de Porto Alegre, Brazil; Veteran Affairs Palo Alto Health Care System and Stanford Univ School of Medicine, CA; et al)
Am J Cardiol 105:677-680, 2010

Exercise-induced (EI) right bundle branch block (RBBB) is an infrequent electrocardiographic phenomenon, and controversy exists regarding its association with cardiovascular disease. We compared the prevalence and prognostic significance of RBBB, abnormal ST depression, and normal electrocardiographic findings in response to exercise testing in 9,623 consecutive veterans who underwent exercise testing from 1987 to 2007. EI RBBB, EI ST depression, and a normal exercise electrocardiographic response occurred in 0.24%, 15.2%, and 71.9% veterans, respectively. After appropriate exclusions, of the 8,047 patients analyzed, 6 patients in the EI RBBB subgroup died. Of these 6 deaths, 3 were cardiovascular deaths during the 9 years of follow-up. The annual death rate was 7.3% (1.4% cardiac deaths), 2.6% (1.2% cardiac deaths), and 1.8% (0.6% cardiac death) among those with EI RBBB, EI ST depression, and a normal ST response, respectively (p <0.0001). The patients with EI RBBB were significantly older, more overweight, and had a greater

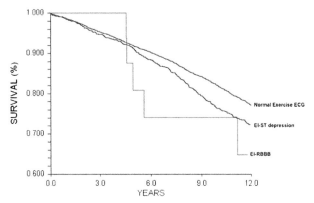

FIGURE 1.—Kaplan-Meier survival curves for all-cause mortality. (Reprinted from Stein R, Nguyen P, Abella J, et al. Prevalence and prognostic significance of exercise-induced right bundle branch block. *Am J Cardiol*. 2010;105:677-680, with permission from Elsevier.)

prevalence of coronary artery disease, heart failure, and hypertension compared to the 2 other subgroups. Patients with EI RBBB had an age-adjusted Cox proportional hazard ratio of 1.13 ($p = 0.75$, 95% confidence interval 0.51 to 2.5) for all-cause mortality and 1.57 ($p = 0.43$, 95% confidence interval 0.51 to 4.8) for cardiovascular mortality, respectively. In conclusion, EI RBBB is a rare occurrence during routine clinical exercise testing that appears to be benign (Fig 1).

▶ One of the hazards of mass ECG screening is that occasionally records appear to depart from normal, and the question arises as to whether this is a harbinger of an adverse prognosis. One rare abnormality is the onset of right bundle branch block (RBB) during an exercise stress test (exercise-induced [EI] RBB). We observed this phenomenon during our studies of Canadian Inuit, and a medical colleague speculated that this might be a reflection of pulmonary hypertension secondary to pulmonary vascular changes induced by repeated exposure of the lungs to extremely cold air.[1] However, the same phenomenon can develop occasionally when performing stress tests in average city-dwelling North Americans. In the present report (based on male veterans, average age 65 years), EI RBB was seen in 0.24% of a large sample. Various studies have linked coronary artery disease[2,3] or heart failure[4] to left bundle branch block; the clinical significance of EI RBB has received much less previous study, although some reports have pointed to similar associations.[5-7] In the present report, the prognosis was indeed poorer in patients with EI RBB than in those with a normal ECG (Fig 1), but the adverse outlook was largely explicable in terms of a greater age. Other contributing factors were a greater body weight and a greater prevalence of coronary artery disease, heart failure, and hypertension. The conclusion seems that little clinical significance should be attached to an EI RBB in an otherwise healthy older patient.

R. J. Shephard, MD (Lond), PhD, DPE

References

1. Shephard RJ, Rode A. *The Health Consequences of Modernisation.* Cambridge: Cambridge University Press; 1996.
2. Schneider JF, Thomas HE, Kreger BE, McNamara PM, Sorlie P, Kannel WB. Newly acquired left bundle branch block: the Framingham Study. *Ann Intern Med.* 1980;92:37-44.
3. Vasey C, O'Donnell J, Morris S, McHenry P. Exercise-induced left bundle branch block and its relation to coronary artery disease. *Am J Cardiol.* 1985;56:892-895.
4. Moran JF, Scurlock B, Henkin R, Scanlon PJ. The clinical significance of exercise-induced bundle branch block. *J Electrocardiol.* 1992;25:229-235.
5. Bounhoure JP, Donzeau JP, Doazan JP, et al. Blocs de branche complets et cours des épreuves d'effort. *Arch Mal Coeur.* 1991;84:167-171.
6. Williams MA, Esterbrooks DJ, Nair CK, Sailors MM, Sketch MH. Clinical significance of exercise-induced bundle branch block. *Am J Cardiol.* 1988;61:346-348.
7. Boran KJ, Oliveros RA, Boulher CA, Beckmann CH, Seaworth JF. Ischemia-associated intraventricular conduction disturbances during exercise testing as a predictor of proximal left anterior descending coronary artery disease. *Am J Cardiol.* 1983;51:1098-1101.

Augmented ST-Segment Elevation During Recovery From Exercise Predicts Cardiac Events in Patients With Brugada Syndrome
Makimoto H, Nakagawa E, Takaki H, et al (Natl Cerebral and Cardiovascular Ctr, Suita, Japan; Osaka City General Hosp, Japan; et al)
J Am Coll Cardiol 56:1576-1584, 2010

Objectives.—The goal of this study was to evaluate the prevalence and the clinical significance of ST-segment elevation during recovery from exercise testing.

Background.—During recovery from exercise testing, ST-segment elevation is reported in some patients with Brugada syndrome (BrS).

Methods.—Treadmill exercise testing was conducted for 93 patients (91 men), 46 ± 14 years of age, with BrS (22 documented ventricular fibrillation, 35 syncope alone, and 36 asymptomatic); and for 102 healthy control subjects (97 men), 46 ± 17 years of age. Patients were routinely followed up. The clinical end point was defined as the occurrence of sudden cardiac death, ventricular fibrillation, or sustained ventricular tachyarrhythmia.

Results.—Augmentation of ST-segment elevation <0.05 mV in V_1 to V_3 leads compared with baseline was observed at early recovery (1 to 4 min at recovery) in 34 BrS patients (37% [group 1]), but was not observed in the remaining 59 BrS patients (63% [group 2]) or in the 102 control subjects. During 76 ± 38 months of follow-up, ventricular fibrillation occurred more frequently in group 1 (15 of 34, 44%) than in group 2 (10 of 59, 17%; $p = 0.004$). Multivariate Cox regression analysis showed that in addition to previous episodes of ventricular fibrillation ($p = 0.005$), augmentation of ST-segment elevation at early recovery was a significant and independent predictor for cardiac events ($p = 0.007$), especially among patients with history of syncope alone (6 of 12 [50%] in group 1 vs. 3 of 23 [13%] in group 2) and among asymptomatic patients (3 of 15 [20%] in group 1 vs. 0 of 21 [0%] in group 2).

Conclusions.—Augmentation of ST-segment elevation during recovery from exercise testing was specific in patients with BrS, and can be a predictor of poor prognosis, especially for patients with syncope alone and for asymptomatic patients (Fig 1).

▶ The Brugada syndrome is a genetically based condition associated with episodes of ventricular fibrillation and sudden unexplained cardiac death in young men.[1,2] It was first described by the Spanish cardiologist Brugada and is particularly prevalent in Asian males. In at least a proportion of cases, genetic anomalies affect the sodium pump and thus cardiac repolarization. Mutations in the genes controlling the calcium pump also cause ST elevation.[3] To date, it has

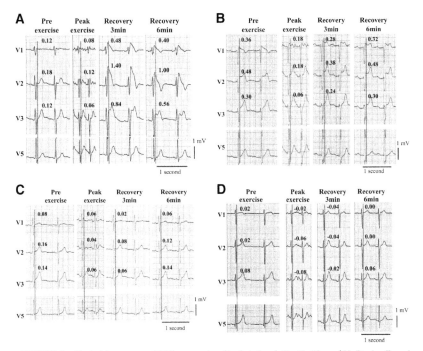

FIGURE 1.—Typical Responses of ST-Segment Amplitude in Leads V_1, V_2, V_3, and V_5 During Exercise Testing in Brugada Syndrome Patients. (**A**) In the group 1 Brugada patient showing saddle-back type ST-segment (lead V_2) at baseline, ST-segment amplitude slightly decreased at peak exercise, but reascended at early recovery (3 min), resulting in typical coved-type ST-segment elevation. (**B, C**) In the group 2 Brugada patient and (**D**) in the control subject, ST-segment amplitude decreased at peak exercise and gradually recovered to the baseline at recovery. It is noteworthy that the peak J-point amplitude in lead V_2 was augmented despite not showing ST-segment augmentation in **A** and **C**. The ST-segment amplitudes are shown as numeric values expressed in millivolts (mV). The **red vertical line** indicates the line from the end point of the QRS interval at electrocardiography lead V_5. For interpretation of the references to color in this figure legend, the reader is referred to web version of this article. (Reprinted from Makimoto H, Nakagawa E, Takaki H, et al. Augmented ST-segment elevation during recovery from exercise predicts cardiac events in patients with Brugada syndrome. *J Am Coll Cardiol.* 2010;56:1576-1584, with permission from the American College of Cardiology Foundation.)

been difficult to identify susceptible individuals prior to an attack of ventricular fibrillation. Makimoto and associates offer a long-term case-control study based on quite a moderately large series (93) of Japanese patients with the syndrome; 22 patients of their sample had previous episodes of ventricular fibrillation, and a further 35 had experienced episodes of syncope; the basis of diagnosis in the remaining patients is not specified, but it apparently included genetic testing. Because the patients were hospitalized, they were presumably relatively high-risk members of the Brugada population. Their recovery electrocardiograms were recorded following progressive treadmill testing to 90% of maximal heart rate. Augmented ST segmental elevation was observed in 34 of the 93 patients (Fig 1). There were relatively few adverse events (25) during the follow-up period. A history of ventricular fibrillation or aborted cardiac arrest was the strongest predictor of an adverse prognosis. However, multiple regression analysis showed that in a proportion of cases, ST elevation during exercise recovery was also a significant and independent predictor of future ventricular fibrillation.

R. J. Shephard, MD (Lond), PhD, DPE

References

1. Nademanee K, Veerakul G, Nimmannit S, et al. Arrhythmogenic marker for the sudden unexplained death syndrome in Thai men. *Circulation.* 1997;96: 2595-2600.
2. Vatta M, Dumaine R, Varghese G, et al. Genetic and biophysical basis of sudden unexplained nocturnal death syndrome (SUNDS), a disease allelic to Brugada syndrome. *Hum Mol Genet.* 2002;11:337-345.
3. Antzelevitch C. Genetic basis of Brugada syndrome. *Heart Rhythm.* 2007;4: 756-757.

Effect of Atrial Fibrillation on Outcome in Patients With Known or Suspected Coronary Artery Disease Referred for Exercise Stress Testing
Bouzas-Mosquera A, Peteiro J, Broullón FJ, et al (Hospital Universitario A Coruña, Spain)
Am J Cardiol 105:1207-1211, 2010

The association of atrial fibrillation (AF) with coronary artery disease (CAD) remains controversial. In addition, the relation of AF to myocardial ischemia and outcomes in patients with known or suspected CAD referred for exercise stress testing has been poorly explored. In this study, 17,100 patients aged ≥50 years with known or suspected CAD who underwent exercise electrocardiography (n = 11,911) or exercise echocardiography (n = 5,189) were evaluated. End points were all-cause mortality, nonfatal myocardial infarction, and coronary revascularization. Overall, 619 patients presented with AF at the time of the tests. Patients with AF who had interpretable electrocardiograms had a lower likelihood of exercise-induced ischemic ST-segment abnormalities (adjusted odds ratio 0.51, 95% confidence interval 0.34 to 0.76, p = 0.001), and those with

AF who underwent exercise echocardiography had a lower likelihood of new or worsening exercise-induced wall motion abnormalities (adjusted odds ratio 0.62, 95% confidence interval 0.44 to 0.87, p = 0.006). During a mean follow-up period of 6.5 ± 3.9 years, 2,364 patients died, 1,311 had nonfatal myocardial infarctions, 1,615 underwent percutaneous coronary intervention, and 922 underwent coronary artery bypass surgery. The 10-year mortality rate was 43% in patients with AF compared to 19% in those without AF (p <0.001). In multivariate analysis, AF remained an independent predictor of all-cause mortality (adjusted hazard ratio 1.45, 95% confidence interval 1.20 to 1.76, p <0.001), but not of nonfatal myocardial infarction or coronary revascularization. In conclusion, despite being associated with an apparently lower likelihood of myocardial ischemia, AF was an independent predictor of all-cause mortality in patients with known or suspected CAD referred for exercise stress testing (Fig 1).

▶ Previous reports have suggested that the prognosis of coronary arterial disease is worsened if there is coexistent atrial fibrillation.[1,2] This report, based on retrospective analysis of a very large sample of patients followed over a period of 10 years, supports this view. During their initial exercise test, patients with atrial fibrillation had less risk of demonstrating ST depression or wall motion anomalies than those individuals with a normal heart rhythm, perhaps because those with fibrillation were referred for exercise testing sooner than was the case for patients with a normal cardiac rhythm. On the other hand,

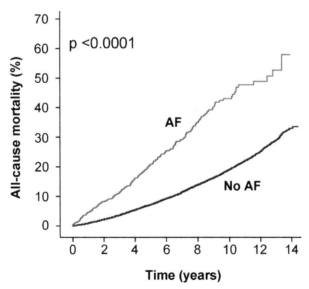

FIGURE 1.—All-cause mortality curves in patients with and without AF. (Reprinted from Bouzas-Mosquera A, Peteiro J, Broullón FJ, et al. Effect of atrial fibrillation on outcome in patients with known or suspected coronary artery disease referred for exercise stress testing. *Am J Cardiol.* 2010;105:1207-1211, with permission from Elsevier.)

over a 10-year follow-up, all-cause mortality (but not the risk of nonfatal infarctions) was substantially worsened if the patient also had atrial fibrillation (Fig 1). The authors stress a number of limitations in their findings, particularly the fact that relatively few patients underwent angiography subsequent to exercise testing and the possible influence of atrial fibrillation on the chronotropic response to exercise and thus the interpretation of the exercise tests. Plainly, there remains scope for further study of this issue.

R. J. Shephard, MD (Lond), PhD, DPE

References

1. Cameron A, Schwartz MJ, Kronmal RA, Kosinski AS. Prevalence and significance of atrial fibrillation in coronary artery disease (CASS registry). *Am J Cardiol.* 1988;61:714-717.
2. Marte T, Saely CH, Schmid F, Koch L, Drexel H. Effectiveness of atrial fibrillation as an independent predictor of death and coronary events in patients having coronary angiography. *Am J Cardiol.* 2009;103:36-40.

Can low risk cardiac patients be 'fast tracked' to Phase IV community exercise schemes for cardiac rehabilitation? A randomised controlled trial
Robinson HJ, Samani NJ, Singh SJ (Univ Hosps of Leicester NHS Trust, England, UK; Univ of Leicester, England, UK)
Int J Cardiol 146:159-163, 2011

Background.—A prospective single blinded randomised controlled trial within a university hospital NHS Trust was undertaken to determine if fast tracking low risk cardiac rehabilitation patients, under the supervision of an exercise instructor, is superior in the medium term to conventional service delivery.

Methods.—100 low risk cardiac rehabilitation patients were randomised to either a conventional Phase III hospital group or to a fast-tracked group in a community scheme led by an exercise instructor. Both groups undertook once weekly supervised exercise sessions for the duration of six weeks. Both groups were also encouraged to continue with Phase IV and were reassessed at six months. The primary outcome measure was Incremental Shuttle Walking Test (ISWT) distance. Secondary health related quality of life measures were also analysed.

Results.—ISWT distance statistically significantly increased over time ($f = 26.80$, $p < 0.001$) for both groups. No between group differences were observed ($f = 0.03$, $p = 0.87$). All domains of the MacNew quality of life questionnaire and five domains of the Short Form 36 showed statistical mean score improvements over time ($p < 0.05$). Continued attendance at Phase IV at six months was statistically significantly higher in the fast track group ($p = 0.04$). At six months all attendees of Phase IV had a clinically and statistically significant mean improvement in ISWT distance in comparison to non-attendees (mean difference 40.38 m, 95%CI 4.20 to 76.57, $p = 0.03$).

TABLE 2.—Incremental Shuttle Walking Test Distance Data

	Pre Rehabilitation	Post Rehabilitation	Six-Month Follow-Up
Hospital	618.22 (165.09)	676.44 (176.84)***	672.00 (177.55)***
Fast track	617.95 (136.90)	677.50 (161.78)***	687.73 (168.26)***

All values expressed as mean metres (SD).
***significant main effect for time from baseline $p < 0.001$.

Conclusions.—The fast track service model of cardiac rehabilitation is effective and offers the additional benefit of greater medium term adherence to exercise (Table 2).

▶ The Toronto cardiac rehabilitation program was long unique in allowing phase III patients to follow supervised exercise sessions once weekly, completing a carefully devised home prescription on the remaining days of the week.[1] We argued that in a major city such as Toronto, the time and hassle involved in daily or thrice-weekly travel to a medically supervised rehabilitation facility provided a negative incentive to program compliance. Compliance rates with our program were unusually high (82.8% engaging in at least 3 sessions per week for 2 years[2,3]), in part because of the reduced commitment of time to driving in heavy traffic. The study of Robinson et al is also based on once-weekly rather than thrice-weekly sessions of exercise, although the phase III classes continued for only 6 weeks, rather than the typical 3 months of a phase III program. Travel demands in the fast-track group were further reduced by arranging local exercise classes, supervised by British Association for Cardiac Rehabilitation—certified exercise instructors. The main criterion of the relative success of the 2 approaches was a simple field test of aerobic power, the incremental shuttle run. Immediate gains on this measure were comparable between hospital and community-based rehabilitation groups, and at 6 months the fast-track community-based group actually had a superior performance (Table 2), associated with a greater continuing program compliance. These observations reinforce the issue that the imposition of unnecessary travel requirements has a negative effect on exercise participation; where possible, exercise should be built into community life. Nevertheless, the authors of this report excluded some 80% of their patients from the randomized trial, and there is a need to see whether a higher proportion of cardiac patients could follow the same fast-track route. Furthermore, the gain in estimated maximal oxygen intake (0.6 metabolic equivalents) at 6 months was only of the order seen in a similar US program[4] and was very modest relative to the gains shown to be possible in some of the patients in Toronto.[2] Can a community-based program eventually realize similar gains without risk to the patient?

R. J. Shephard, MD (Lond), PhD, DPE

References

1. Kavanagh T, Shephard RJ, Doney H, Pandit V. Intensive exercise in coronary rehabilitation. *Med Sci Sports.* 1973;5:34-39.

2. Shephard RJ. *Ischemic Heart Disease and Exercise*. London, UK: Croom Helm; 1981.
3. Shephard RJ, Corey P, Kavanagh T. Exercise compliance and the prevention of recurrence myocardial infarction. *Med Sci Sports Exerc*. 1981;13:1-5.
4. Carlson JJ, Johnson JA, Franklin BA, VanderLaan RL. Program participation, exercise adherence, cardiovascular outcomes and program cost of traditional versus modified cardiac rehabilitation. *Am J Cardiol*. 2000;86:17-23.

Longer Time Spent in Light Physical Activity Is Associated With Reduced Arterial Stiffness in Older Adults

Gando Y, Yamamoto K, Murakami H, et al (Natl Inst of Health and Nutrition, Tokyo, Japan; et al)
Hypertension 56:540-546, 2010

Habitual moderate-to-vigorous—intensity physical activity attenuates arterial stiffening. However, it is unclear whether light physical activity also attenuates arterial stiffening. It is also unclear whether light physical activity has the same effects in fit and unfit individuals. This cross-sectional study was performed to determine the relationships between amount of light physical activity determined with a triaxial accelerometer and arterial stiffness. A total of 538 healthy men and women participated in this study. Subjects in each age category were divided into either high-light or low-light physical activity groups based on daily time spent in light physical activity. Arterial stiffness was measured by carotid-femoral pulse wave velocity. Two-way ANOVA indicated a significant interaction between age and time spent in light physical activity in determining carotid-femoral pulse wave velocity ($P < 0.05$). In the older group, carotid femoral pulse wave velocity was higher in the low-light physical activity level group than in the high-light physical activity level group (945 ± 19 versus 882 ± 16 cm/s; $P < 0.01$). The difference remained significant after normalizing carotid-femoral pulse wave velocity for amounts of moderate and vigorous physical activity. The carotid-femoral pulse wave velocity ($r = -0.47$; $P < 0.01$) was correlated with daily time spent in light physical activity in older unfit subjects. No relationship was observed in older fit subjects. These results suggested that longer time spent in light physical activity is associated with attenuation of arterial stiffening, especially in unfit older people (Fig 2).

▶ We have previously demonstrated[1] a graded relationship between the stiffness of the central elastic vessels (but not the peripheral arteries) in an elderly free-living Japanese population aged 65 to 85 years; others, also, have noted such an association in younger populations.[2,3] In our study, the association was relatively weak, and the optimal elasticity was observed in subjects who recorded a daily step count of greater than 6600 and/or engaged in more than 16 minutes of activity per day at an intensity greater than 3 metabolic equivalents (METs) (moderately vigorous exercise for this age group). This study is interesting in demonstrating a cross-sectional association between

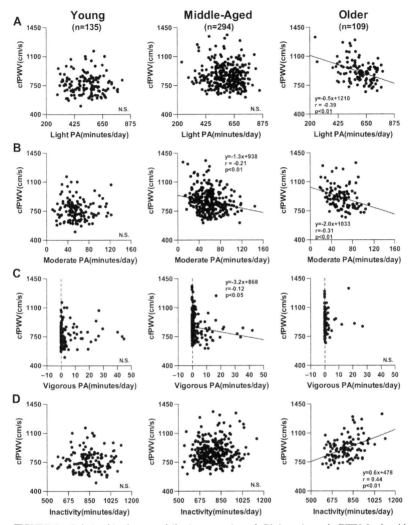

FIGURE 2.—Relationships between daily time spent in each PA intensity and cfPWV. In the older group, cfPWV was significantly related to the daily time spent in light PA ($r=-0.39$; $P<0.01$), moderate PA ($r=-0.31$; $P<0.01$), and inactivity ($r=0.44$; $P<0.01$). (Reprinted from Gando Y, Yamamoto K, Murakami H, et al. Longer time spent in light physical activity is associated with reduced arterial stiffness in older adults. *Hypertension.* 2010;56:540-546.)

central arterial elasticity and involvement in very light physical activity (less than 3 METs) (Fig 2). Gando and associates argue that this may not have been seen before because earlier studies were based either on questionnaire assessments of physical activity or the use of uniaxial accelerometers (which have difficulty in capturing light activities performed with the arms). A further factor may be the fitness of the subjects examined because the association is seen mainly in elderly and unfit subjects. Given the cross-sectional nature of this study, it remains unclear whether there is an immediate effect from the light activity or whether it is serving as a marker of more vigorous activity at a younger age. However, the practical message for the unfit elderly seems that any amount of physical activity is better than none.

R. J. Shephard, MD (Lond), PhD, DPE

References

1. Aoyagi Y, Park H, Kakiyama T, Park S, Yoshiuchi K, Shephard RJ. Yearlong physical activity and regional stiffness of arteries in older adults: the Nakanojo Study. *Eur J Appl Physiol.* 2010;109:455-464.
2. Sugawara J, Otsuki T, Tanabe T, Hayashi K, Maeda S, Matsuda M. Physical activity duration, intensity, and arterial stiffening in postmenopausal women. *Am J Hypertens.* 2006;19:1032-1036.
3. Kozakova M, Palombo C, Mhamdi L, Konrad T, Nilsson P, Staehr PB, et al. Habitual physical activity and vascular aging in a young to middle-age population at low cardiovascular risk. *Stroke.* 2007;38:2549-2555.

The effects of aerobic interval training on the left ventricular morphology and function of VLCAD-deficient mice
Riggs CE Jr, Michaelides MA, Parpa KM, et al (Univ of Arkansas, Fayetteville)
Eur J Appl Physiol 110:915-923, 2010

This study examined the effect of aerobic interval training on cardiac adaptations in VLCAD-deficient mice and determined the effects of the deficiency on the morphology and function of the left ventricle among 53 knockout homozygous VLCAD−/−, 28 heterozygous VLCAD ±, and 39 controls VLCAD+/+ male mice (129 SvJ/C57BL6). Echocardiographic images were used to determine the left ventricular (LV) wall thicknesses, during systole and diastole, acquired at a depth setting of 20 mm. Cardiac hypertrophy (as evidenced by increased wall thickness, and decreased left ventricular dimension in diastole and systole) appeared to be a major finding in the VLCAD−/− mouse with, however, normal %FS. The trained mice from all three genotypes exhibited lower body weight compared with their controls. The echocardiographic data of this study demonstrated structural but not functional differences among the three genotypes. This study demonstrated that VLCAD ± deficient mice handled interval training similarly to the non-deficient mice. Four VLCAD−/− deficient mice died unexpectedly on the treadmill during the early stages of training. The VLCAD−/− deficient mice that survived adapted to the aerobic interval training similarly to the non-deficient mice. It is unclear whether aerobic interval training is an appropriate training tool for the VLCAD-deficient humans (Table 2).

▶ In humans, very long chain acyl-CoA dehydrogenase (VLCAD) deficiency invariably leads to cardiac abnormalities, sometimes dilated cardiomyopathy and sometimes hypertrophic cardiomyopathy,[1] often with ventricular tachycardia during exercise and other forms of sympathetic stimulation.[2] This is an

TABLE 2.—Descriptive Statistics and Cardiac Measurements

Genotype	VLCAD−/−		VLCAD−/+		VLCAD+/+	
	Trained	Control	Trained	Control	Trained	Control
Variable	$n = 25$	$n = 28$	$n = 18$	$n = 10$	$n = 25$	$n = 14$
HR (bpm)	572 ± 64	583 ± 60	581 ± 51	561 ± 79	547 ± 82	528 ± 50
Wt (g)	27.55 ± 2.19	30.05 ± 3.60	26.68 ± 2.60	31.37 ± 3.26	24.51 ± 2.72	25.49 ± 2.13
HWt (g)	0.18 ± 0.02	0.17 ± 0.01	0.17 ± 0.02	0.16 ± 0.01	0.15 ± 0.02	0.14 ± 0.02
IVSd (cm)	0.14 ± 0.03	0.14 ± 0.03	0.12 ± 0.03	0.12 ± 0.03	0.10 ± 0.03	0.12 ± 0.04
LVIDd (cm)	0.28 ± 0.04	0.26 ± 0.05	0.31 ± 0.03	0.31 ± 0.04	0.32 ± 0.04	0.30 ± 0.04
LVPWd (cm)	0.12 ± 0.03	0.12 ± 0.03	0.10 ± 0.02	0.10 ± 0.03	0.09 ± 0.03	0.10 ± 0.03
IVSs (cm)	0.20 ± 0.03	0.20 ± 0.03	0.19 ± 0.03	0.18 ± 0.04	0.17 ± 0.03	0.18 ± 0.05
LVIDs (cm)	0.13 ± 0.05	0.13 ± 0.04	0.15 ± 0.05	0.15 ± 0.05	0.16 ± 0.06	0.16 ± 0.06
LVPWs (cm)	0.18 ± 0.03	0.18 ± 0.04	0.16 ± 0.04	0.15 ± 0.05	0.15 ± 0.04	0.15 ± 0.04
COI (cc/min)	11.00 ± 4.89	10.13 ± 5.96	15.19 ± 4.77	14.98 ± 6.15	14.88 ± 5.23	12.17 ± 3.55
FS% (%)	56 ± 12	53 ± 14	52 ± 14	49 ± 17	51 ± 14	47 ± 15
HWT/BW	0.58 ± 0.02	0.55 ± 0.07	0.56 ± 0.05	0.56 ± 0.03	0.62 ± 0.09	0.58 ± 0.09
LVMd (g)	0.13 ± 0.04	0.13 ± 0.03	0.12 ± 0.03	0.12 ± 0.03	0.11 ± 0.03	0.12 ± 0.04
LVMs (g)	0.11 ± 0.06	0.10 ± 0.05	0.13 ± 0.07	0.12 ± 0.07	0.14 ± 0.09	0.14 ± 0.10

Data are mean ± SD

COI cardiac output index, *FS%* fractional shortening, *HR* heart rate, *IVS* intraventricular septum, *LV* left ventricular, *LVID* LV internal dimension, *LVM* LV mass, *LVPW* LV posterior wall, *s* systolic, *d* diastolic, *bpm* beats per minute, *cm* centimeters, *g* grams, *EF* ejection fraction, *HWt* heart weight, *HWT/BW* heart-to-bodyweight.

interesting study because one would certainly be nervous about assessing the response of humans with known hypertrophic cardiomyopathy to various types of physical training; likely responses can be inferred from the study of genetically manipulated mice, although there is no guarantee that humans would have responded in identical fashion. One reason for caution is that the difference in heart weight between normal and VLCAD-deficient mice was relatively small (about 9%; Table 2). Moreover, it was necessary to conduct echocardiography under anesthesia, and this is likely to have modified cardiac function. Although, in general, the VLCAD-deficient mice seemed to respond quite well to aerobic interval training (enforced treadmill running), 4 of 29 animals died during training; this would plainly be an unacceptable mortality rate for a human experiment.

R. J. Shephard, MD (Lond), PhD, DPE

References

1. Mathur A, Sims HF, Gopalakrishnan D, et al. Molecular heterogeneity in very-long-chain acyl-CoA dehydrogenase deficiency causing pediatric cardiomyopathy and sudden death. *Circulation.* 1999;99:1337-1343.
2. Exil VJ, Roberts RL, Sims H, et al. Very-long-chain acyl-coenzyme a dehydrogenase deficiency in mice. *Circ Res.* 2003;93:448-455.

Physical Activity and Albuminuria

Robinson ES, Fisher ND, Forman JP, et al (Brigham and Women's Hosp, Boston, MA)
Am J Epidemiol 171:515-521, 2010

Higher urinary albumin excretion predicts future cardiovascular disease, hypertension, and chronic kidney disease. Physical activity improves endothelial function so activity may reduce albuminuria. Among diabetics, physical activity decreases albuminuria. In nondiabetics, prior studies have shown no association. The authors explored the cross-sectional association between physical activity and albuminuria in 3,587 nondiabetic women in 2 US cohorts, the Nurses' Health Study I in 2000 and the Nurses' Health Study II in 1997. Physical activity was expressed as metabolic equivalents per week. The outcome was the top albumin/creatinine ratio (ACR) decile. Multivariate logistic regression was used. Secondary analyses explored the ACR association with strenuous activity and walking. The mean age was 58.6 years. Compared with women in the lowest physical activity quintile, those in the highest quintile had a multivariate-adjusted odds ratio for the top ACR decile of 0.65 (95% confidence interval (CI): 0.46, 0.93). The multivariate-adjusted odds ratio for the top ACR decile for those with greater than 210 minutes per week of strenuous activity compared with no strenuous activity was 0.61 (95% CI: 0.37, 0.99), and for those in the highest quintile of walking compared with the lowest quintile, it was 0.69 (95% CI: 0.47, 1.02). Greater physical activity is associated with a lower ACR in nondiabetic women (Table 3).

▶ Proteinuria is well recognized as an accompaniment of vigorous exercise. However, the chronic excretion of albumin is a sign of cardiovascular disease and associated deterioration in renal function.[1-3] One might anticipate that regular physical activity would reduce the risk of cardiovascular disease and thus the likelihood of chronic proteinuria. Perhaps because of weaknesses in

TABLE 3.—Age- and Multivariate-adjusted Odds Ratio of Being in the Top Decile of the Albumin/Creatinine Ratio by Category of Strenuous Activity in the Nurses' Health Study I, United States, 2000, and the Nurses' Health Study II, United States, 1997

	None (n = 1,618)	Categories of Strenuous Activity, minutes/week							
		>0−60 (n = 616)		>60−120 (n = 423)		>120−210 (n = 370)		>210 (n = 287)	
Cases, no.	187	616		38		28		20	
	Odds Ratio (Referent)	Odds Ratio	95% Confidence Interval	Odds Ratio	95% Confidence Interval	Odds Ratio	95% Confidence Interval	Odds Ratio	95% Confidence Interval
Age adjusted	1.0	0.84	0.61, 1.14	0.78	0.54, 1.12	0.64	0.42, 0.97	0.59	0.37, 0.96
Multivariate adjusted[a]	1.0	0.84	0.62, 1.15	0.77	0.53, 1.11	0.66	0.44, 1.01	0.61	0.37, 0.99

[a]Adjusted for age, estimated glomerular filtration rate, body mass index, hypertension, smoking, and walking.

the physical activity assessment, previous studies failed to show such an association,[4,5] but this has now been demonstrated in an analysis of results from the US Nurses Health Study, particularly when data are classed in terms of the minutes per week spent in strenuous physical activity (Table 3). The authors attribute benefit to the maintenance of endothelial function in active individuals. An albumin excretion as low as 5 mg/g of creatinine is a warning sign of vascular disease, hypertension, major cardiovascular events, and all-cause mortality.

R. J. Shephard, MD (Lond), PhD, DPE

References

1. Gerstein HC, Mann JF, Yi Q, et al. Albuminuria and risk of cardiovascular events, death, and heart failure in diabetic and nondiabetic individuals. *JAMA.* 2001;286: 421-426.
2. Forman JP, Fisher ND, Schopick EL, Curhan GC. Higher levels of albuminuria within the normal range predict incident hypertension. *J Am Soc Nephrol.* 2008;19:1983-1988.
3. Klausen K, Borch-Johnsen K, Feldt-Rasmussen B, et al. Very low levels of micro-albuminuria are associated with increased risk of coronary heart disease and death independently of renal. *Am J Epidemiol.* 2010;171:515-521.
4. Finkelstein J, Joshi A, Hise MK. Association of physical activity and renal function in subjects with and without metabolic syndrome: a review of the Third National Health and Nutrition Examination Survey (NHANES III). *Am J Kidney Dis.* 2006; 48:372-382.
5. Metcalf PA, Baker JR, Scragg RK, Dryson E, Scott AJ, Wild CJ. Albuminuria in people at least 40 years old: effect of alcohol consumption, regular exercise, and cigarette smoking. *Clin Chem.* 1993;39:1793-1797.

Metabolic Modulator Perhexiline Corrects Energy Deficiency and Improves Exercise Capacity in Symptomatic Hypertrophic Cardiomyopathy
Abozguia K, Elliott P, McKenna W, et al (Univ of Birmingham, Edgbaston, UK; Univ College London Hosps, UK; et al)
Circulation 122:1562-1569, 2010

Background.—Hypertrophic cardiomyopathy patients exhibit myocardial energetic impairment, but a causative role for this energy deficiency in the pathophysiology of hypertrophic cardiomyopathy remains unproven. We hypothesized that the metabolic modulator perhexiline would ameliorate myocardial energy deficiency and thereby improve diastolic function and exercise capacity.

Methods and Results.—Forty-six consecutive patients with symptomatic exercise limitation (peak $\dot{V}_{O_2}$ <75% of predicted) caused by nonobstructive hypertrophic cardiomyopathy (mean age, 55 ± 0.26 years) were randomized to perhexiline 100 mg (n = 24) or placebo (n = 22). Myocardial ratio of phosphocreatine to adenosine triphosphate, an established marker of cardiac energetic status, as measured by P magnetic resonance spectroscopy, left ventricular diastolic filling (heart rate normalized time to peak filling) at rest and during exercise using radionuclide ventriculography, peak $\dot{V}_{O_2}$, symptoms, quality of life, and serum metabolites were assessed at baseline and study end (4.6 ± 1.8 months). Perhexiline improved myocardial ratios of phosphocreatine to adenosine triphosphate (from 1.27 ± 0.02 to 1.73 ± 0.02 versus 1.29 ± 0.01 to 1.23 ± 0.01; $P = 0.003$) and normalized the abnormal prolongation of heart rate normalized time to peak filling between rest and exercise (0.11 ± 0.008 to -0.01 ± 0.005 versus 0.15 ± 0.007 to 0.11 ± 0.008 second; $P = 0.03$). These changes were accompanied by an improvement in primary end point (peak $\dot{V}_{O_2}$) (22.2 ± 0.2 to 24.3 ± 0.2 versus 23.6 ± 0.3 to 22.3 ± 0.2 mL $\cdot$ kg^{-1} $\cdot$ min^{-1}; $P = 0.003$) and New York Heart Association class ($P < 0.001$) (all P values ANCOVA, perhexiline versus placebo).

Conclusions.—In symptomatic hypertrophic cardiomyopathy, perhexiline, a modulator of substrate metabolism, ameliorates cardiac energetic impairment, corrects diastolic dysfunction, and increases exercise capacity. This study supports the hypothesis that energy deficiency contributes to the pathophysiology and provides a rationale for further consideration of metabolic therapies in hypertrophic cardiomyopathy.

Clinical Trial Registration.—URL: http://www.clinicaltrials.gov. Unique identifier: NCT00500552 (Table 2).

▶ One of the interesting aspects of hypertrophic cardiomyopathy is the range of genetic abnormalities found in those affected by this group of disorders; more than 400 mutations have been implicated.[1] In about one-third of cases, there is an outflow obstruction that is susceptible to surgical correction.[2] However, in some cases, the problem seems an excessive use of energy by the cardiac sarcomeres, with an associated slowing of diastolic relaxation.[3] The drug perhexiline is thought to increase metabolic efficiency by shifting the metabolism

TABLE 2.—Effects of Placebo and Perhexiline on Metabolic Exercise Parameters, Myocardial Energetic, Symptomatic Status, and LV Systolic Function at Rest and During Exercise

Parameter	Perhexiline Group Baseline	Perhexiline Group Follow-Up	Placebo Group Baseline	Placebo Group Follow-Up	P, ANCOVA
Metabolic exercise parameters					
Peak $\dot{V}_{O_2}$, mL $\cdot$ kg^{-1} $\cdot$ min^{-1}	22.2 ± 0.2	24.3 ± 0.2	23.6 ± 0.3	22.3 ± 0.2	0.003*
$\dot{V}_{O_2}$-AT, mL $\cdot$ kg^{-1} $\cdot$ min^{-1}	16 ± 0.11	15 ± 0.1	17 ± 0.23	16 ± 0.15	0.85
$\dot{V}_E / \dot{V}_{CO_2}$ slope	30 ± 0.12	32 ± 0.12	30 ± 0.23	32 ± 0.3	0.99
Myocardial energetic status					
PCr/ATP ratio	1.27 ± 0.02	1.73 ± 0.02	1.29 ± 0.01	1.23 ± 0.01	0.003*
Symptomatic status					
MLHFQ score	36 ± 0.94	28 ± 0.75	37 ± 1.21	34 ± 1.25	<0.001*
LV systolic function (at rest and during exercise), %[†]					
Resting EF	68 ± 0.51	67 ± 0.49	66 ± 0.46	65 ± 0.42	0.22
Exercise EF	72 ± 0.75	69 ± 0.45	73 ± 0.56	75 ± 0.39	0.07

AT indicates anaerobic threshold; $\dot{V}_E / \dot{V}_{CO_2}$ slope, minute ventilation–carbon dioxide production relationship; MLHFQ, Minnesota Living With Heart Failure Questionnaire; and EF, ejection fraction. ANCOVA P values represent the significant difference between perhexiline and placebo responses.
* Statistically significant.
[†] Measured with radionuclide ventriculography.

of the heart muscle to the consumption of carbohydrates.[4] This randomized controlled trial supports the use of this type of drug therapy in appropriate cases, showing a normalization of the phosphocreatine/adenosine triphosphate ratio and the diastolic filling time, with a clinically significant improvement of aerobic power in response to the administration of perhexiline (100 mg/d) (Table 2). Quality of life was improved for those receiving the active treatment, although longer studies will be needed to evaluate any changes in prognosis.

R. J. Shephard, MD (Lond), PhD, DPE

References

1. Seidman JG, Seidman C. The genetic basis for cardiomyopathy; from mutation identification to mechanistic paradigms. *Cell.* 2001;104:557-567.
2. Sorraja JJ, Valeti U, Nishimura RA, et al. Outcome of alcoholic septal ablation for obstructive hypertrophic cardiomyopathy. *Circulation.* 2008;118:131-139.
3. Ashrafian H, Redwood C, Blair E, Watkins H. Hypertrophic cardiomyopathy; a paradigm for myocardial energy depletion. *Trends Genet.* 2003;19:263-268.
4. Jeffrey FM, Alvarez L, Diczku V, Sherry AD, Malloy CR. Direct evidence that perhexiline modifies myocardial substrate utilization from fatty acids to lactate. *J Cardiovasc Pharmacol.* 1995;25:469-472.

Occupational, Commuting, and Leisure-Time Physical Activity in Relation to Heart Failure Among Finnish Men and Women

Wang Y, Tuomilehto J, Jousilahti P, et al (Pennington Biomedical Res Ctr, Baton Rouge, LA; Univ of Helsinki, Finland; Natl Inst for Health and Welfare, Helsinki, Finland; et al)
J Am Coll Cardiol 56:1140-1148, 2010

Objectives.—The purpose of this study was to examine the association of different levels of occupational, commuting, and leisure-time physical activity and heart failure (HF) risk.

Background.—The role of different types of physical activity in explaining the risk of HF is not properly established.

Methods.—Study cohorts included 28,334 Finnish men and 29,874 women who were 25 to 74 years of age and free of HF at baseline. Baseline measurement of different types of physical activity was used to predict incident HF.

Results.—During a mean follow-up of 18.4 years, HF developed in 1,868 men and 1,640 women. The multivariate adjusted (age; smoking; education; alcohol consumption; body mass index; systolic blood pressure; total cholesterol; history of myocardial infarction, valvular heart disease, diabetes, lung disease, and use of antihypertensive drugs; and other types of physical activity) hazard ratios of HF associated with light, moderate, and active occupational activity were 1.00, 0.90, and 0.83 (p = 0.005, for trend) for men and 1.00, 0.80, and 0.92 (p = 0.007, for trend) for women, respectively. The multivariate adjusted hazard ratios of HF associated with low, moderate, and high leisure-time physical activity were 1.00, 0.83, and 0.65 (p < 0.001, for trend) for men and

1.00, 0.84, and 0.75 (p < 0.001, for trend) for women, respectively. Active commuting had a significant inverse association with HF risk in women, but not in men, before adjustment for occupational and leisure-time physical activity. The joint effects of any 2 types of physical activity on HF risk were even greater.

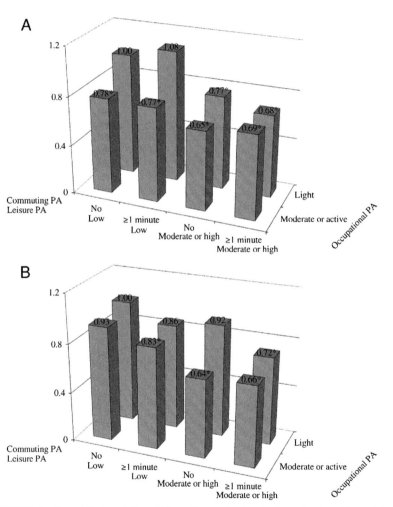

FIGURE 1.—Hazard Ratios of Heart Failure. Bar graphs showing hazard ratios of heart failure according to joint categories of occupational, commuting, and leisure-time physical activity (PA) among (A) men and (B) women, adjusted for age, study year, education, smoking, alcohol consumption, history of myocardial infarction, history of valvular heart disease, history of diabetes, history of using antihypertensive drugs, history of lung disease, body mass index, systolic blood pressure, and total cholesterol. *p < 0.05. (Reprinted from the Journal of the American College of Cardiology, Wang Y, Tuomilehto J, Jousilahti P, et al. Occupational, commuting, and leisure-time physical activity in relation to heart failure among Finnish men and women. *J Am Coll Cardiol.* 2010;56:1140-1148. Copyright 2010, with permission from the American College of Cardiology.)

Conclusions.—Moderate and high levels of occupational or leisure-time physical activity are associated with a reduced risk of HF (Fig 1).

▶ The long-term cardiovascular outcome of habitual physical activity has usually been assessed in terms of deaths from ischemic heart disease or overall mortality, but given the prevalence of heart failure (currently 5 million cases in the United States alone[1]), this also seems an important yardstick. The report of Wang and associates covers a very large sample of Finnish men and women over a very long follow-up period averaging more than 18 years. Although there have been few previous studies, they have focused simply on leisure activity, and the results have been inconsistent.[2-4] The present investigation looks at each leisure, occupational, and commuting activity alone and in combination (Fig 1). Assessments were based on a self-administered questionnaire (applied only once, at baseline), with the upper 2 levels of commuting reflecting 1 to 29 minutes and more than 30 minutes of cycling or walking per day. In contrast to North America, a large proportion of those surveyed engaged in some active commuting. Leisure and occupational activity had a significant impact on the risk of future heart failure in both sexes, but commuting activity had a significant influence only in women. This may be because the relative cost of cycling and walking tends to be somewhat greater in women than in men, and commuting is thus more likely to modify a woman's fitness level. The significant influence of occupational activity in both men and women implies that the risk of heart failure will increase in the future unless the population can be persuaded to replace diminishing occupational activity by more physically active leisure pursuits.

R. J. Shephard, MD (Lond), PhD, DPE

References

1. Schocken DD, Benjamin EJ, Fonarow GC, et al. Prevention of heart failure: a scientific statement from the American Heart Association Councils on Epidemiology and Prevention, Clinical Cardiology, Cardiovascular Nursing, and High Blood Pressure Research; Quality of Care and Outcomes Research Interdisciplinary Working Group; and Functional Genomics and Translational Biology Interdisciplinary Working Group. *Circulation.* 2008;117:2544-2565.
2. He J, Ogden LG, Bazzano LA, Vupputuri S, Loria C, Whelton PK. Risk factors for congestive heart failure in US men and women: NHANES I epidemiologic follow-up study. *Arch Intern Med.* 2001;161:996-1002.
3. Kenchaiah S, Sesso HD, Gaziano JM. Body mass index and vigorous physical activity and the risk of heart failure among men. *Circulation.* 2009;119:44-52.
4. Djoussé L, Driver JA, Gaziano JM. Relation between modifiable lifestyle factors and lifetime risk of heart failure. *JAMA.* 2009;302:394-400.

Physical Activity and Onset of Acute Ischemic Stroke: The Stroke Onset Study

Mostofsky E, Laier E, Levitan EB, et al (Beth Israel Deaconess Med Ctr, Boston, MA; et al)
Am J Epidemiol 173:330-336, 2011

Regular physical activity is known to decrease the risk of cardiovascular disease, but the risk of ischemic stroke immediately following moderate or vigorous physical activity remains unclear. The authors evaluated the risk of acute ischemic stroke immediately following physical activity and examined whether the risk was modified by regular physical activity. In a multicenter case-crossover study, the authors interviewed 390 ischemic stroke patients (209 men, 181 women) at 3 North American hospitals between January 2001 and November 2006. Physical activity during the hour before stroke symptoms arose was compared with usual frequency of physical activity over the prior year. Of the 390 subjects, 21 (5%) reported having engaged in moderate or vigorous physical activity during the hour before ischemic stroke onset, and 6 subjects had lifted an object weighing at least 50 pounds ($\geq$23 kg) during that hour. The rate ratio for ischemic stroke was 2.3 (95% confidence interval (CI): 1.5, 3.7; $P < 0.001$)

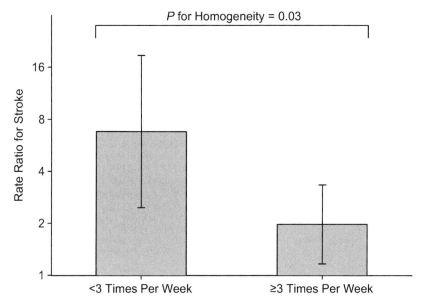

FIGURE 1.—Impact of habitual physical activity on the rate ratio for stroke onset following an isolated bout of moderate or vigorous physical activity, Stroke Onset Study, 2001–2006. Bars, 95% confidence interval. (Reprinted from Mostofsky E, Laier E, Levitan EB, et al. Physical activity and onset of acute ischemic stroke: the stroke onset study. *Am J Epidemiol.* 2011;173(3):330-336, by permission of Oxford University Press.)

for moderate or vigorous physical activity in the previous hour and 2.6 (95% CI: 1.1, 5.9; $P = 0.02$) for lifting 50 pounds or more. People who reported engaging in moderate or vigorous physical activity at least 3 times per week experienced a 2-fold increased risk (95% CI: 1.2, 3.3) with each bout of physical activity, as compared with a 6.8-fold risk (95% CI: 2.5, 18.8) among more sedentary subjects (P for homogeneity $= 0.03$) (Fig 1).

▶ Stroke risk is reduced among physically active compared with inactive populations,[1,2] but little is known about the acute risk of ischemic stroke onset following physical activity in trained and untrained individuals. Each bout of physical activity causes increased sympathetic nervous system activity, heart rate, and systolic blood pressure, and individuals at risk for stroke may experience stroke onset during or soon after physical activity. This study showed that isolated episodes of physical activity transiently increased the risk of ischemic stroke, but that this risk was greatly attenuated by habitual physical activity (Fig 1). This study reinforces the importance of habitual physical activity in preventing stroke both before and after physical activity bouts.

D. C. Nieman, DrPH

References

1. Wendel-Vos GC, Schuit AJ, Feskens EJ, et al. Physical activity and stroke. A meta-analysis of observational data. *Int J Epidemiol.* 2004;33:787-798.
2. Lee CD, Folsom AR, Blair SN. Physical activity and stroke risk: a meta-analysis. *Stroke.* 2003;34:2475-2481.

Plasma Pentraxin 3 Concentration Increases in Endurance-Trained Men
Miyaki A, Maeda S, Otsuki T, et al (Univ of Tsukuba, Ibaraki, Japan; Ryutsu Keizai Univ, Ryugasaki, Ibaraki, Japan)
Med Sci Sports Exerc 43:12-17, 2011

Introduction.—Pentraxin 3 (PTX3), which is mainly produced by endothelial cells, macrophages, and smooth muscle cells in the atherosclerotic region, has a cardioprotective effect. Endurance exercise training has also been known to offer cardioprotection. However, the effect of regular endurance exercise on PTX3 is unknown. This study aimed to investigate whether plasma PTX3 concentrations increase in endurance-trained men. Ten young endurance-trained men and 12 age-and gender-matched sedentary controls participated in this study.

Methods.—We measured plasma PTX3 concentrations of the participants in each group. We also determined systemic arterial compliance (SAC) by using simultaneous M-mode ultrasound and arterial applanation tonometry of the common carotid artery and used HDL cholesterol (HDLC) as an index of cardioprotective effect.

Results.—Maximal oxygen uptake was significantly higher in the endurance-trained men than that in the sedentary controls. SAC and

HDLC were significantly higher in the endurance-trained men than that in the sedentary controls (SAC $= 1.74 \pm 0.11$ vs 1.41 ± 0.09 mL·mm Hg^{-1}, $P < 0.05$; HDLC $= 70 \pm 5$ vs 57 ± 4 mg·dL^{-1}, $P < 0.05$). Plasma PTX3 concentrations were markedly higher in the endurance-trained men than that in the sedentary controls $(0.93 \pm 0.11$ vs 0.68 ± 0.06 ng·mL^{-1}, $P < 0.05$). Relationships between plasma PTX3 concentrations and SAC and HDLC were linear.

Conclusions.—This is the first study revealing that endurance-trained individuals had higher levels of circulating PTX3 than sedentary controls. PTX3 may play a partial role in endurance exercise training–induced cardioprotection.

▶ Pentraxin 3, a substance produced by endothelial cells, macrophages, and smooth muscle in regions of atherosclerosis,[1,2] has attracted growing attention as a substance that protects against atherosclerosis[3] and can promote vascular healing by activation of tissue factor.[4] It thus seems a reasonable hypothesis that pentraxin 3 might contribute to the cardioprotective effect of regular physical activity. Miyaki et al here show in a small-scale cross-sectional comparison that levels of pentraxin 3 are substantially higher in young endurance-trained men (maximal oxygen intake, 60 mL min^{-1} kg^{-1}) than in sedentary controls (maximal oxygen intake, 45 mL min^{-1} kg^{-1}) of similar age (Fig 3 in the original article). The advantage of the active individuals was also seen in terms of systemic arterial compliance and high-density lipoprotein cholesterol concentrations, and these variables were linearly related to pentraxin 3 values. More surprisingly, despite the intergroup difference, and perhaps because of the small sample size, pentraxin 3 was not directly related to maximal oxygen intake. There remains scope to find out more about pentraxin 3—on the basis of present information, it seems to fine-tune pro- and anti-inflammatory factors in a manner that is beneficial to cardiac health.

R. J. Shephard, MD (Lond), PhD, DPE

References

1. Ortega-Hernandez OD, Bassi N, Shoenfeld Y, Anaya JM. The long pentraxin 3 and its role in autoimmunity. *Semin Arthritis Rheum.* 2009;39:38-54.
2. Rolph MS, Zimmer S, Bottazzi B, Garlanda C, Mantovani A, Hansson GK. Production of the long pentraxin PTX3 in advanced atherosclerotic plaques. *Arterioscler Thromb Vasc Biol.* 2002;22:e10-e14.
3. Norata GD, Marchesi P, Pulakazhi Venu VK, et al. Deficiency of the long pentraxin PTX3 promotes vascular inflammation and atherosclerosis. *Circulation.* 2009;120:699-708.
4. Napoleone E, di Santo A, Peri G, et al. The long pentraxin PTX3 up-regulates tissue factor in activated monocytes: another link between inflammation and clotting activation. *J Leukoc Biol.* 2004;76:203-209.

Physical Activity, Stress, and Self-Reported Upper Respiratory Tract Infection

Fondell E, Lagerros YT, Sundberg CJ, et al (Karolinska Institutet, Stockholm, Sweden; et al)
Med Sci Sports Exerc 43:272-279, 2011

Purpose.—Upper respiratory tract infection (URTI) is the most common reason for seeking primary care in many countries. Still, little is known about potential strategies to reduce susceptibility. We investigated the relationships between physical activity level, perceived stress, and incidence of self-reported URTI.

Methods.—We conducted a population-based prospective cohort study of 1509 Swedish men and women aged 20–60 yr with a follow-up period of 4 months. We used a Web-based questionnaire to assess disease status and lifestyle factors at the start of the study. We assessed physical activity and inactivity as total MET-hours (MET task) per day and perceived stress by the 14-item Perceived Stress Scale. Participants were contacted every 3 wk via e-mail to assess incidence of URTI. They reported a total of 1181 occurrences of URTI. We used Poisson regression models to control for age, sex, and other potential confounding factors.

Results.—We found that high levels of physical activity (≥ 55 $MET \cdot h \cdot d^{-1}$) were associated with an 18% reduced risk (incidence rate ratio (IRR) = 0.82, 95% confidence interval (CI) = 0.69–0.98) of self-reporting URTI compared with low levels of physical activity (≥ 45 $MET \cdot h \cdot d^{-1}$). This association was stronger among those reporting high levels of stress (IRR = 0.58, 95% CI = 0.43–0.78), especially among men (IRR = 0.37, 95% CI = 0.24–0.59), but absent in the group with low levels of stress.

Conclusions.—We found that high physical activity was associated with a lower risk of contracting URTI for both men and women. In addition, we found that highly stressed people, particularly men, appear to benefit more from physical activity than those with lower stress levels (Table 3).

▶ The relationship between exercise and training intensity is widely considered to be U shaped.[1,2] The adverse immune effects of excessive physical activity are quite well documented. The benefits of moderate activity are less clearly established in empirical studies,[3-5] although immune responses to pathogens do seem to be enhanced.[6] One difficulty in the analysis is that an individual's incidence of respiratory infections is relatively low (typically 1-2 episodes per year). Thus, a substantial population sample must be followed for a prolonged period, and this in turn commonly implies using a questionnaire to assess habitual physical activity. Often, as in the study of Fondell and associates, the ascertainment of upper respiratory tract infections has been based on questionnaire responses. Good points in this study are a large sample and a 4-month follow-up period. Physical activity is expressed in $MET \cdot h \cdot d^{-1}$ (MET, metabolic equivalent task). The 3-category classification of activity appears to correspond with average energy expenditures of < 1.8, 1.8-2.3, and > 2.3 METs throughout a 24-hour

TABLE 3.—Physical Activity and IRR of URTI

Physical Activity (MET·h·d^{-1})	No. of Cases	Person-Weeks	Adjusted for Age and Sex		Multivariable Model	
			IRR	95% CI	IRR[a]	95% CI
All URTI cases						
Low (<45)[b]	648	8646	1.00		1.00	
Medium (45 to <55)	273	4267.5	0.86	0.75−0.98	0.84	0.73−0.97
High (≥55)	169	2866.5	0.81	0.69−0.96	0.82	0.69−0.98
Nonsystemic URTI cases[c]						
Low (<45)[b]	502	8865	1.00		1.00	
Medium (45 to <55)	204	4371	0.85	0.72−0.99	0.82	0.69−0.97
High (≥55)	121	2938.5	0.75	0.62−0.91	0.75	0.61−0.93
Systemic URTI cases[d]						
Low (<45)[b]	146	9399	1.00		1.00	
Medium (45 to <55)		4573.5	0.90	0.68−1.20	0.94	0.70−1.26
High (≥55)	48	3048	1.02	0.74−1.41	1.10	0.78−1.55

[a]Adjusted for age (20−29, 30−39, 40−49, and 50−60 yr) sex, body mass index (low, normal, overweight, and obese), asthma (yes/no), weakened immune system (yes/no), perceived stress (below and above median), contact with children at home or work (yes/no), regular contact with large crowds at leisure time (yes/no), education level (secondary school or less and university), and intake of vitamin D, vitamin E, and selenium (energy-adjusted intakes in four categories) and month (February to May).
[b]Reference category.
[c]Only including URTI cases with no fever.
[d]Only including URTI cases with fever.

day (although the authors speak of vigorous activity as > 6 METs, and moderate activity as 3-5 METs, these intensities presumably being sustained over a much shorter portion of the day). The data show a 16% decrease in the prevalence of infection for moderate physical activity and an 18% decrease for more vigorous activity (Table 3). This benefit persists after multivariate adjustment for age, sex, history of asthma, contact with children, vitamin intake, stress level, and other potentially confounding variables. Plainly, the margin of benefit is sufficient to be considered seriously when advocating moderate exercise to our patients. In contrast with some previous reports,[7,8] perceived stress did not seem to influence the risk of infection, although admittedly none of the groups were complaining of severe stress.

R. J. Shephard, MD (Lond), PhD, DPE

References

1. Nieman DC. Exercise, upper respiratory tract infection, and the immune system. *Med Sci Sports Exerc.* 1994;26:128-139.
2. Shephard RJ. *Physical activity, training and the immune system.* Carmel, IN: Cooper Publications; 1997.
3. Nieman DC, Henson DA, Gusewitch G, et al. Physical activity and immune function in elderly women. *Med Sci Sports Exerc.* 1993;25:823-831.
4. Matthews CE, Ockene IS, Freedson PS, Rosal MC, Merriam PA, Hebert JR. Moderate to vigorous physical activity and risk of upper-respiratory tract infection. *Med Sci Sports Exerc.* 2002;34:1242-1248.
5. Hemilä H, Virtamo J, Albanes D, Kaprio J. Physical activity and the common cold in men administered vitamin E and beta-carotene. *Med Sci Sports Exerc.* 2003;35:1815-1820.
6. Martin SA, Pence BD, Woods JA. Exercise and respiratory tract viral infections. *Exerc Sport Sci Rev.* 2009;37:157-164.

7. Takkouche B, Regueira C, Gestal-Otero JJ. A cohort study of stress and the common cold. *Epidemiology.* 2001;12:345-349.
8. Cohen S. Keynote Presentation at the Eight International Congress of Behavioral Medicine: the Pittsburgh common cold studies: psychosocial predictors of susceptibility to respiratory infectious illness. *Int J Behav Med.* 2005;12:123-131.

Swimming-induced pulmonary edema in triathletes

Miller CC III, Calder-Becker K, Modave F (Texas Tech Univ Health Sciences Ctr at El Paso Paul L. Foster School of Medicine; Cap Cities Triathalon, Montreal, Quebec, Canada; Univ of Texas at El Paso WA)
Am J Emerg Med 28:941-946, 2010

Background.—Pulmonary edema related to water immersion has been reported in military trainees and scuba and breath-hold divers, but rarely in the community. To date, no risk factors for this phenomenon have been identified by epidemiological methods. Recently, sporadic reports of swimming-induced pulmonary edema (SIPE) have emerged in the triathlon community. We surveyed the population of a national North American triathlon organization (USA Triathlon) to determine prevalence of and risk factors for symptoms compatible with SIPE.

Methods.—We surveyed the population of USA Triathlon through the organization's monthly newsletter distribution channel. We evaluated prevalence of symptoms compatible with pulmonary edema, and then followed up with a case-control study that included additional cases we had identified previously, to identify risk factors for this condition among triathletes.

Results.—Symptom history compatible with SIPE was identified in 1.4% of the population. Associated factors identified in multivariable analysis included history of hypertension, course length of half-Ironman distance or greater, female gender and use of fish oil supplements. Of the 31 cases reported, only 4 occurred in the absence of any associated factors.

Conclusions.—The identification of hypertension and fish oil in particular as risk factors raise questions about the role of cardiac diastolic function in the setting of water-immersion cardiac preload, as well as the hematologic effects of fish oil. Mechanistic studies of these risk factors in a directly observed prospective cohort are indicated (Table 2).

▶ A number of previous reports have found evidence of transient impairment of cardiac function following participation in ultraendurance events, such as a triathlon competition; sometimes, findings have been linked to the release of cardiac troponin after such events. In general, the finding has been regarded as benign, with the transient cardiac dysfunction perhaps even an essential part of the process of developing the enlarged heart of the endurance athlete. However, further enquiry has been stimulated recently by newspaper reports of a substantial number of swimming-related deaths in triathletes,[1] 8 in the

TABLE 2.—Multiple Logistic Regression Risk Factors for SIPE

Variable	Parameter Estimate	Adjusted Odds Ratio	95% C.I.	P
Intercept	−5.1506			
Hypertension	1.6821	5.38	2.15-13.48	.0003
Female Gender	1.0114	2.75	1.26-6.02	.02
Long Course	1.1938	3.30	1.50-7.27	.003
Fish Oil	0.9792	2.66	1.28-5.54	.009

Hypertension is self-reported history of hypertension.
Diabetes is self-reported Type 1 or Type 2 diabetes.
Long course is half-Ironman distance or greater.
Hot climate is self reported perception of climate.

United States of America during 2008 and 18 of 23 deaths during 2004-2008 occurring during the swimming component of the triathlon. One surprising feature was that most deaths occurred early during the swim. Possible factors include unfamiliarity with swimming in a wet suit in open water, collisions with other contestants, and unexpected coldness of the water. Miller and associates report a case-control study, where cases of swimming-induced pulmonary edema were identified through an internet questionnaire focusing on a cough with pink frothy or blood-tinged secretions that was circulated to 104 887 triathletes, data being retained from those over the age of 20 years; there were 1400 respondents, and all those without symptoms served as controls. The prevalence of appropriate symptoms among respondents was 1.4% (20/1400); others have previously made similar estimates of prevalence in combat swimmers and scuba divers.[2,3] Another 11 cases were added from other sources to look at correlates of edema; the condition appeared to be associated with a history of hypertension, fish oil use, and a long course distance (Table 2). A horizontal posture, water pressure, the wearing of wet suits, and cold exposure may all increase central blood volume, and these factors together with hypertension seem likely precursors of pulmonary edema. The association with fish oil ingestion is a little more surprising, perhaps reflecting the antiplatelet and vasodilatory action of omega fatty acids. Another potential issue, which did not emerge in this analysis, is an excessive prerace hydration. The prevalence of the problem seems to be sufficient to merit further investigation of causal factors and methods of prevention.

R. J. Shephard, MD (Lond), PhD, DPE

References

1. Aschwanden C. Deaths draw attention to triathlon swim. *The New York Times.* July 31, 2008 http://www.nytimes.com/2008/07/31/fashion/31fitness.html.
2. Ludwig BB, Mahon RT, Schwartzman EL. Cardiopulmonary function after recovery from swimming-induced pulmonary edema. *Clin J Sport Med.* 2006; 16:348-351.
3. Adir Y, Shupak A, Gil A, et al. Swimming-induced pulmonary edema: clinical presentation and serial lung function. *Chest.* 2004;126:394-399.

Comparative Effects of Caffeine and Albuterol on the Bronchoconstrictor Response to Exercise in Asthmatic Athletes

VanHaitsma TA, Mickleborough T, Stager JM, et al (Univ of Utah, Salt Lake City; Indiana Univ, Blooomington; et al)
Int J Sports Med 31:231-236, 2010

The main aim of this study was to evaluate the comparative and additive effects of caffeine and albuterol (short-acting β_2-agonist) on the severity of EIB. Ten asthmatic subjects with EIB (exercise-induced bronchoconstriction) participated in a randomized, double-blind, double-dummy crossover study. One hour before an exercise challenge, each subject was given 0, 3, 6, or 9 mg/kg of caffeine or placebo mixed in a flavored sugar drink. Fifteen minutes before the exercise bout, an inhaler containing either albuterol (180 µg) or placebo was administered to each subject. Pulmonary function tests were conducted pre- and post-exercise. Caffeine at a dose of 6 and 9 mg/kg significantly reduced (p < 0.05) the mean maximum % fall in post-exercise FEV_1 to $-9.0 \pm 9.2\%$ and $-6.8 \pm 6.5\%$ respectively compared to the double-placebo ($-14.3 \pm 11.1\%$) and baseline ($-18.4 \pm 7.2\%$). There was no significant difference (p > 0.05) in the post-exercise % fall in FEV_1 between albuterol (*plus caffeine placebo*) ($-4.0 \pm 5.2\%$) and the 9 mg/kg dose of caffeine ($-6.8 \pm 6.5\%$). Interestingly, there was no significant difference (p > 0.05) in the post-exercise % fall in FEV_1 between albuterol (*plus caffeine placebo*) ($-4.0 \pm 5.2\%$) and albuterol with 3, 6 or 9 mg/kg of caffeine (-4.4 ± 3.8, -6.8 ± 5.6, $-4.4 \pm 6.0\%$ respectively). Similar changes were observed for the post-exercise % fall in FVC, $FEF_{25-75\%}$

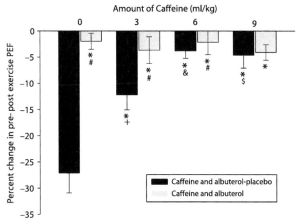

FIGURE 4.—The percent change in PEF from pre- to post-exercise for the different caffeine doses with and without albuterol. * p < 0.05, significantly different from double-placebo; $ p < 0.05, significantly different from 3 mg/kg caffeine dose; & p < 0.05, significantly different from 3 ml/kg caffeine dose; + p < 0.05, significantly different from 9 ml/kg caffeine dose; # p < 0.05, albuterol treatment significantly different from albuterol plus caffeine treatment. (Reprinted from VanHaitsma TA, Mickleborough T, Stager JM, et al. Comparative effects of caffeine and albuterol on the bronchoconstrictor response to exercise in asthmatic athletes. *Int J Sports Med.* 2010;31:231-236.)

and PEF. These data indicate that moderate (6 mg/kg) to high doses (9 mg/kg) of caffeine provide a significant protective effect against EIB. It is feasible that the negative effects of daily use of short-acting β_2-agonists by asthmatic athletes could be reduced simply by increasing caffeine consumption prior to exercise (Fig 4).

▶ Beta-2 agonists, such as albuterol, are initially quite effective in treating exercise-induced asthma, probably because the relaxation of smooth muscle that they induce counters the mediators of bronchoconstriction that cold dry air releases from mast cells.[1] However, if such drugs are taken routinely before every bout of exercise, there is a progressive decline in their effectiveness,[2,3] and there is also some risk of a build-up of lymphoid aggregates in the bronchial mucosa. This small-scale, double-blind, double-dummy trial confirms earlier reports that a moderate or large dose of caffeine may offer a helpful alternative treatment (Fig 4). Caffeine lessens exercise-induced bronchoconstriction in a dose-responsive manner; a large dose (9 mg/kg, equivalent to 4-5 cups of coffee) taken 1 hour before exercise is as effective as albuterol, and no additional benefit is seen if albuterol is given in combination with this amount of caffeine. The last finding is surprising because caffeine exerts its action via a different pathway to albuterol. One attraction of caffeine is that currently, there are no antidoping restrictions on the ingestion of this substance, whereas a therapeutic exemption would be required if competitors wished to use a beta-2 agonist to counter exercise-induced bronchospasm.

R. J. Shephard, MD (Lond), PhD, DPE

References

1. Anderson SD, Caillaud C, Brannan JD. Beta2-agonists and exercise-induced asthma. *Clin Rev Allergy Immunol.* 2006;31:163-180.
2. Hancox RJ, Subbarao P, Kamada D, Watson RM, Hargreave FE, Inman MD. Beta2-agonist tolerance and exercise-induced bronchospasm. *Am J Respir Crit Care Med.* 2002;165:1068-1070.
3. Nelson JA, Strauss L, Skowronski M, Ciufo R, Novak R, McFadden ER Jr. Effect of long-term salmetarol treatment on exercise-induced asthma. *N Engl J Med.* 1998;339:141-146.

Exercise but not mannitol provocation increases urinary Clara cell protein (CC16) in elite swimmers
Romberg K, Bjermer L, Tufvesson E (Lund Univ, Sweden)
Respir Med 105:31-36, 2011

Elite swimmers have an increased risk of developing asthma, and exposure to chloramine is believed to be an important trigger factor. The aim of the present study was to explore pathophysiological mechanisms behind induced bronchoconstriction in swimmers exposed to chloramine, before and after swim exercise provocation as well as mannitol provocation. Urinary Clara cell protein (CC16) was used as a possible marker for epithelial stress.

101 elite aspiring swim athletes were investigated and urinary samples were collected before and 1 h after completed exercise and mannitol challenge. CC16, 11β-prostaglandin (PG)$F_{2\alpha}$ and leukotriene E_4 (LTE_4) were measured.

Urinary levels of CC16 were clearly increased after exercise challenge, while no reaction was seen after mannitol challenge. Similar to CC16, the level of 11β-$PGF_{2\alpha}$ was increased after exercise challenge, but not after mannitol challenge, while LTE_4 was reduced after exercise. There was no significant difference in urinary response between those with a negative compared to positive challenge, but a tendency of increased baseline levels of 11β-$PGF_{2\alpha}$ and LTE_4 in individuals with a positive mannitol challenge.

The uniform increase of CC16 after swim exercise indicates that CC16 is of importance in epithelial stress, and may as such be an important pathogenic factor behind asthma development in swimmers. The changes seen in urinary levels of 11β-$PGF_{2\alpha}$ and LTE_4 indicate a pathophysiological role in both mannitol and exercise challenge (Fig 1).

▶ Physicians are divided on their opinions on the role of swimming pools in the treatment of patients with asthma.[1] Some hospitals have heated swimming pools, believing that the warm moist air will allow exercise without the risk of provoking bronchospasm. However, others caution that pools kept at a high temperature require high concentrations of chlorine to restrict bacterial proliferation, and this chlorine can itself serve as a respiratory irritant.

The immediate effects of chlorination seem relatively small; swimming sessions of sufficient duration to boost cardiorespiratory fitness did not increase symptoms in asthmatic children.[2] However, correlations have been observed between the frequency of pool attendance, damage to pulmonary epithelium

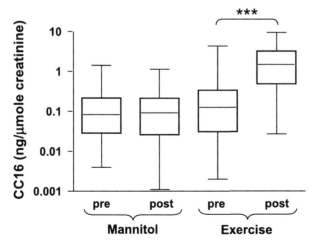

FIGURE 1.—Urinary levels of CC16 in swimmers before (pre) and 1 h after (post) mannitol or swim exercise challenge. *** = $p < 0.001$. (Reprinted from Romberg K, Bjermer L, Tufvesson E. Exercise but not mannitol provocation increases urinary Clara cell protein (CC16) in elite swimmers. *Respir Med.* 2011;105:31-36, with permission from Elsevier.)

(as estimated from lung proteins in the serum), and serum levels of IgE.[3] The prevalence of airway hyperresponsiveness and airway inflammation is certainly high in adult swimmers, and their sputum shows increased levels of eosinophils, eosinophil peroxidase, and neutrophil lipocalin.[4-9] On the other hand, airway responsiveness may disappear after a competitive career is ended,[8] and some studies of elite swimmers have found no evidence of either pulmonary inflammation[10] or increased postswim nasal concentration of nitric oxide (usually considered a marker of inflammation).[11]

The article of Romberg and associates uses the urinary levels of Clara cell protein as a measure of stress imposed on the cells lining the respiratory bronchioles (although it may itself play a protective role). It shows a substantial increase in this substance following a pool challenge (600-m swim at 90% of capacity) but not following a mannitol challenge (inhalation of increasing doses until a 15% drop in one second forced expiratory volume was observed) (Fig 1). These findings, obtained on a substantial sample of swimmers (55 males and 46 females aged 13-23 years, elite category, training an average of 18 h/wk), suggest that in those who are training hard, chlorine derivatives may produce bronchiolar damage in addition to bronchospasm. Further studies using plasma rather than urinary concentration and examining the extent of pathological change in the bronchi seem desirable.

R. J. Shephard, MD (Lond), PhD, DPE

References

1. Shephard RJ. Lifestyle and the respiratory health of children. *Am J Lifestyle Med.* 2010; 10.1177/1559827610378337.
2. Weisgerber MC, Guill M, Weisgerber JM, Butler H. Benefits of swimming in asthma: effect of a session of swimming lessons on symptoms and PFTs with review of the literature. *J Asthma.* 2003;40:453-464.
3. Bernard A, Carbonnelle S, Michel O, et al. Lung hyperpermeability and asthma prevalence in schoolchildren: unexpected associations with the attendance at indoor chlorinated swimming pools. *Occup Environ Med.* 2003;60:385-394.
4. Helenius IJ, Tikkanen HO, Sarna S, Haahtela T. Asthma and increased bronchial responsiveness in elite athletes: atopy and sport event as risk factors. *J Allergy Clin Immunol.* 1998;101:646-652.
5. Potts J. Factors associated with respiratory problems in swimmers. *Sports Med.* 1996;21:256-261.
6. Mustchin PA, Pickering CAC. "Coughing water;" bronchial hyperreactivity induced by swimming in a chlorinated pool. *Thorax.* 1979;34:682-683.
7. Katelaris CH, Carrozzi FM, Burke TV, Byth K. Patterns of allergic reactivity and disease in Olympic athletes. *Clin J Sport Med.* 2006;16:401-405.
8. Helenius IJ, Rytilä P, Sarna S, et al. Effect of continuing or finishing high-level sports on airway inflammation, bronchial hyperresponsiveness, and asthma: a 5-year prospective follow-up study of 42 highly trained swimmers. *J Allergy Clin Immunol.* 2002;109:962-968.
9. Zwick H, Popp W, Budik G, Wanke T, Rauscher H. Increased sensitization to aeroallergens in competitive swimmers. *Lung.* 1990;168:111-115.
10. Pedersen L, Lund TK, Barnes PJ, Kharitonov SA, Backer V. Airway responsiveness and inflammation in adolescent elite swimmers. *J Allergy Clin Immunol.* 2008;122:322-327.
11. Clearie KL, Vaidyanathan SW, Williamson PA, et al. Effects of chlorine and exercise on the unified airway in adolescent elite Scottish swimmers. *Allergy.* 2010;65: 269-273.

Effects of Aerobic Training on Airway Inflammation in Asthmatic Patients

Mendes FAR, Almeida FM, Cukier A, et al (Univ of São Paulo, Brazil)
Med Sci Sports Exerc 43:197-203, 2011

Purpose.—There is evidence suggesting that physical activity has anti-inflammatory effects in many chronic diseases; however, the role of exercise in airway inflammation in asthma is poorly understood. We aimed to evaluate the effects of an aerobic training program on eosinophil inflammation (primary aim) and nitric oxide (secondary aim) in patients with moderate or severe persistent asthma.

Methods.—Sixty-eight patients randomly assigned to either control (CG) or aerobic training (TG) groups were studied during the period between medical consultations. Patients in the CG (educational program + breathing exercises; $N = 34$) and TG (educational program + breathing exercises + aerobic training; $N = 34$) were examined twice a week during a 3-month period. Before and after the intervention, patients underwent induced sputum, fractional exhaled nitric oxide (FeNO), pulmonary function, and cardiopulmonary exercise testing. Asthma symptom-free days were quantified monthly, and asthma exacerbation was monitored during 3 months of intervention.

Results.—At 3 months, decreases in the total and eosinophil cell counts in induced sputum ($P = 0.004$) and in the levels of FeNO ($P = 0.009$) were observed after intervention only in the TG. The number of asthma symptom-free days and $\dot{V}O_{2max}$ also significantly improved ($P < 0.001$), and lower asthma exacerbation occurred in the TG ($P < 0.01$). In addition, the TG presented a strong positive relationship between baseline FeNO and eosinophil counts as well as their improvement after training ($r = 0.77$ and $r = 0.9$, respectively).

Conclusions.—Aerobic training reduces sputum eosinophil and FeNO in patients with moderate or severe asthma, and these benefits were more significant in subjects with higher levels of inflammation. These

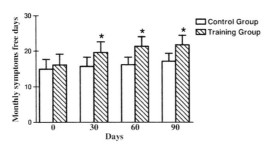

FIGURE 4.—Asthma symptoms during the study period. Values are expressed as the mean number of symptom-free days per month with a 95% CI. Time points are as follows: 0 d, 1 month before intervention; 30 d, first month of intervention; 60 d, second month of intervention; 90 d, third month of intervention. *$P < 0.05$ when compared with baseline and CG values (two-way repeated-measure ANOVA test). (Reprinted from Mendes FAR, Almeida FM, Cukier A, et al. Effects of aerobic training on airway inflammation in asthmatic patients. *Med Sci Sports Exerc.* 2011;43:197-203, with permission from the American College of Sports Medicine.)

results suggest that aerobic training might be useful as an adjuvant therapy in asthmatic patients under optimized medical treatment (Fig 4).

▶ This is the first study to demonstrate that aerobic training by asthmatic patients reduces airway inflammation. This effect was strongest among patients with the highest prestudy inflammation levels. Also, as summarized in Fig 4, improvement in aerobic capacity increased the number of asthma symptom—free days reported by the patients 1 month into the exercise training program, and this was maintained until the end of the program. The authors concluded that aerobic training is useful as an adjuvant therapy in asthmatic patients under optimized medical treatment.

D. C. Nieman, DrPH

The Asthmatic Athlete: Inhaled Beta-2 Agonists, Sport Performance, and Doping
McKenzie DC, Fitch KD (Univ of British Columbia, Vancouver, Canada; The Univ of Western Australia, Perth, Australia)
Clin J Sport Med 21:46-50, 2011

The asthmatic athlete has a long history in competitive sport in terms of success in performance and issues related to doping. Well documented are detailed objective tests used to evaluate the athlete with symptoms of asthma or airway hyperresponsiveness and the medical management. Initiated at the 2002 Salt Lake City Games, the International Olympic Committee's Independent Asthma Panel required testing to justify the use of inhaled beta-2 agonists (IBAs) in Olympic athletes and has provided valuable guidelines to the practicing physician. This program was educational and documented the variability in prevalence of asthma and/or airway hyperresponsiveness and IBA use between different sports and different countries. It provided a standard of care for the athlete with respiratory symptoms and led to the discovery that asthmatic Olympic athletes outperformed their peers at both Summer and Winter Olympic Games from 2002 to 2010. Changes to the World Anti-Doping Agency's Prohibited List in 2010 permitted the use of 2 IBA produced by the same pharmaceutical company. All others remain prohibited. However, there is no pharmacological difference between the permitted and prohibited IBAs. As a result of these changes, asthmatic athletes are being managed differently based on a World Anti-Doping Agency directive that has no foundation in pharmacological science or in clinical practice.

▶ Although several laboratory studies have suggested that physical performance is not enhanced by the inhalation of beta-2 adrenergic agents, even if they are administered in very large doses,[1-6] the question of allowing the use of such agents in competition has remained controversial among bodies regulating doping and international sport. The issue has considerable practical importance, given that a substantial proportion of the athletes who are involved in endurance and winter sports seem vulnerable to exercise-induced broncho-spasm.[7] What is in effect a therapeutic use exemption has been required by the International Olympic Committee from 2002, and 7%-8% of Olympic athletes currently receive permission to use such drugs. However, the situation became even more complicated in 2010, when the World Anti-Doping Agency decided to permit the declared use of salbutamol and salmeterol but somewhat illogi-cally prohibited the administration of other inhaled beta-blockers with similar pharmacological properties[8] unless a physician provided clear evidence that a beta-blocker was medically necessary and that neither salbutamol nor salme-terol was an appropriate treatment for the athlete in question. One particularly puzzling feature of recent statistics, as noted by McKenzie and Fitch, is that despite the lack of benefit in the laboratory, athletes who are treated with inhaled beta-2 blockers consistently outperform their peers in the Olympic Games (Fig in the original article). Is this because they train harder and thus make themselves more vulnerable to respiratory irritants? Or is the marginal gain of performance enough to give victory but too small to detect in the labo-ratory? This seems an important question to resolve in the near future.

R. J. Shephard, MD (Lond), PhD, DPE

References

1. Meeuwisse WH, McKenzie DC, Hopkins SR, Road JD. The effect of salbutamol on performance in elite nonasthmatic athletes. *Med Sci Sports Exerc.* 1992;24: 1161-1166.
2. Carlsen KH, Hem E, Stensrud T, et al. Can asthma treatment in sports be doping? The effect of the rapid onset, long-acting inhaled beta2-agonist formoterol upon endurance performance in healthy well-trained athletes. *Respir Med.* 2001;95: 571-576.
3. Kindermann W. Do inhaled beta(2)-agonists have an ergogenic potential in non-asthmatic competitive athletes? *Sports Med.* 2007;37:95-102.
4. Norris SR, Petersen SR, Jones RL. The effect of salbutamol on performance in endurance cyclists. *Eur J Appl Physiol.* 1996;73:364-368.
5. Stewart IB, Labreche JM, McKenzie DC. Acute formoterol administration has no ergogenic effect in nonasthmatic athletes. *Med Sci Sports Exerc.* 2002;34:213-217.
6. Sporer BC, Sheel AW, McKenzie DC. Dose response of inhaled salbutamol on exer-cise performance and urine concentrations. *Med Sci Sports Exerc.* 2008;40: 149-157.
7. Fitch KD, Sue-Chu M, Anderson SD, et al. Asthma and the elite athlete: summary of the International Olympic Committee's Consensus Conference, Lausanne, Switzerland, January 22-24, 2008. *J Allergy Clin Immunol.* 2008;122:254-260.
8. *Minutes of the WADA Executive Committee Meeting.* Montreal, Canada: World Anti-Doping Agency; May 9, 2009. http://www.wada-ama.org/en/Science-Medicine/TUE/QA-on-Therapeutic-Use-Exemption-TUE; May 9, 2009. Accessed February 7, 2011.

The role of the bronchial provocation challenge tests in the diagnosis of exercise-induced bronchoconstriction in elite swimmers

Castricum A, Holzer K, Brukner P, et al (Royal Melbourne Hosp, Australia)
Br J Sports Med 44:736-740, 2010

Background.—The International Olympic Committee—Medical Commission (IOC-MC) accepts a number of bronchial provocation tests for the diagnosis of exercise-induced bronchoconstriction (EIB) in elite athletes, none of which have been studied in elite swimmers. With the suggestion of a different pathogenesis involved in the development of EIB in swimmers, there is a possibility that the recommended test for EIB in elite athletes, the eucapnic voluntary hyperpnoea (EVH) challenge, may be missing the diagnosis in elite swimmers.

Objective.—The aim of this study was to assess the effectiveness of the EVH challenge, the field swim challenge and the laboratory cycle challenge in the diagnosis of EIB in elite swimmers.

Design.—33 elite swimmers were evaluated on separate days for the presence of EIB using 3 different bronchial provocation challenge tests: an 8 minute field swim challenge, a 6 minute laboratory EVH challenge, and an 8 minute laboratory cycle challenge.

Main Outcome Measurements.—Change in forced expiratory volume in 1 second (FEV_1) pre and post test protocol. A fall in FEV_1 from baseline of $\geq 10\%$ post challenge was diagnostic of EIB.

Results.—Only 1 of the 33 subjects (3%) had a positive field swim challenge with a fall in FEV_1 of 16% from baseline. 18 of the 33 subjects (55%) had a positive EVH challenge, with a mean fall in FEV_1 of 20.4 (SD 11.7)% from baseline. 4 of the subjects (12%) had a positive laboratory cycle challenge, with a mean fall in FEV_1 of 14.8 (4.7)% from baseline. Only 1 of the 33 subjects was positive to all 3 challenges.

Conclusions.—These results suggest that the EVH challenge is a highly sensitive challenge for identifying EIB in elite swimmers, in contrast to the laboratory and field-based exercise challenge tests, which significantly underdiagnose the condition. The EVH challenge, a well-established and standardised test for EIB in elite winter and summer land-based athletes, should thus be used for the diagnosis of EIB in elite swimmers, as recommended by the IOC-MC (Table 1).

▶ Swimmers seem particularly vulnerable to exercise-induced bronchospasm (EIB), perhaps in part because people with asthma are encouraged to swim[1] and in part because of the chlorine metabolites that tend to accumulate at the surface of the pool, causing chronic damage to the airways.[2-4] The prevalence of EIB in swimmers approaches 50% of competitors.[1] The International Olympic Committee (IOC) accepts various objective indices of significant EIB, including a positive response to a number of bronchial challenges and a positive response to eucapnic voluntary hyperpnea (EVH). Most of these tests fail to include chlorine exposure, so that one might expect field swim challenge to induce a higher frequency of positive diagnoses. It is quite surprising that in fact

TABLE 1.—Subject Baseline Spirometry and Fall in FEV_1 in Response to the EVH, Swim and Cycle Challenges

Subject	FEV_1 (litres) (% pred)	FVC (litres/s) (% pred)	FEV_1/FVC%	EVH Fall in FEV_1 (%)	Swim Fall in FEV_1 (%)	Cycle Fall in FEV_1 (%)
1*	4.70 (96)	7.36 (125)	64	36	7	8
2	4.97 (104)	6.67 (117)	75	33	7	5
3	3.95 (110)	5.13 (120)	71	12	6	up 1
4	4.95 (105)	6.50 (116)	76	10	2	4
5	3.90 (122)	4.43 (117)	88	6	8	8
6	4.67 (98)	6.13 (104)	76	11	1	up 7
7*	2.94 (82)	4.13 (94)	71	43	16	15
8	3.78 (118)	4.40 (116)	86	25	5	3
9	4.34 (124)	5.03 (120)	86	2	up 1	3
10	4.71 (98)	6.11 (105)	77	13	3	2
11	4.30 (113)	5.29 (115)	81	12	2	9
12	3.72 (133)	4.21 (128)	88	9	3	3
13	5.57 (119)	7.04 (126)	79	7	3	5
14	3.83 (98)	4.50 (95)	85	6	2	5
15	4.54 (134)	4.72 (115)	96	3	6	2
16	3.54 (126)	3.78 (115)	94	11	no change	up 1
17	3.57 (101)	4.10 (96)	87	5	4	up 1
18*	3.53 (101)	4.36 (109)	81	9	1	up 4
19	3.46 (101)	4.32 (104)	80	11	1	4
20	3.34 (120)	4.23 (129)	79	34	6	13
21	5.75 (127)	6.48 (118)	89	9	1	1
22	6.18 (125)	7.50 (124)	82	13	3	4
23	5.17 (115)	5.79 (109)	89	5	1	5
24	4.21 (115)	5.44 (123)	77	12	3	1
25	4.38 (130)	4.66 (116)	94	6	2	3
26	5.57 (119)	7.40 (130)	75	5	3	up 2
27	5.38 (117)	6.37 (116)	84	2	5	no change
28	4.07 (146)	4.33 (132)	94	15	3	3
29	5.44 (126)	6.58 (129)	83	8	up 1	1
30	5.39 (120)	6.58 (123)	82	10	up 1	3
31	5.65 (144)	6.30 (133)	90	5	5	11
32	3.19 (107)	3.46 (99)	92	38	2	21
33	4.00 (92)	5.50 (107)	73	29	6	6

EIB-positive swimmers identified in bold. pred, predicted.
*Subjects 1, 7 and 18 had a positive bronchodilator response for asthma.

EVH induces EIB in 18 of 33 swimmers, whereas in the field swim test the diagnostic threshold (a 10% decrease of forced expiratory volume in 1 second) was reached in only 1 individual (Table 1). The ventilation is not monitored during the swim test, and it may be that it does not attain a high enough level to provoke EIB; in contrast, ventilation is closely monitored in EVH. Another factor is that the air inhaled in the swimming test had a much higher water content than that used in EVH. Although the IOC accepts the EVH results, in the case of swimmers, the response observed when inhaling moist air from the pool surface may provide a fairer measure of any incapacitation that the athlete will experience in competition. One interesting aspect of this study is that EVH induced a high proportion of positive tests, although the inspired air was free of chlorine derivatives; any adverse effects of chlorine upon the airways must therefore be long term in nature.

R. J. Shephard, MD (Lond), PhD, DPE

References

1. Bar-Or O, Inbar O. Swimming and asthma. Benefits and deleterious effects. *Sports Med.* 1992;14:397-405.
2. Drobnic F, Freixa A, Casan P, Sanchis J, Guardino X. Assessment of chlorine exposure in swimmers during training. *Med Sci Sports Exerc.* 1996;28:271-274.
3. Helenius IJ, Rytilä P, Metso T, Haahtela T, Venge P, Tikkanen HO. Respiratory symptoms, bronchial responsiveness, and cellular characteristics of induced sputum in elite swimmers. *Allergy.* 1998;53:346-352.
4. Zwick H, Popp W, Budik G, Wanke T, Rauscher H. Increased sensitization to aeroallergens in competitive swimmers. *Lung.* 1990;168:111-115.

Wheat dependent exercise induced anaphylaxis: is this an appropriate terminology?

Wong GKY, Huissoon AP, Goddard S, et al (Birmingham Heartlands Hosp, UK)
J Clin Pathol 63:814-817, 2010

Background.—The presentation of wheat dependent exercise induced anaphylaxis (WDEIA) can be variable. A high index of clinical suspicion is required to initiate the investigation pathway. Double blind placebo controlled food-exercise challenge is the gold standard investigation but the practicality of this test limits its application.

Aim.—To critically analyse the symptoms of WDEIA and their correlation with serum specific IgE (sIgE) to rω-5-gliadin.

Methods.—17 patients were tested for serum sIgE to rω-5-gliadin. The clinical response to a diet/exercise intervention protocol was used to assess specificity of a positive sIgE to rω-5-gliadin. Length of time to diagnosis, clinical likelihood scores, exercise intensity involved and the severity of allergic reactions were examined retrospectively.

Result.—8/10 patients with positive sIgE to rω-5-gliadin had a confirmed diagnosis of WDEIA. Half of the WDEIA patients had a prolonged time lag to diagnosis (32–62 months) and were initially diagnosed with idiopathic anaphylaxis or chronic idiopathic urticaria and angioedema. Only three patients had experienced life threatening symptoms (Mueller grading 4). A close association was observed between requirements of lower exercise intensity to provoke a reaction and diagnostic delay.

Conclusion.—Specific IgE to rω-5-gliadin can provide supportive evidence for WDEIA without the need of a food-exercise challenge. The wheat-exercise association is not obvious in many patients, highlighting the need to consider WDEIA in the differential diagnosis of all patients presenting with idiopathic systemic reactions. The term anaphylaxis may be inappropriate and it is therefore worth considering an alternative terminology such as 'activity dependent wheat allergy' to describe this condition (Table 2).

▶ Exercise-induced anaphylaxis is relatively rare, but it can be a disturbing disorder. Severe cases show asphyxiating airway obstruction, marked urticaria,

TABLE 2.—Characteristic of Subjects

Patient No.	Gender	Age of Presentation	*Clinical Likelihood Scores (Total of 2)	Total IgE (kU/l)	Specific IgE to ω-5-Gliadin (kUa/l)	No. of Allergic Reactions Per 6/12 Before Modified Exercise Dietary Test	No. of Allergic Reactions Per 6/12 After Modified Exercise Dietary Test	Diagnosis
1	M	25	4/3 (7)	323	29.6	4	1	WDEIA
2	M	41	3/1 (4)	358	17.7	2	0	WDEIA
3	F	47	2/4 (6)	3617	17.9	4	0	WDEIA
4	M	53	3/3 (6)	203	6.46	12	1	WDEIA
5	F	31	4/4 (8)	176	12.0	26	2	WDEIA
6	M	52	3/3 (6)	Not done	3.89	12	0	WDEIA
7	M	30	4/4 (8)	100	5.96	3	1	WDEIA
8	M	20	3/2 (5)	46	0.96	24	6	WDEIA
9	M	44	2/3 (5)	1172	6.62	8	6	EIA
10	F	26	1/1 (2)	109	0.53	6	5	CIUA
11	F	22	3/4 (7)	Not done	0.14	—	—	Prawn allergy
12	F	25	1/1 (2)	21	0.00	—	—	CIU
13	M	51	2/3 (5)	986	0.02	—	—	IA
14	F	8	1/1 (2)	Not done	0.00	—	—	IBS
15	F	24	1/3 (4)	283	0.03	—	—	Wheat allergy
16	M	20	3/3 (6)	1947	0.05	—	—	IA
17	F	17	1/1 (2)	134	0.00	—	—	CIUA

CIUA, chronic idiopathic urticaria and angiodema; CIU, chronic idiopathic urticaria; EIA, exercise induced anaphylaxis; IA, idiopathic anaphylaxis; WDEIA, wheat dependent exercise induced anaphylaxis; ≥0.35 kUa/l, positive sIgE to rω-5-gliadin.

*The scoring system for clinical likelihood score is as follows: (1) will not consider as a differential diagnosis at all; (2) will consider as an unlikely differential diagnosis and will adopt a 'wait and watch' policy; (3) will consider as the top three differential diagnosis and will actively investigate for the condition; or (4) highly suggestive.

hypotension, nausea, vomiting, and diarrhea.[1-5] Symptoms typically appear if exercise is taken 1 to 2 hours after ingesting a triggering food product such as peanuts, wheat protein, shellfish, celery, or certain antibiotics. Susceptible individuals have an above-average proportion of helper-2-type T cells, and ingestion of the allergen causes a correspondingly large production of immunoglobulin E, with the release of histamine from circulating mast cells.[6] Many of the food items concerned can cause some narrowing of the airways in the absence of exercise, and it seems likely that in such patients, exercising simply exacerbates mediator release, bringing what would otherwise have been a mild allergic reaction to a dangerous level. The study of Wong et al found 17 cases of bronchospasm that were thought to be triggered by a combination of exercise and the ingestion of wheat products. The IgE response to the critical agent (rω-5-gliadin) was monitored, thus avoiding the need to establish the diagnosis by undergoing a combined food/exercise test. Although the IgE response to this antigen usually provides a good clinical test of exercise-induced wheat allergies, sensitivity can be further improved by also examining the IgE responses to wheat glutenin. The authors of this report established a diagnosis of wheat-induced exercise anaphylaxis in 8 of their 17 cases, but the condition was life threatening in only 3 of these cases. Two important conclusions from their study are the time required to establish a diagnosis (longer than 32 months in 4 of the 8 cases) and the fact that reactions occurred with mild rather than very heavy exercise. In terms of practical treatment, if neither the food product nor exercise cause a problem on their own, it seems sufficient to delay exercise until at least 4 hours after a meal (Table 2).

R. J. Shephard, MD (Lond), PhD, DPE

References

1. Bochner BS, Lichtenstein LM. Anaphylaxis. *N Engl J Med*. 1991;324:1785-1790.
2. Yunginger JW, Sweeney KG, Sturner WQ, et al. Fatal food-induced anaphylaxis. *JAMA*. 1988;260:1450-1452.
3. Sampson HA, Mendelson L, Rosen JP. Fatal and near-fatal anaphylactic reactions to food in children and adolescents. *N Engl J Med*. 1992;327:380-384.
4. Canadian Pediatric Society. Position Statement. Fatal anaphylactic reactions to food in children. *CMAJ*. 1994;150:337-339.
5. Shephard RJ. Lifestyle and the respiratory health of children. Am J Lifestyle Med, in press. doi:10.1177/1559827610378377.
6. Sheffer AL, Tong AK, Murphy GF, Lewis RA, McFadden ER Jr, Austin KE. Exercise-induced anaphylaxis: a serious form of physical allergy associated mast cell degranulation. *J Allergy Clin Immunol*. 1985;75:479-484.

Effects of Aerobic Training on Airway Inflammation in Asthmatic Patients
Mendes FAR, Almeida FM, Cukier A, et al (Univ of São Paulo, Brazil)
Med Sci Sports Exerc 43:197-203, 2011

Purpose.—There is evidence suggesting that physical activity has anti-inflammatory effects in many chronic diseases; however, the role of exercise in airway inflammation in asthma is poorly understood. We aimed to evaluate the effects of an aerobic training program on eosinophil inflammation (primary aim) and nitric oxide (secondary aim) in patients with moderate or severe persistent asthma.

Methods.—Sixty-eight patients randomly assigned to either control (CG) or aerobic training (TG) groups were studied during the period between medical consultations. Patients in the CG (educational program + breathing exercises; $N = 34$) and TG (educational program + breathing exercises + aerobic training; $N = 34$) were examined twice a week during a 3-month period. Before and after the intervention, patients underwent induced sputum, fractional exhaled nitric oxide (FeNO), pulmonary function, and cardiopulmonary exercise testing. Asthma symptom-free days were quantified monthly, and asthma exacerbation was monitored during 3 months of intervention.

Results.—At 3 months, decreases in the total and eosinophil cell counts in induced sputum ($P = 0.004$) and in the levels of FeNO ($P = 0.009$) were observed after intervention only in the TG. The number of asthma symptom-free days and $\dot{V}O_{2max}$ also significantly improved ($P < 0.001$), and lower asthma exacerbation occurred in the TG ($P < 0.01$). In addition, the TG presented a strong positive relationship between baseline FeNO and eosinophil counts as well as their improvement after training ($r = 0.77$ and $r = 0.9$, respectively).

Conclusions.—Aerobic training reduces sputum eosinophil and FeNO in patients with moderate or severe asthma, and these benefits were more significant in subjects with higher levels of inflammation. These results suggest that aerobic training might be useful as an adjuvant therapy in asthmatic patients under optimized medical treatment.

▶ In children, the association between asthma and physical inactivity or a low level of aerobic fitness is contentious[1]; any observed negative associations reflect as much an imposed restriction of physical activity by those treating the asthma as a causal relationship. In adults, spurious associations may also arise because exercise habits increase exposure to cold or allergenic pollens. Nevertheless, some studies suggest the therapeutic value from programs of moderate physical activity. Exercise-induced bronchoconstriction is reduced,[2] as is the use of corticosteroid medication.[2,3] Physical activity is also recognized as having an anti-inflammatory action in healthy individuals and those with other chronic conditions.[4-6] This study is based on adults aged 20 to 50 years with moderate or severe persistent asthma. The findings of reduced sputum eosinophil counts (Fig 2 in the original article) and fractional exhaled nitric oxide after 3 months of training (30 minutes, twice per week, at 60%-70% of maximal oxygen intake) are plainly at variance with 2 previous trials in children[7,8] where the intensity of training was less carefully monitored and probably was lower. Mendes and associates noted that an average 14% increase in symptom-limited peak treadmill oxygen intake among respondent patients was associated with an increase in the number of asthma-free days. However, the findings may not apply to all individuals with asthma; of 160 apparently eligible patients, only 68 were randomized, and only 51 of these completed the trial. Conclusions are based on this reduced sample, rather than the more usual intention to treat analysis. Moreover, not all of the experimental group showed a decrease in inflammatory markers; paradoxically, the best response was seen in those with the most marked symptoms after normal pharmacological treatment.

R. J. Shephard, MD (Lond), PhD, DPE

References

1. Shephard RJ. Lifestyle and the respiratory health of children [published online ahead of print September 14, 2010]. *Am J Lifestyle Med.* 2010; 10.1177/15598 27610378337
2. Fanelli A, Cabral ALB, Neder JA, Martins MA, Carvalho CR. Exercise training on disease control and quality of life in asthmatic children. *Med Sci Sports Exerc.* 2007;39:1474-1480.
3. Neder JA, Nery LE, Silva AC, Cabral AL, Fernandes AL. Short term effects of aerobic training in the clinical management of moderate to severe asthma in children. *Thorax.* 1999;54:202-206.
4. Gleeson M. Immune function in sport and exercise. *J Appl Physiol.* 2007;103: 693-699.
5. Handschin C, Spiegelman BM. The role of exercise and PGC1alpha in inflammation and chronic disease. *Nature.* 2008;454:463-469.
6. Mathur N, Pedersen BK. Exercise as a mean to control low-grade systemic inflammation. *Mediators Inflamm.* 2008;2008:109-502.
7. Bonsignore MR, La Grutta S, Cibella F, et al. Effects of exercise training and montelukast in children with mild asthma. *Med Sci Sports Exerc.* 2008;40:405-412.
8. Morreira A, Delgado L, Haahtela T, et al. Physical training does not increase allergic inflammation in asthmatic children. *Eur Respir J.* 2008;32:1570-1575.

Effects of exercise training on airway responsiveness and airway cells in healthy subjects
Scichilone N, Morici G, Zangla D, et al (Univ of Palermo, Italy; et al)
J Appl Physiol 109:288-294, 2010

Airway responsiveness to methacholine (Mch) in the absence of deep inspirations (DIs) is lower in athletes compared with sedentary individuals. In this prospective study, we tested the hypothesis that a training exercise program reduces the bronchoconstrictive effect of Mch. Ten healthy sedentary subjects (M/F: 3/7; mean ± SD age: 22 ± 3 yr) entered a 10-wk indoor rowing exercise program on rowing ergometer and underwent Mch bronchoprovocation in the absence of DIs at baseline, at *weeks 5* and *10*, as well as 4−6 wk after the training program was completed. Exercise-induced changes on airway cells and markers of airway inflammation were also assessed by sputum induction and venous blood samples. Mean power output during the 1,000 m test was 169 ± 49 W/stroke at baseline, 174 ± 49 W/stroke at 5 wk, and 200 ± 60 W/stroke at 10 wk of training ($P < 0.05$). The median Mch dose used at baseline was 50 mg/ml (range 25−75 mg/ml) and remained constant per study design. At the pretraining evaluation, the percent reduction in the primary

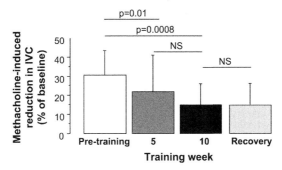

FIGURE 2.—Single-dose methacholine-induced reductions in IVC from baseline in the absence of deep inspirations, at baseline, after 5 and 10 wk of rowing exercise, and 4–6 wk after the exercise program had ended (recovery). Bars represent means ± SD. NS, not significant. (Reprinted from Scichilone N, Morici G, Zangla D, et al. Effects of exercise training on airway responsiveness and airway cells in healthy subjects. *J Appl Physiol.* 2010;109:288-294, used with permission.)

outcome, the inspiratory vital capacity (IVC) after inhalation of Mch in the absence of DIs was 31 ± 13%; *at week 5*, the Mch-induced reduction in IVC was 22 ± 19%, P = 0.01, and it further decreased to 15 ± 11% at *week 10* (P = 0.0008). The percent fall in IVC 4–6 wk after the end of training was 15 ± 11% (P = 0.87 vs. end of training). Changes in airway cells were not associated with changes in airway responsiveness. Our data show that a course of exercise training can attenuate airway responsiveness against Mch inhaled in the absence of DIs in healthy subjects and suggest that a sedentary lifestyle may favor development of airways hyperresponsiveness (Fig 2).

▶ Other recent reports have suggested that a sedentary lifestyle may be a factor in the development of airway hyperresponsiveness.[1-3] The changes induced by the vigorous training of sedentary individuals (Fig 2) offer some support for this suggestion. However, there are several aspects of this study that need further evaluation. Firstly, the technique adopted, exposure to methacholine without deep inhalation, is a little unusual. Moreover, there was no control group, so it is just possible that some unmeasured environmental change may have led to the change in airway responsiveness with training (although the observed change is rather large to explain in this way). It also remains to be demonstrated how long the effects of training persisted after completion of the 10-week training program; conceivably, if the subjects had persisted with the vigorous training, this may have led to long-term airway irritation.[4-6] Finally, the subjects were healthy individuals; there is no known benefit from a reduced methacholine response of this type in those who are healthy. The findings cannot necessarily be transferred to those with asthma, although the same group of investigators have recently suggested that training can reduce bronchial responsiveness in children with mild asthma.[7]

R. J. Shephard, MD (Lond), PhD, DPE

References

1. Shaaban R, Leynaert B, Soussan D, et al. Physical activity and bronchial hyperresponsiveness: European Community Respiratory Health Survey II. *Thorax.* 2007; 62:403-410.
2. Shore SA, Fredberg JJ. Obesity, smooth muscle, and airway hyperresponsiveness. *J Allergy Clin Immunol.* 2005;115:925-927.
3. Scichilone N, Morici G, Marchese R, et al. Reduced airway responsiveness in nonelite runners. *Med Sci Sports Exerc.* 2005;37:2019-2025.
4. Bonsignore MR, Morici G, Vignola AM, et al. Increased airway inflammatory cells in endurance athletes: what do they mean? *Clin Exp Allergy.* 2003;33:14-21.
5. Karjalainen EM, Laitinen A, Sue-Chu M, Altraja A, Bjermer L, Laitinen LA. Evidence of airway inflammation and remodeling in ski athletes with and without bronchial hyperresponsiveness to methacholine. *Am J Respir Crit Care Med.* 2000; 161:2086-2091.
6. Sue-Chu M, Larsson L, Moen T, Rennard SI, Bjermer L. Bronchoscopy and bronchoalveolar lavage findings in cross-country skiers with and without "ski asthma". *Eur Respir J.* 1999;13:626-632.
7. Bonsignore MR, La Grutta S, Cibella F, et al. Effects of exercise training and montelukast in children with mild asthma. *Med Sci Sports Exerc.* 2008;40:405-412.

Effects of Ipratropium on Exercise-Induced Bronchospasm
Boaventura LC, Araujo AC, Martinez JB, et al (Univ of São Paulo, Ribeirão Preto, Brazil)
Int J Sports Med 31:516-520, 2010

Exercise-induced bronchospasm (EIB) is the transient narrowing of the airways that follows vigorous exercise. Ipratropium bromide may be used to prevent EIB, but its effect varies among individuals. We hypothesized that time of administration of ipratropium interferes with its action. This was a prospective, double-blind, cross-over study carried out to evaluate the bronchoprotective and bronchodilatory effect of ipratropium at different times of day. The study consisted of 4 exercise challenge tests (2 at 7 am and 2 at 6 pm). In the morning, one of the tests was performed after placebo administration and the other one after ipratropium (80 µg) and the two tests (placebo and ipratropium) were repeated in the evening. Twenty-one patients with severe or moderate asthma and previous confirmation of EIB were enrolled in this prospective trial. The bronchodilatory effect of ipratropium was 0.25 ± 0.21 L or $13.11 \pm 10.99\%$ ($p = 0.001$ compared to baseline values) in the morning, and 0.14 ± 0.25 L or $7.25 \pm 11.37\%$ ($p > 0.05$) in the evening. In the morning, EIB was 0.58 ± 0.29 L on the placebo day and 0.38 ± 0.22 L on the treatment day ($p = 0.01$). In the evening, EIB was 0.62 ± 0.28 L on the placebo day and 0.51 ± 0.35 L on the treatment day ($p > 0.05$). We suggest that the use of ipratropium for the treatment of asthma and EIB should take into consideration the time of administration (Fig 2).

▶ Given the efficacy of beta-adrenergic agonists, one might wonder at the need to consider treating exercise-induced bronchospasm (EIB) with cholinergic

Effect of ipratropium on exercise-induced bronchospasm

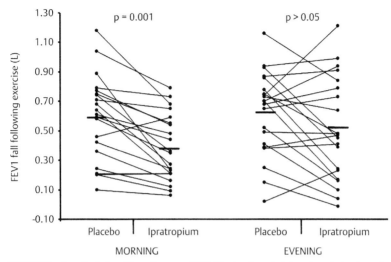

FIGURE 2.—Exercise-induced bronchospasm (EIB) 30 min after administration of placebo and after administration of ipratropium bromide (80 mcg), 36 h to 7 days apart, in 21 asthmatic patients at 7 am and 6 pm. (Reprinted from Boaventura LC, Araujo AC, Martinez JB, et al. Effects of ipratropium on exercise-induced bronchospasm. *Int J Sports Med.* 2010;31:516-520.)

antagonists such as ipratropium (Atrovent), agents that induce a local block of cholinergic receptors in the bronchial muscle but have minimal systemic effects on the brain or via the blood stream. One reason for considering this option is that some athletes develop significant side effects from beta-agonists, such as tachycardia, arrhythmia, and tremor.[1] Boaventura and associates here suggest that arguments about the effectiveness of ipratropium in the treatment of EIB[2] reflect a circadian rhythm of autonomic function. In the asthmatic individual, lung function reaches its nadir at 4 AM and its peak at 4 PM.[3,4] The present data suggest that there is an opposite type of rhythm in the response to an 80-μg dose of ipratropium (Fig 2). It would be interesting to test responses to ipratropium over the course of an entire day, and also to examine whether there is a similar circadian differential in the response to beta-agonists. It should be underlined that although side effects from inhalation of ipratropium are generally slight, there have been occasional reports of dry mouth, tachycardia, nausea, palpitations, and headache with such treatment.

R. J. Shephard, MD (Lond), PhD, DPE

References

1. National Institutes of Health. *Global Strategy for Asthma Management and Prevention: Global Initiative for Asthma (GINA).* Bethesda, MD: National Herat, Lung & Blood Institute; 2002.
2. Poppius H, Salorinne Y. Comparative trial of Salbutamol and an anticholinergic drug (SCH 1000) in the prevention of exercise-induced asthma. *Scand J Respir Dis.* 1973;54:142-147.

3. Hetzel MR, Clark TJ. Comparison of normal and asthmatic circadian rhythms in peak expiratory flow rate. *Thorax.* 1980;35:732-738.
4. Martin RJ. Location of airway inflammations in asthma and the relation to circadian change in lung function. *Chronobiol Int.* 1999;16:623-630.

Community based physiotherapeutic exercise in COPD self-management: A randomised controlled trial

Effing T, Zielhuis G, Kerstjens H, et al (Medisch Spectrum Twente, Enschede, The Netherlands; Radboud Univ Nijmegen, The Netherlands; Univ of Groningen, The Netherlands)
Respir Med 105:418-426, 2011

Little is known about effects of community-based physiotherapeutic exercise programmes incorporated in COPD self-management programmes. In a randomised trial, the effect of such a programme (COPE-active) on exercise capacity and various secondary outcomes including daily activity as a marker of behaviour change was evaluated.

All patients attended four 2-h self-management sessions. In addition the intervention group participated in the COPE-active programme offered by physiotherapists of private practices, consisting of a 6-month "compulsory" period (3 sessions/week) and subsequently a 5-month "optional" period (2 sessions/week). Because COPE-active was intended to change behaviour with regard to exercise, one session/week in both periods consisted of unsupervised home-based exercise training.

Of 153 patients, 74 intervention and 68 control patients completed the one-year follow-up. Statistically significant between-group differences in incremental shuttle walk test-distance (35.1 m; 95% CI (8.4; 61.8)) and daily activity (1190 steps/day; 95% CI (256; 2125)) were found in favour of the intervention group. Over the 12-month period a significant difference of the chronic respiratory questionnaire (CRQ) dyspnoea-score (0.33 points; 95% CI (0.01; 0.64)) and a non-significant difference of the endurance shuttle walk test (135 m (95% CI (−29; 298)) was found. No differences were found in the other CRQ-components, anxiety and depression scores and percentage of fat free mass.

This study demonstrates that a community-based reactivation programme improves exercise capacity in patients with moderately to severe COPD. Even more important, the programme improves actual daily activity after one-year which indicates behaviour change with regard to daily exercise (Fig 2).

▶ Most community-based chronic disease management programs include a large self-management component. This study examines the benefits of a physiotherapy exercise program added to the typical self-management strategies. The authors conducted a randomized controlled trial on the subject. The strength of this study is that the outcomes were measured at 7 months (1 month after intervention) and at 12 months, and both objective (shuttle

Incremental Shuttle Walk Test: intention to treat analysis

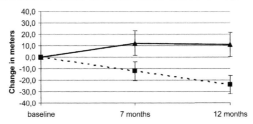

Incremental Shuttle Walk Test: per protocol analysis

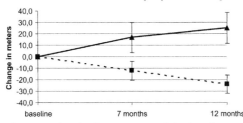

FIGURE 2.—Mean change (SE) from baseline in incremental shuttle walk test walking distance (m) at 7 and 12 months after baseline measurements of the COPE-active (▲) and control (■) group using an intention to treat analysis (number of patients at baseline: COPE-active: 77; control: 74) and a per protocol analysis (number of patients at baseline: COPE-active: 51; control: 74). (Reprinted from Effing T, Zielhuis G, Kerstjens H, et al. Community based physiotherapeutic exercise in COPD self-management: a randomised controlled trial. *Respir Med.* 2011;105:418-426, with permission from Elsevier Ltd.)

walk test) and subjective patient-reported outcomes were included. Typically, there is a decline in health over time for patients with chronic obstructive pulmonary disease. This study showed that the addition of a community-based physiotherapy program, such as shuttle walk test walking distance (Fig 2), daily activity, and dyspnea score, improved outcomes for these patients. Cost-effectiveness studies need to be done to justify widespread implementation of these programs.

D. E. Feldman, PT, PhD

Cost-saving effect of supervised exercise associated to COPD self-management education program
Ninot G, Moullec G, Picot MC, et al (Univ Montpellier, France)
Respir Med 105:377-385, 2011

Background.—Although the benefits of comprehensive pulmonary rehabilitation have been demonstrated in patients with COPD, the effects of exercise sessions within self-management programs remain unclear. We hypothesized that 8 supervised exercise sessions incorporated in a 1-month self-management education program in COPD patients would be effective to improve health outcomes and to reduce direct medical costs after one year, compared to usual care.

Methods.—In this randomized controlled trial, 38 moderate-to-severe COPD patients were assigned either to an intervention group or to a usual care group. The hospital-based intervention program provided a combination of 8 sessions of supervised exercise with 8 self-management education sessions over a 1-month period. The primary end-point was the 6-min walking distance (6MWD), with secondary outcomes being health-related quality of life (HRQoL) — using the St. George's Respiratory Questionnaire (SGRQ) and Nottingham Health Profile (NHP), maximal exercise capacity and healthcare utilization. Data were collected before and one year after the program.

Results.—After 12 months, we found statistically significant between-group differences in favor of the intervention group in 6MWD (+50.5 m (95%CI, 2 to 99), in two domains of NHP (*energy*, −19.8 (−38 to −1); *emotional reaction*, −10.4 (−20 to 0)); in SGRQ-*symptoms* (−14.0 (−23 to −5)), and in cost of COPD medication (−480.7 € (CI, −891 to −70) per patient per year).

Conclusion.—The present hospital-based intervention combining supervised exercise with self-management education provides significant improvements in patient's exercise tolerance and HRQoL, and significant decrease of COPD medication costs, compared to usual care (Table 2).

▶ The benefits of exercise rehabilitation have long been recognized in chronic obstructive pulmonary disease (COPD). The program examined by Ninot and associates emphasized self-management, and it incorporated an extensive educational component. The authors criticize previous studies on the basis that the exercise component of earlier programs did not meet the generally accepted minimal demands of an effective course of rehabilitation. In this randomized controlled study, patients older than 40 years with stable COPD and a forced expiratory volume in 1 second/forced vital capacity ratio < 0.70 exercised in the laboratory at their personal ventilatory threshold; sessions lasted 30 to 45 minutes and twice per week, and participants were also encouraged to incorporate exercise into the home management of their condition. After 1 month of hospital visits, persistence of the home program was encouraged by telephone calls. At 1 year, the experimental group participants had better scores for emotional reactions and energy and were also walking further on a 6-minute test but had no advantage in a laboratory cycle ergometer test of peak aerobic power (Table 2). They showed a substantial reduction in expenditures on medications relative to those receiving usual care. Expenses for hospitalization did not differ from those in the control group, but this may be because few in either group were hospitalized. Reduction of hospital costs is plainly an important goal that needs further exploration; there is one published study showing such an effect.[1] As is often the case, one weakness of this investigation is that a rather small proportion of patients were included in the randomized trial. Of an initial sample of 101 individuals, 56 did not meet all of the study criteria and 16 demanded financial compensation. A further 7 did not complete the study, leaving a total of 18 control and 20 experimental

TABLE 2.—6MWD, Dyspnea, Peak Work Rate, Peak VO$_2$, Voorrips Score, NHP Score, SGRQ Score and HealthCare Use Differences from Baseline to 12 month

Variable	Within-Group Differences from Baseline (Median, 25th to 75th Percentile)				Between-Group Difference (Intervention Minus Usual Care Group)		
	Usual Care Group ($n=18$) 1 yr	P	Intervention Group ($n=20$) 1 yr	P	Univariate Analysis P	Linear Regression β (95%CI)	P
6-min walking distance, m	12.5 (−15 to 48)	0.52	30.0 (5 to 80)	<0.01	0.15	50.5 (2−99)	0.04
Dyspnea VAS score (end of 6MWD)	0.0 (−1 to 1.50)	0.90	−1.0 (−3.25 to 0.75)	0.06	0.18	−0.5 (−2 to 1)	0.52
Peak work rate, W	8.0 (0 to 20)	<0.01	0.0 (−4 to 11)	0.45	0.14	−6.3 (−15 to 3)	0.17
Peak VO$_2$, mL^{-1} kg^{-1} min^{-1}	0.1 (−0.1 to 0.1)	0.90	−0.1 (−0.2 to 0.1)	0.50	0.40	−0.03 (−0.2 to 0.1)	0.76
Voorrips total	1.4 (0.6 to 2.3)	<0.001	4.1 (2.5 to 6.7)	<0.001	<0.001	2.7 (1.1−4.3)	<0.01
NHP score							
Energy	0.0 (−39 to 0)	0.18	−13.3 (−63 to 0)	0.03	0.47	−19.8 (−38 to −1)	0.04
Pain	0.0 (−10 to 6)	0.97	−5.7 (−12 to 5)	0.11	0.21	−4.7 (−14 to 5)	0.32
Emotional reaction	0.0 (−8 to 0)	0.66	−8.2 (−18 to 0)	0.03	0.11	−10.4 (−20 to 0)	0.04
Sleep	0.0 (0−20)	0.17	0.0 (−1 to 0)	0.68	0.16	−12.2 (−26 to 1)	0.07
Isolation	0.0 (−17 to 0)	0.68	0.0 (0−25)	0.84	0.49	−8.5 (−20 to 3)	0.15
Mobility	0.0 (−3 to 1)	0.99	0.0 (−13 to 5)	0.23	0.53	−2.2 (−10 to 6)	0.58
SGRQ score							
Symptoms	3.7 (−8 to 18)	0.31	−7.0 (−19 to 1)	0.02	0.02	−14.0 (−23 to −5)	<0.01
Activity	−6.7 (−13 to 0)	0.03	−6.7 (−16 to −5)	<0.01	0.61	−2.8 (−13 to 7)	0.58
Impacts	−5.6 (−9 to 9)	0.52	−6.3 (−24 to 0)	0.04	0.18	−8.9 (−19 to 1)	0.08
Total	−4.7 (−11 to 4)	0.33	−7.6 (−18 to −1)	<0.01	0.15	−8.0 (−16 to 0)	0.06
COPD-related hospital LOS#, day	0.0 (−1 to 0)	0.50	0.0 (−3 to 0)	0.64	1.00	1.7 (−1 to 4)	0.18
All cause hospital LOS#, day	0.0 (0−2)	0.94	0.0 (−3 to 0.5)	0.71	0.61	1.2 (−1 to 4)	0.34
Cost of COPD medication#, €	−9.6 (−17 to 157)	0.76	−6.5 (−179 to 0)	0.025	0.30	−480.7 (−891 to −70)	0.02
Cost of COPD-related hospitalizations#, €	0.0 (−1017 to 0)	0.44	0.0 (−2879 to 49)	0.67	0.89	1690.8 (−812 to 4194)	0.18
Cost of all cause hospitalizations#, €	0.0 (0−2035)	0.94	0.0 (−2905 to 509)	0.62	0.56	1110.0 (−1551 to 3771)	0.40

Results presented as: † = mean (95% confidence interval) or ‡ = median (25th to 75th percentile); # = per patient and per year; LOS = length of stay. Regression coefficient β (95% confidence interval) of variable 'group', adjusted for the baseline value of the outcome measure concerned.

subjects. This leaves the study potentially open to attrition bias and limits both the statistical significance and potential for generalization of the results.

R. J. Shephard, MD (Lond), PhD, DPE

Reference

1. Bourbeau J, Julien M, Maltais F, et al. Reduction of hospital utilization in patients with chronic obstructive pulmonary disease: a disease-specific self-management intervention. *Arch Intern Med.* 2003;163:585-591.

Exercise induced skeletal muscle metabolic stress is reduced after pulmonary rehabilitation in COPD

Calvert LD, Singh SJ, Morgan MD, et al (Univ Hosps of Leicester NHS Trust, UK)
Respir Med 105:363-370, 2011

In COPD, skeletal muscle ATP resynthesis may be insufficient to meet demand during exercise due to excessive anaerobic and reduced oxidative (mitochondrial) energy production, leading to metabolic stress. We investigated the effect of outpatient pulmonary rehabilitation (PR) on the metabolic response (measured by exercise-induced accumulation of plasma ammonia) and determined whether this response predicted functional improvement following PR.

25 subjects with stable COPD [mean (SD) age 67 (8)years and FEV_1 47 (18)% predicted] performed maximal cycling ergometry before and after PR. Plasma ammonia was measured at rest, during exercise and 2 min post-exercise.

Following PR, there were significant increases in peak cycle WR and ISWT performance (Mean (SEM) changes 13.1 (2.0) W and 93 (15) m respectively, $p < 0.001$). Mean (SEM) rise in plasma ammonia was reduced at peak (Pre vs Post-PR: 29.0 (4.5) vs 20.2 (2.5) µmol/l, $p < 0.05$) and isotime (Pre vs Post-PR: 29.0 (4.5) vs 10.6 (1.7) µmol/l, $p < 0.001$) exercise. Improvements in exercise performance after PR were similar among subgroups who did versus those who did not show a rise in ammonia at baseline.

The results suggest that muscle cellular energy production was better matched to the demands of exercise following PR. We conclude that a pragmatic outpatient PR programme involving high intensity walking exercise results in significant adaptation of the skeletal muscle metabolic response with a reduction in exercise-related metabolic stress. However, the outcome of PR could not be predicted from baseline metabolic response (Fig 1).

▶ Calvert and colleagues found improved exercise capacity and reduced plasma ammonia and lactate accumulation in response to outpatient pulmonary rehabilitation in women and men with mild to moderate chronic obstructive pulmonary

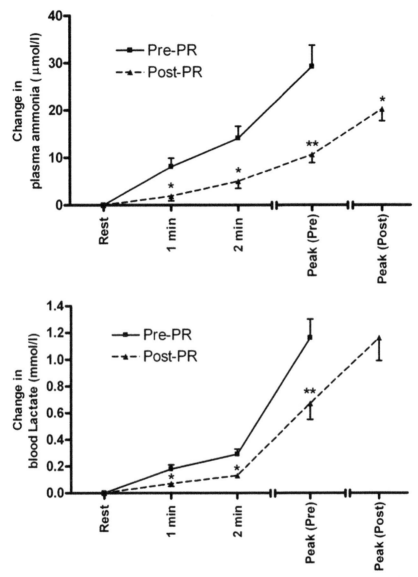

FIGURE 1.—Change in plasma ammonia (upper panel) and blood lactate (lower panel) from resting values during maximal cycling exercise before (solid lines) and after (dashed lines) Pulmonary Rehabilitation (PR). *$p < 0.05$, **$p < 0.001$ between pre-PR and post-PR analysis. (Reprinted from Calvert LD, Singh SJ, Morgan MD, et al. Exercise induced skeletal muscle metabolic stress is reduced after pulmonary rehabilitation in COPD. *Respir Med.* 2011;105:363-370, copyright 2011, with permission from Elsevier.)

disease (COPD) (Fig 1). Exercise capacity of patients with COPD is limited by the early onset of anaerobic metabolism within skeletal muscle. In COPD, the supply of adenosine triphosphate (ATP) is not replenished sufficiently to meet the demands of muscle contraction, thereby leading to deamination of adenosine monophosphate and release of ammonia into the circulation. The change in ammonia concentration during exercise is a sign of metabolic stress. In this study, plasma ammonia and lactate were measured during a peak cycle ergometer test before and after 7 weeks of outpatient pulmonary rehabilitation. The training comprised progressive walking and strength training exercises for 1 hour on 2 days per week. The walking intensity was set at 85% of peak Vo_2 predicted from a walk test at baseline. Performance on intermittent and endurance walk tests improved significantly. About half of the patients had a clinically significant increase in walking performance. Measures of exercise metabolic stress before training did not predict the improvements in walking capacity or peak exercise after training. There is no established metabolic stress criterion to refer patients to pulmonary rehabilitation. To further elucidate the metabolic stress mechanisms in peripheral skeletal muscle of patients with COPD, muscle biopsies with measurement of ATP and deamination products will be needed.

C. M. Jankowski, PhD

Feasibility of physical and occupational therapy beginning from initiation of mechanical ventilation
Pohlman MC, Schweickert WD, Pohlman AS, et al (Univ of Chicago, IL)
Crit Care Med 38:2089-2094, 2010

Objective.—Physical and occupational therapy are possible immediately after intubation in mechanically ventilated medical intensive care unit patients. The objective of this study was to describe a protocol of daily sedative interruption and early physical and occupational therapy and to specify details of intensive care unit-based therapy, including neurocognitive state, potential barriers, and adverse events related to this intervention.

Design and Patients.—Detailed descriptive study of the intervention arm of a trial of mechanically ventilated patients receiving early physical and occupational therapy.

Setting.—Two tertiary care academic medical centers participating in a randomized controlled trial.

Intervention.—Patients underwent daily sedative interruption followed by physical and occupational therapy every hospital day until achieving independent functional status. Therapy began with active range of motion and progressed to activities of daily living, sitting, standing, and walking as tolerated.

Measurements and Main Results.—Forty-nine mechanically ventilated patients received early physical and occupational therapy occurring a median of 1.5 days (range, 1.0−2.1 days) after intubation. Therapy was provided on 90% of MICU days during mechanical ventilation. While endotracheally intubated, subjects sat at the edge of the bed in 69% of all physical and occupational therapy sessions, transferred from bed to chair in 33%, stood in 33%, and ambulated during 15% (n = 26 of 168) of all physical and occupational therapy sessions (median distance of 15 feet; range, 15–20 feet). At least one potential barrier to mobilization during mechanical ventilation (acute lung injury, vasoactive medication administration, delirium, renal replacement therapy, or body mass index ≥ 30 kg/m^2) was present in 89% of patient encounters. Therapy was interrupted prematurely in 4% of all sessions, most commonly for patient-ventilator asynchrony and agitation.

Conclusion.—Early physical and occupational therapy is feasible from the onset of mechanical ventilation despite high illness acuity and presence of life support devices. Adverse events are uncommon, even in this high-risk group.

▶ These authors have previously published a randomized controlled trial on the benefits of physical and occupational therapies in critically ill patients who are on mechanical ventilation.[1] This article describes the intervention and the activities accomplished by the patients at the various stages of hospitalization and, in a large part, in the intensive care unit. They also discuss safety issues related to the intervention. The importance of this article is that it underscores the feasibility, safety, and potential barriers to treatment. It also describes the protocol with respect to sedative interruption and the safety screen they used to permit patients to receive the intervention along with the sedative interruption. They also include in the appendix, contraindications to initiating physical or occupational therapy and adverse events that would call for discontinuation of these therapies. Fortunately, the frequency of adverse events was low (16%). The detail in the article permits a similar protocol to be replicated elsewhere.

D. E. Feldman, PT, PhD

Reference

1. Schweickert WD, Pohlman MC, Pohlman AS, et al. Early physical and occupational therapy in mechanically ventilated, critically ill patients: a randomised controlled trial. *Lancet.* 2009;373:1874-1882.

7 Other Medical Problems

Submaximal Cardiopulmonary Exercise Testing Predicts Complications and Hospital Length of Stay in Patients Undergoing Major Elective Surgery
Snowden CP, Prentis JM, Anderson HL, et al (Freeman Hosp, Newcastle Upon Tyne, UK; Sunderland Royal Hosp, UK)
Ann Surg 251:535-541, 2010

Objective.—To investigate the null hypothesis that an objective, noninvasive technique of measuring cardiorespiratory reserve, does not improve the preoperative assessment of patient risk of postoperative complications, when compared with a standard questionnaire-based assessment of functional capacity.

Summary Background Data.—Postoperative complications may be increased in patients with reduced cardiorespiratory function. Activity questionnaires are subjective, whereas cardiopulmonary exercise testing (CPET) provides an objective definition of cardiorespiratory reserve. The use of preoperative CPET to predict postoperative complications is not fully defined.

Method.—CPET and an algorithm-based activity assessment (Veterans Activity Questionnaire Index [VASI]) were performed on consecutive patients (n = 171) with low subjective functional capacity (metabolic equivalent score [METS] < 7), being assessed for major surgery. A morbidity survey determined postoperative day 7 complications. Logistic regression defined independent predictors of complication group. Receiver-operating curve (ROC) analysis defined the predictive value of CPET to outcome. $P < 0.05$ value demonstrated significance.

Results.—Objective cardiorespiratory reserve did not differ between operated (n = 116) and nonoperated patients (n = 55). Median complication rate on postoperative day 7 was 1. Patients with >1 complication had an increase in hospital LOS compared to the group with ≤1 complication (26 vs. 10 days; $P < 0.001$). Anaerobic threshold (AT) was higher in the group with ≤1 complication (11.9 vs. 9.1 mL/kg/min; $P = 0.001$) and demonstrated high accuracy (AUC = 0.85), sensitivity (88%), and specificity (79%), at an optimum AT of 10.1 mL/kg/min (defined by the furthest left point on the ROC curve). AT, VASI, and surgical reintervention were independent predictors of complication group. Preoperative

TABLE 3.—Univariate and Multivariate Logistic Regression Analysis With Dependent Variable as Postoperative Complication Group (≤1 Complication vs. >1 Complication)

Variables	OR	β	95% CI	Wald	Significance
Univariate regression					
Age (yr)	1.05	0.050	1.000–1.100	4.30	0.04
Revised Cardiac Risk Index	1.23	0.203	0.813–1.840	0.941	0.33
Body mass index (BMI)	1.01	0.011	0.941–1.087	0.096	0.76
Serum creatinine (μmol/L)	1.01	0.006	0.991–1.022	0.653	0.42
Emergency surgical reoperation	15.4	2.734	1.778–133.3	6.164	0.01
POSSUM physiology score	1.11	0.104	0.987–1.246	1.25	0.08
POSSUM morbidity	1.02	0.022	0.994–1.052	2.423	0.12
Veterans activity score index (VASI)	0.49	−0.715	0.343–0.698	15.53	<0.0001
CPET variables					
AT (mL/min/kg)	0.47	−0.748	0.346–0.648	21.902	<0.0001
Peak VO_2 (mL/min/kg)	0.77	−0.260	0.669–0.889	12.79	<0.0001
VE/VCO_2	1.00	0.003	0.950–1.058	0.01	0.92
Multivariate regression					
Overall model					
Veterans Activity Score Index (VASI)	0.557	−0.586	0.347–0.894	5.865	0.02
Surgical reintervention	94.23	4.546	3.558–2495.6	7.394	0.07
AT	0.441	−0.818	0.302–0.644	17.92	<0.0001
Preoperative model					
Veterans Activity Score Index (VASI)	0.553	−0.593	0.349–0.876	6.372	0.01
AT	0.424	−0.859	0.285–0.629	18.107	<0.0001

AT significantly improved outcome prediction when compared with the use of VASI alone.

Conclusion.—An objective measure of cardiorespiratory reserve was an independent predictor of a major surgical group with increased postoperative complications and hospital LOS. AT measurement significantly improved outcome prediction compared with an algorithm-based activity assessment (Table 3).

▶ Assessment of the suitability of an older patient for major surgery is often based on supplementing a clinical examination by a resting or an exercise electrocardiogram, although the added value of such organ-specific examination has been questioned.[1,2] At best, it provides a limited indication of the risk of postoperative complications.[3-5] This study began from the premise that a questionnaire assessment of habitual physical activity and a laboratory measurement of anaerobic threshold might provide the surgeon with helpful indications of overall cardiorespiratory reserve and thus indicate the level of postoperative risk. The value of the 2 assessments was tested in a substantial sample of surgical patients with a low subjective functional capacity (<7 metabolic equivalents). A multiple regression approach in a carefully blinded trial demonstrated independent prediction of the risk of postsurgical complications from each of the 2 assessments (Table 3). The data suggest that there may be a need to rethink the American College of Cardiology/American Heart Association verdict that a cardiopulmonary assessment is not helpful as a preliminary assessment to noncardiac surgery.[6]

R. J. Shephard, MD (Lond), PhD, DPE

References

1. Halm EA, Browner WS, Tubau JF, Tateo IM, Mangano DT. Echocardiography for assessing cardiac risk in patients having noncardiac surgery. Study of Perioperative Ischemia Research Group. *Ann Intern Med.* 1996;125:433-441.
2. Mangano DT, London MJ, Tubau JF, et al. Dipyridamole thallium-201 scintigraphy as a preoperative screening test. A reexamination of its predictive potential. Study of Perioperative Ischemia Research Group. *Circulation.* 1991;84:493-502.
3. Kertai MD, Boersma E, Bax JJ, et al. A meta-analysis comparing the prognostic accuracy of six diagnostic tests for predicting perioperative cardiac risk in patients undergoing major vascular surgery. *Heart.* 2003;89:1327-1334.
4. Schouten O, Bax JJ, Poldermans D. Assessment of cardiac risk before non-cardiac general surgery. *Heart.* 2006;92:1866-1872.
5. Ridley S. Cardiac scoring systems—what is their value? *Anaesthesia.* 2003;58: 985-991.
6. Fleisher LA, Beckman JA, Brown KA, et al. ACC/AHA 2007 Guidelines on Perioperative Cardiovascular Evaluation and Care for Noncardiac Surgery: Executive Summary: A Report of the American College of Cardiology/American Heart Association Task Force on Practice Guidelines (Writing Committee to Revise the 2002 Guidelines on Perioperative Cardiovascular Evaluation for Noncardiac Surgery) Developed in Collaboration With the American Society of Echocardiography, American Society of Nuclear Cardiology, Heart Rhythm Society, Society of Cardiovascular Anesthesiologists, Society for Cardiovascular Angiography and Interventions, Society for Vascular Medicine and Biology, and Society for Vascular Surgery. *J Am Coll Cardiol.* 2007;50:1707-1732.

American College of Sports Medicine Roundtable on Exercise Guidelines for Cancer Survivors

Schmitz KH, Courneya KS, Matthews C, et al (American College of Sports Medicine)
Med Sci Sports Exerc 42:1409-1426, 2010

Early detection and improved treatments for cancer have resulted in roughly 12 million survivors alive in the United States today. This growing population faces unique challenges from their disease and treatments, including risk for recurrent cancer, other chronic diseases, and persistent adverse effects on physical functioning and quality of life. Historically, clinicians advised cancer patients to rest and to avoid activity; however, emerging research on exercise has challenged this recommendation. To this end, a roundtable was convened by American College of Sports Medicine to distill the literature on the safety and efficacy of exercise training during and after adjuvant cancer therapy and to provide guidelines. The roundtable concluded that exercise training is safe during and after cancer treatments and results in improvements in physical functioning, quality of life, and cancer-related fatigue in several cancer survivor groups. Implications for disease outcomes and survival are still unknown. Nevertheless, the benefits to physical functioning and quality of life are sufficient for the recommendation that cancer survivors follow the 2008 Physical Activity Guidelines for Americans, with specific exercise programming adaptations based on disease and treatment-related adverse effects. The

TABLE 2.—Preexercise Medical Assessments and Exercise Testing

Cancer Site	Breast	Prostate	Colon	Adult Hematologic (No HSCT)	Adult HSCT	Gynecologic
General medical assessments recommended before exercise	Recommend evaluation for peripheral neuropathies and musculoskeletal morbidities secondary to treatment regardless of time since treatment. If there has been hormonal therapy, recommend evaluation of fracture risk. Individuals with known metastatic disease to the bone will require evaluation to discern what is safe before starting exercise. Individuals with known cardiac conditions (secondary to cancer or not) require medical assessment of the safety of exercise before starting. There is always a risk that metastasis to the bone or cardiac toxicity secondary to cancer treatments will be undetected. This risk will vary widely across the population of survivors. Fitness professionals may want to consult with the patient's medical team to discern this likelihood. However, requiring medical assessment for metastatic disease and cardiotoxicity for all survivors before exercise is not recommended because this would create an unnecessary barrier to obtaining the well-established health benefits of exercise for the majority of survivors, for whom metastasis and cardiotoxicity are unlikely to occur.					
Cancer site–specific medical assessments recommended before starting an exercise program	Recommend evaluation of arm/shoulder morbidity before upper body exercise.	Evaluation of muscle strength and wasting.	Patient should be evaluated as having established consistent and proactive infection prevention behaviors for an existing ostomy before engaging in exercise training more vigorous than a walking program.	None	None	Morbidly obese patients may require additional medical assessment for the safety of activity beyond cancer-specific risk. Recommend evaluation for lower extremity lymphedema before vigorous aerobic exercise or resistance training.
Exercise testing recommended	No exercise testing required before walking, flexibility, or resistance training. Follow ACSM guidelines for exercise testing before moderate to vigorous aerobic exercise training. One-repetition maximum testing has been demonstrated to be safe in breast cancer survivors with and at risk for lymphedema.					
Exercise testing mode and intensity considerations	As per outcome of medical assessments and following ACSM guidelines for exercise testing.					
Contraindications to exercise testing and reasons to stop exercise testing	Follow ACSM guidelines for exercise testing.					

TABLE 3.—. Exercise Prescription for Cancer Survivors

	Breast	Prostate	Colon	Adult Hematologic (No HSCT)	Adult HSCT	Gynecologic
Objectives/goals of exercise prescription	1. To regain and improve physical function, aerobic capacity, strength and flexibility. 2. To improve body image and QOL. 3. To improve body composition. 4. To improve cardiorespiratory, endocrine, neurological, muscular, cognitive, and psychosocial outcomes. 5. Potentially, to reduce or delay recurrence or a second primary cancer. 6. To improve the ability to physically and psychologically withstand the ongoing anxiety regarding recurrence or a second primary cancer. 7. To reduce, attenuate, and prevent long-term and late effects of cancer treatment. 8. To improve the physiologic and psychological ability to withstand any current or future cancer treatments. These goals will vary according to where the survivor is in the continuum of cancer experience, as depicted in Figure 1.					
General contraindications for starting an exercise program common across all cancer sites	Allow adequate time to heal after surgery. The number of weeks required for surgical recovery may be as high as 8. Do not exercise individuals who are experiencing extreme fatigue, anemia, or ataxia. Follow ACSM guidelines for exercise prescription concerning cardiovascular and pulmonary contraindications for starting an exercise program. However, the potential for an adverse cardiopulmonary event might be higher among cancer survivors than age-matched comparisons given the toxicity of radiotherapy and chemotherapy and long-term/late effects of cancer surgery.					
Cancer-specific contraindications for starting an exercise program	Women with immediate arm or shoulder problems secondary to breast cancer treatment should seek medical care to resolve those issues before exercise training with the upper body.	None	Physician permission recommended for patients with an ostomy before participation in contact sports (risk of blow) and weight training (risk of hernia).	None	None	Women with swelling or inflammation in the abdomen, groin, or lower extremity should seek medical care to resolve these issues before exercise training with the lower body.
Cancer-specific reasons for stopping an exercise program. (Note: General ACSM guidelines for stopping exercise remain in place for this population.)	Changes in arm/shoulder symptoms or swelling should result in reductions or avoidance of upper body exercise until after appropriate medical evaluation and treatment resolves the issue.	None	Hernia, ostomy-related systemic infection.	None	None	Changes in swelling or inflammation of the abdomen, groin, or lower extremities should result in reductions or avoidance of lower body exercise until after appropriate medical evaluation and treatment resolves the issue.

(Continued)

TABLE 3. (*continued*)

	Breast	Prostate	Colon	Adult Hematologic (No HSCT)	Adult HSCT	Gynecologic
General injury risk issues in common across cancer sites	Patients with bone metastases may need to alter their exercise program concerning intensity, duration, and mode given increased risk for skeletal fractures. Infection risk is higher for patients who are currently undergoing chemotherapy or radiation treatment or have compromised immune function after treatment. Care should be taken to reduce infection risk in fitness centers frequented by cancer survivors. Exercise tolerance of patients currently in treatment and immediately after treatment may vary from exercise session-to-exercise session about exercise tolerance, depending on their treatment schedule. Individuals with known metastatic disease to the bone will require modifications and increased supervision to avoid fractures. Individuals with cardiac conditions (secondary to cancer or not) will require modifications and may require increased supervision for safety.					
Cancer-specific risk of injury and emergency procedures	The arms/shoulders should be exercised, but proactive injury prevention approaches are encouraged, given the high incidence of arm/shoulder morbidity in breast cancer survivors. Women with lymphedema should wear a well-fitting compression garment during exercise. Be aware of risk for fracture among those treated with hormonal therapy, a diagnosis of osteoporosis, or bony metastases.	Be aware of risk for fracture among patients treated with ADT, a diagnosis of osteoporosis or bony metastases	Advisable to avoid excessive intra-abdominal pressures for patients with an stomp.	Multiple myeloma patients should be treated as if they have osteoporosis.	None	The lower body should be exercised, but proactive injury prevention approaches are encouraged, given the potential for lower extremity swelling or inflammation in this population. Women with lymphedema should wear a well-fitting compression garment during exercise. Be aware of risk for fractures among those treated with hormonal therapies, with diagnosed osteoporosis, or with bony metastases.

advice to "avoid inactivity," even in cancer patients with existing disease or undergoing difficult treatments, is likely helpful (Tables 2 and 3).

▶ A panel of experts in cancer and exercise convened a roundtable to develop exercise testing and training recommendations for cancer survivors. The American College of Sports Medicine (ACSM) roundtable expert panel surveyed peer-reviewed published studies of exercise interventions for cancer survivors. The vast majority of these studies were conducted in patients with breast cancer, with a small collection of studies in patients with prostate, colon, adult hematologic, and gynecologic cancers. The basic message of the ACSM roundtable is that cancer survivors should remain as active as possible during and after completion of cancer treatment. However, it was also recognized that exercise programs need to be adapted to the individual survivor, taking into consideration his/her health status, including noncancer comorbidities, treatments received, and anticipated disease trajectory. The guidelines include recommendations for preexercise medical screening (Table 2) and exercise prescription (Table 3). These recommendations address site-specific side effects of cancer treatments, such as upper extremity lymphedema in breast cancer survivors and infection prevention in survivors of colon cancer. The risk-to-benefit ratio of exercise training during and after cancer treatment tips well toward benefit, although more studies reporting adverse events are needed. Individual risks can be further reduced by evaluating comorbidities, such as cardiovascular disease in the older prostate or colon cancer survivor. The overall evidence level for these recommendations are National Heart, Lung, and Blood Institute level B (few randomized controlled trials exist or they are small and results are inconsistent). The effects of exercise to improve cardiovascular fitness and muscular strength of cancer survivors have been consistent. There is less consistency when the outcomes are depression, anxiety, fatigue, body composition, or physical function. Because exercise intervention studies have been quite small, the generalizability of results to the cancer population is questionable. Further research is needed to improve the evidence level and modify the expert panel's recommendations. Nonetheless, exercise can be safely undertaken by cancer survivors with some input from primary care providers and oncologists. More exercise programs dedicated to the evaluation and exercise training of cancer survivors will be needed, and these programs will need to be staffed by competent exercise professionals.

C. M. Jankowski, PhD

American College of Sports Medicine Roundtable on Exercise Guidelines for Cancer Survivors
Schmitz KH, Courneya KS, Matthews C, et al (American College of Sports Medicine)
Med Sci Sports Exerc 42:1409-1426, 2010

Early detection and improved treatments for cancer have resulted in roughly 12 million survivors alive in the United States today. This growing population faces unique challenges from their disease and treatments, including risk for recurrent cancer, other chronic diseases, and persistent adverse effects on physical functioning and quality of life. Historically, clinicians advised cancer patients to rest and to avoid activity; however, emerging research on exercise has challenged this recommendation. To this end, a roundtable was convened by American College of Sports Medicine to distill the literature on the safety and efficacy of exercise training during and after adjuvant cancer therapy and to provide guidelines. The roundtable concluded that exercise training is safe during and after cancer treatments and results in improvements in physical functioning, quality of life, and cancer-related fatigue in several cancer survivor groups. Implications for disease outcomes and survival are still unknown. Nevertheless, the benefits to physical functioning and quality of life are sufficient for the recommendation that cancer survivors follow the

TABLE 1.—Persistent Changes Resulting from the Most Commonly Used Curative Therapies

	Surgery	Chemotherapy	Radiation	Hormonal Therapy, Oophorectomy or Orchiectomy	Targeted Therapies
Second cancers		✓	✓		
Fatigue	✓	✓	✓	✓	✓
Pain	✓	✓	✓	✓	✓
Cardiovascular changes: damage or increased CVD risk		✓	✓	✓	✓
Pulmonary changes	✓	✓	✓		
Neurological changes: Peripheral neuropathy		✓			
Cognitive changes	✓	✓	✓	✓	✓
Endocrine changes Reproductive changes (e.g., infertility, early menopause, impaired sexual function)	✓	✓	✓	✓	✓
Body weight changes (increases or decreases)	✓	✓		✓	
Fat mass increases	✓	✓		✓	
Lean mass losses	✓	✓		✓	
Worsened bone health		✓	✓	✓	
Musculoskeletal soft tissues: changes or damage	✓		✓	✓	
Immune system Impaired immune function and/or anemia		✓	✓	✓	✓
Lymphedema	✓		✓		
Gastrointestinal system: changes or impaired function	✓	✓	✓	✓	✓
Organ function changes	✓				
Skin changes			✓	✓	✓

2008 Physical Activity Guidelines for Americans, with specific exercise programming adaptations based on disease and treatment-related adverse effects. The advice to "avoid inactivity," even in cancer patients with existing disease or undergoing difficult treatments, is likely helpful (Table 1).

▶ It is useful to have a consensus summary of the quality of the evidence supporting the emerging viewpoints that exercise is often helpful during the treatment of malignancies, and that cancer survivors should subsequently adopt a similar volume of physical activity to that recommended for the general population. Nevertheless, this recommendation must have due regard for any residual complications of treatment (Table 1) that may impinge on the ability to perform particular types of physical activity or that may benefit from specific types of corrective exercise. In general, exercise programs posttreatment have to date proven very safe, the one exception being swelling from the onset or worsening of lymphedema in a substantial proportion of patients undertaking arm exercises after mastectomy. Most of the trials reported to date have been in patients successfully treated for breast and prostate cancers; there remains a pressing need for data on the safety and effectiveness of exercise programs after the successful treatment of other common cancers such as those of the colon.

R. J. Shephard, MD (Lond), PhD, DPE

Influence of Cardiorespiratory Fitness on Lung Cancer Mortality

Sui X, Lee D-C, Matthews CE, et al (Univ of South Carolina, Columbia; Natl Cancer Inst, Rockville, MD; et al)
Med Sci Sports Exerc 42:872-878, 2010

Purpose.—Previous studies have suggested that higher levels of physical activity may lower lung cancer risk; however, few prospective studies have evaluated lung cancer mortality in relation to cardiorespiratory fitness (CRF), an objective marker of recent physical activity habits.

Methods.—Thirty-eight thousand men, aged 20–84 yr, without history of cancer, received a preventive medical examination at the Cooper Clinic in Dallas, Texas, between 1974 and 2002. CRF was quantified as maximal treadmill exercise test duration and was grouped for analysis as low (lowest 20% of exercise duration), moderate (middle 40%), and high (upper 40%).

Results.—A total of 232 lung cancer deaths occurred during follow-up (mean = 17 yr). After adjustment for age, examination year, body mass index, smoking, drinking, physical activity, and family history of cancer, hazard ratios (95% confidence intervals) for lung cancer deaths across low, moderate, and high CRF categories were 1.0, 0.48 (0.35–0.67), and 0.43 (0.28–0.65), respectively. There was an inverse association between CRF and lung cancer mortality in former (P for trend = 0.005) and current smokers (P for trend < 0.001) but not in never smokers (trend $P = 0.14$). Joint analysis of smoking and fitness status revealed a significant 12-fold higher risk of death in current smokers (hazard ratio = 11.9, 95% confidence interval = 6.0−23.6) with low CRF as compared with never smokers who had high CRF.

Conclusions.—Although the potential for some residual confounding by smoking could not be eliminated, these data suggest that CRF is inversely associated with lung cancer mortality in men. Continued study of CRF in relation to lung cancer, particularly among smokers, may further our understanding of disease etiology and reveal additional strategies for reducing its burden (Table 2).

▶ Some authors (including Dr Blair and his associates) have argued that the assessment of an individual's aerobic fitness provides a better estimate of physical activity than the questionnaire methods used in most epidemiological surveys because measurements of maximal aerobic power can be made with greater precision. There are a number of caveats to this conclusion, particularly in the context of long-term illnesses such as cancer. Firstly, maximal aerobic power can change substantially with a few weeks of activity or inactivity; thus, it does not give information on long-term patterns of physical activity. Secondly, a part of the usual score (maximal oxygen intake per kg of body mass or the simpler treadmill endurance time as used in this study) reflects a combination of genetic endowment and body mass rather than recent habitual physical activity. It is also not clear why one would adjust data for physical

TABLE 2.—Event Rates and Hazard Ratios for Lung Cancer Mortality by Cardiorespiratory Fitness (CRF) Groups, ACLS, Dallas, Texas, 1974−2003

	Deaths for Lung Caner	Event Rate[a]	HR[b]	95% CI[b]	HR[c]	95% CI[c]
All men (N = 38,000)						
Low CRF	86	7.3	1.00	Referent		
Moderate CRF	86	3.1	0.48	0.35−0.67		
High CRF	60	2.3	0.43	0.28−0.65		
P linear trend		<0.001		<0.001		
Never smoker (n = 6245)						
Low CRF	7	2.0			1.00	Referent
Moderate CRF	15	1.3			0.93	0.29−2.96
High CRF	13	1.0			0.76	0.21−2.79
P linear trend		0.14				0.62
Former smoker (n = 15,024)						
Low CRF	29	7.3			1.00	Referent
Moderate CRF	35	3.4			0.44	0.26−0.74
High CRF	33	3.3			0.44	0.24−0.81
P linear trend		0.005				0.02
Current smoker (n = 16,731)						
Low CRF	50	12.1			1.00	Referent
Moderate CRF	36	6.3			0.48	0.30−0.76
High CRF	14	5.1			0.38	0.18−0.79
P linear trend		<0.001				0.001

HR, hazard ratio; CI, conference interval; CRF, cardiorespiratory fitness; BMI, body mass index.
[a]Event rate is expressed as per 10,000 person-years and adjusted for age.
[b]Adjusted for age, examination year, smoking status (never, past, or current), alcohol intake (drinks per week), physical inactivity (yes or no), BMI ($kg \cdot m^{-2}$), and family history of cancer (present or not).
[c]Adjusted for age, examination year, cigarettes per day (for former and current smoker), alcohol intake (drinks per week), physical inactivity (yes or not), BMI ($kg \cdot m^{-2}$), and family history of cancer (present or not).

inactivity if one is using the score on the treadmill test as a measure of habitual activity. With these caveats, the present data show a negative association between lung cancer mortality and physical fitness in current and former smokers but not in those who have never smoked (Table 2). If there were a true effect of physical activity, one would expect benefit in nonsmokers as well as smokers, and because the pattern of smoking (daily consumption, pack years, inhalation, etc) was not analyzed, it may be that active smokers consume fewer cigarettes or work in less hazardous occupations than those who are inactive. However, as the authors point out, other explanations of why there was no association in nonsmokers include a very small number of cases of cancer in this group and possible differences in the type of cancer.[1,2] Possible mechanisms of benefit, if the association proves to be causal, could include an increase of natural killer cell activity,[3] a decrease of C-reactive protein levels,[4] or enhanced antioxidant defenses.[5]

R. J. Shephard, MD (Lond), PhD, DPE

References

1. Thune I, Lund E. The influence of physical activity on lung-cancer risk: A prospective study of 81,516 men and women. *Int J Cancer.* 1997;70:57-62.
2. Wakelee HA, Chang ET, Gomez SL, Keegan TH, Feskanich D, Clarke CA. Lung cancer incidence in never smokers. *J Clin Oncol.* 2007;25:472-478.
3. Shephard RJ, Shek PN. Associations between physical activity and susceptibility to cancer: possible mechanisms. *Sports Med.* 1998;26:293-315.
4. Kasapis C, Thompson PD. The effects of physical activity on serum C-reactive protein and inflammatory markers: a systematic review. *J Am Coll Cardiol.* 2005;45:1563-1569.
5. Rundle A. Molecular epidemiology of physical activity and cancer. *Cancer Epidemiol Biomarkers Prev.* 2005;14:227-236.

Combined Resistance and Aerobic Exercise Program Reverses Muscle Loss in Men Undergoing Androgen Suppression Therapy for Prostate Cancer Without Bone Metastases: A Randomized Controlled Trial

Galvão DA, Taaffe DR, Spry N, et al (Edith Cowan Univ, Joondalup, Western Australia; Sir Charles Gairdner Hosp, Western Australia; Univ of Western Australia, Nedlands; et al)
J Clin Oncol 28:340-347, 2010

Purpose.—Androgen suppression therapy (AST) results in musculoskeletal toxicity that reduces physical function and quality of life. This study examined the impact of a combined resistance and aerobic exercise program as a countermeasure to these AST-related toxicities.

Patients and Methods.—Between 2007 and 2008, 57 patients with prostate cancer undergoing AST (commenced > 2 months prior) were randomly assigned to a program of resistance and aerobic exercise (n = 29) or usual care (n = 28) for 12 weeks. Primary end points were whole body and regional lean mass. Secondary end points were muscle strength and function, cardiorespiratory capacity, blood biomarkers, and quality of life.

TABLE 3.—Muscle Strength and Endurance Absolute Values and Change Over 12 Weeks Exercise Training

Measure	Baseline				12 Weeks				Adjusted Group Difference in Mean Change Over 12 Weeks		P*
	Exercise		Control		Exercise		Control				
	Mean	SD	Mean	SD	Mean	SD	Mean	SD	Mean	95% CI	
Muscle strength, one repetition maximal, kg											
Chest press	34.6	11.2	34.7	13.6	38.4	11.3	35.2	12.1	2.8	0.50 to 5.1	.018
Seated row	40.1	7.6	39.2	8.0	45.8	8.8	40.0	8.9	5.1	3.3 to 7.0	< .001
Leg press	98.4	43.0	102.6	54.1	134.6	52.8	109.6	53.3	30.8	20.1 to 41.6	< .001
Leg extension	38.1	14.9	40.0	15.7	50.1	15.4	41.6	16.9	11.5	7.2 to 15.8	< .001
Muscle endurance											
Chest press											
At baseline test 70% of 1-RM (rep)	10.9	3.9	11.9	4.1	16.0	5.2	11.3	4.2	5.2	3.0 to 7.5	< .001
At post-test 70% of 1-RM (rep)	10.9	3.9	11.9	4.1	11.7	5.1	10.3	3.3	2.5	0.11 to 4.9	.041
Leg press											
At baseline test 70% of 1-RM (rep)	17.8	7.3	16.8	6.4	30.0	8.8	19.5	9.2	10.8	7.1 to 14.6	< .001
At post-test 70% of 1-RM (rep)	17.8	7.3	16.8	6.4	21.5	8.4	17.3	8.3	3.4	−0.96 to 7.8	.124

Abbreviations: SD, standard deviation; 1-RM, one repetition maximal; rep, number of repetitions.
*Between group change by analysis of covariance (adjusted for baseline, androgen suppression therapy time, use of antiandrogen, number of medications, and education).

Results.—Analysis of covariance was used to compare outcomes for groups at 12 weeks adjusted for baseline values and potential confounders. Patients undergoing exercise showed an increase in lean mass compared with usual care (total body, $P = .047$; upper limb, $P < .001$; lower limb, $P = .019$) and similarly better muscle strength ($P < .01$), 6-meter walk time ($P = .024$), and 6-meter backward walk time ($P = .039$). Exercise also improved several aspects of quality of life including general health ($P = .022$) and reduced fatigue ($P = .021$) and decreased levels of C-reactive protein ($P = .008$). There were no adverse events during the testing or exercise intervention program.

Conclusion.—A relatively brief exposure to exercise significantly improved muscle mass, strength, physical function, and balance in hypogonadal men compared with normal care. The exercise regimen was well tolerated and could be recommended for patients undergoing AST as an effective counter-measure to these common treatment-related adverse effects (Table 3).

▶ There is a growing use of androgen suppressants for a period of 2 to 3 years following standard radiotherapy treatment of prostate cancers.[1] Although the risk of a recurrence appears to be reduced by this tactic, there are unfortunate side effects to the administration of androgen suppressants, including muscle wasting, osteoporosis, and an increased risk of fractures. Such side effects can have a substantial negative effect on the patient's quality of life and (in older individuals) may be sufficiently severe as to compromise independence.[2,3] It seems logical to attempt to counter these complications by a program of resistance and/or aerobic exercise, and these authors obtained some evidence of benefit from such an initiative in a previous uncontrolled trial. This encouraged them to organize this randomized controlled study where experimental subjects undertook 15 to 20 minutes of aerobic exercise plus resistance exercises twice per week for 12 weeks. Relative to the usual treatment controls, the experimental group showed substantial increases of lean muscle mass and muscle strength (Table 3); there were also gains in the quality of life, as assessed by the SF-36 questionnaire, but gains of walking speed, rising from a chair, and stair climbing were less impressive. The observed benefits were achieved without adverse changes in levels of prostate serum antigen. Gains would probably have been larger if the exercise regimen had continued throughout the period of androgen suppression. Problems in controlling the bladder and/or the bowel are an issue in some patients after prostate surgery or irradiation; moreover, vigorous exercise may aggravate such symptoms. However, this article does not discuss this issue.

R. J. Shephard, MD (Lond), PhD, DPE

References

1. Shahinian VB, Kuo YF, Freeman JL, et al. Increasing use of gonadotropin-releasing hormone agonists for the treatment of localized prostate carcinoma. *Cancer.* 2005; 103:1615-1624.
2. Galvão DA, Taaffe DR, Spry N, Joseph D, Turner D, Newton RU. Reduced muscle strength and functional performance in men with prostatic cancer undergoing

androgen suppression: a comprehensive cross-sectional investigation. *Prostate Cancer Prostatic Dis.* 2009;12:198-203.

3. Shahinian VB, Kuo YF, Freeman JL, Goodwin JS. Risk of fracture after androgen deprivation for prostate cancer. *N Engl J Med.* 2005;352:154-164.

Beyond Recreational Physical Activity: Examining Occupational and Household Activity, Transportation Activity, and Sedentary Behavior in Relation to Postmenopausal Breast Cancer Risk

George SM, Irwin ML, Matthews CE, et al (Natl Cancer Inst, Rockville, MD; Yale School of Public Health, New Haven, CT; et al)
Am J Public Health 100:2288-2295, 2010

Objectives.—We prospectively examined nonrecreational physical activity and sedentary behavior in relation to breast cancer risk among 97039 postmenopausal women in the National Institutes of Health–AARP Diet and Health Study.

Methods.—We identified 2866 invasive and 570 in situ breast cancer cases recorded between 1996 and 2003 and used Cox proportional hazards regression to estimate multivariate relative risks (RRs) and 95% confidence intervals (CIs).

Results.—Routine activity during the day at work or at home that included heavy lifting or carrying versus mostly sitting was associated with reduced risk of invasive breast cancer (RR = 0.62; 95% CI = 0.42, 0.91; P_{trend} = .024).

Conclusions.—Routine activity during the day at work or home may be related to reduced invasive breast cancer risk. Domains outside of recreation time may be attractive targets for increasing physical activity and reducing sedentary behavior among postmenopausal women.

▶ The 2008 Physical Activity Guidelines (PAG) divided bodily movement into 2 categories: (1) Baseline activity or the light-intensity activities of daily life, such as standing, walking slowly, and lifting lightweight objects, and (2) Health-enhancing physical activities, such as brisk walking, jumping rope, swimming, or cycling, which when added to baseline activity, produce health benefits.[1] No specific guidelines for baseline activity were given in the 2008 PAG because "we don't understand enough about whether doing more baseline activity results in health benefits." Data from this large epidemiological study of postmenopausal women indicate that independent of recreational moderate-vigorous physical activity level, increases in routine or baseline activity during the day at work or home and, possibly, active commuting may be protective against invasive but not in situ breast cancer. The authors opined that "given that many postmenopausal women may not be capable of meeting US physical activity guidelines for cancer prevention through recreational moderate–vigorous physical activity alone, domains outside of recreation time may be attractive targets for increasing physical activity and reducing sedentary behavior."

D. C. Nieman, DrPH

Reference

1. Physical Activity Guidelines Advisory Committee. *Physical Activity Guidelines Advisory Committee Report, 2008*. Washington, DC: U.S. Department of Health and Human Services; 2008.

Physical activity, sedentary behaviours, and the prevention of endometrial cancer

Moore SC, Gierach GL, Schatzkin A, et al (Natl Cancer Inst, Bethesda, MD)

Br J Cancer 103:933-938, 2010

Physical activity has been hypothesised to reduce endometrial cancer risk, but this relationship has been difficult to confirm because of a limited number of prospective studies. However, recent publications from five cohort studies, which together comprise 2663 out of 3463 cases in the published literature for analyses of recreational physical activity, may help resolve this question. To synthesise these new data, we conducted a meta-analysis of prospective studies published through to December 2009. We found that physical activity was clearly associated with reduced risk of endometrial cancer, with active women having an approximately 30% lower risk than inactive women. Owing to recent interest in sedentary behaviour, we further investigated sitting time in relation to endometrial cancer risk using data from the NIH-AARP Diet and Health Study. We found that, independent of the level of moderate–vigorous physical activity, greater sitting time was associated with increased endometrial cancer risk. Thus, limiting time in sedentary behaviours may complement increasing level of moderate–vigorous physical activity as a means of reducing endometrial cancer risk. Taken together with the established biological plausibility of this relation, the totality of evidence now convincingly indicates that physical activity prevents or reduces risk of endometrial cancer (Fig 1).

▶ As much as 50% of endometrial cancer has been blamed upon obesity,[1] so a relationship of risk to habitual physical activity seems likely. Physical activity is known to reduce serum levels of estradiol and to increase levels of sex hormone–binding globulin, perhaps by reducing body fat stores. Regular physical activity also counters hyperinsulinemia and thus reduces the rate of endometrial proliferation. However, until recently, experts have concluded that evidence for the preventive role of physical activity was probable rather than convincing because conclusions were based mainly on case-control studies (subject to recall bias) rather than on large prospective trials, the latter being one of the currently accepted criteria for a satisfactory proof.[2] A number of large prospective trials have recently been published,[3-7] and Moore et al have thus conducted a meta-analysis that incorporates this new information. Their analysis includes data from 9 studies of recreational activity and 5 of occupational activity, for a total subject pool of 3463 cases. In addition to confirming the preventive

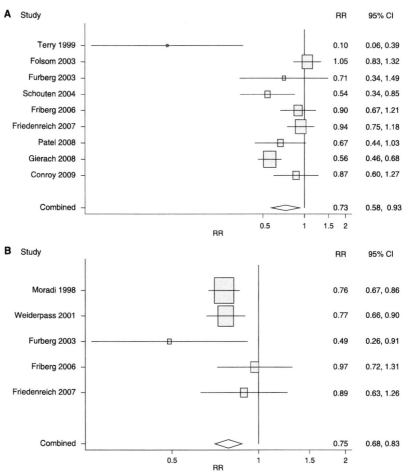

FIGURE 1.—(A) Relative risk (RR) and 95% confidence intervals (CI) of endometrial cancer according to the highest *vs* the lowest level of recreational physical activity. Relative risks were obtained from multivariate adjusted models, except Folsom *et al* (2003), which presented only age-adjusted results. For Friberg *et al* (12), Patel *et al* (14), and Gierach *et al* (15), we used results from models without adjustment for BMI, although BMI-adjusted results were available in separate models in these publications. In a sensitivity analysis, we examined results when using only RRs adjusted for BMI (including all studies, except Folsom *et al*). In these models, there was modest attenuation of relative risks, but an inverse association was still evident (pooled RR = 0.78; 95% CI = 0.63, 0.95). (B) Relative risk (RR) and 95% confidence intervals (CI) of endometrial cancer according to the highest *vs* lowest level of occupational physical activity. Editor's Note: Please refer to original journal article for full references. (Reprinted from Moore SC, Gierach GL, Schatzkin A, et al. Physical activity, sedentary behaviours, and the prevention of endometrial cancer. *Br J Cancer.* 2010;103:933-938.)

role of both leisure and occupational physical activity (Fig 1), the analysis supports previous assertions[3,5] that too much sitting time may compound the adverse effects of limited physical activity. A possible independent adverse effect of sedentary behavior is an important current topic of discussion among epidemiologists. It is difficult to disentangle sitting from the continuum of physical activity; thus, in my view sitting is probably not an independent risk factor. The questionnaire assessments of physical activity and sitting time are relatively weak, and use of the 2 pieces of information is likely giving a more accurate picture of a person's attitude toward a physically active lifestyle.

R. J. Shephard, MD (Lond), PhD, DPE

References

1. Calle EE, Kaaks R. Overweight, obesity and cancer: epidemiological evidence and proposed mechanisms. *Nat Rev Cancer.* 2004;4:579-591.
2. World Cancer Research Fund and American Institute for Cancer Research. *Food, Nutrition, Physical Activity, and the Prevention of Cancer: A Global Perspective.* Washington, DC: American Institute for Cancer Research; 2007.
3. Friberg E, Mantzoros CS, Wolk A. Physical activity and risk of endometrial cancer: a population-based prospective cohort study. *Cancer Epidemiol Biomarkers Prev.* 2006;15:2136-2140.
4. Friedenreich C, Cust A, Lahmann PH, et al. Physical activity and risk of endometrial cancer: the European prospective investigation into cancer and nutrition. *Int J Cancer.* 2007;121:347-355.
5. Patel AV, Feigelson HS, Talbot JT, et al. The role of body weight in the relationship between physical activity and endometrial cancer: results from a large cohort of US women. *Int J Cancer.* 2008;123:1877-1882.
6. Conroy MB, Sattelmair JR, Cook NR, Manson JE, Buring JE, Lee IM. Physical activity, adiposity, and risk of endometrial cancer. *Cancer Causes Control.* 2009; 20:1107-1115.
7. Gierach GL, Chang SC, Brinton LA, et al. Physical activity, sedentary behavior, and endometrial cancer risk in the NIH-AARP Diet and Health Study. *Int J Cancer.* 2009;124:2139-2147.

Physical activity, sedentary behaviours, and the prevention of endometrial cancer
Moore SC, Gierach GL, Schatzkin A, et al (Natl Cancer Inst, Bethesda, MD)
Br J Cancer 103:933-938, 2010

Physical activity has been hypothesised to reduce endometrial cancer risk, but this relationship has been difficult to confirm because of a limited number of prospective studies. However, recent publications from five cohort studies, which together comprise 2663 out of 3463 cases in the published literature for analyses of recreational physical activity, may help resolve this question. To synthesise these new data, we conducted a meta-analysis of prospective studies published through to December 2009. We found that physical activity was clearly associated with reduced risk of endometrial cancer, with active women having an approximately 30% lower risk than inactive women. Owing to recent interest in sedentary behaviour, we further investigated sitting time in relation to endometrial cancer risk using data from the NIH-AARP Diet and Health Study. We found that, independent of the level of moderate–vigorous physical activity, greater sitting time was associated with increased endometrial cancer risk. Thus, limiting time in sedentary behaviours may complement increasing level of moderate–vigorous physical activity as a means of reducing endometrial cancer risk. Taken together with the established biological plausibility of this relation, the totality of evidence now convincingly indicates that physical activity prevents or reduces risk of endometrial cancer.

▶ Endometrial cancer is the fourth most common incident cancer in US women and the eighth leading cancer killer. As with breast cancer, estrogen exposure is a strong risk factor for endometrial cancer. Factors that increase estrogen exposure include menopausal estrogen therapy (without use of progestin), being overweight/obese, late menopause, never having children, and a history of polycystic ovary syndrome. Endometrial cancer is more common in westernized nations, and 40% to 50% of endometrial cancers may be due to too much body fat.[1] Whether physical activity, a key factor in the regulation of energy balance, also contributes to endometrial cancer risk is less clear. This meta-analysis supports a link between higher levels of physical activity and reduced endometrial cancer risk. Excessive sitting time may also contribute to endometrial cancer risk. Physical activity is hypothesized to decrease endometrial cancer risk through alterations in serum estradiol and insulin levels, and sex hormone binding globulin. Taken together, there is sufficient evidence to support a convincing causal relationship between physical activity and endometrial cancer.

D. C. Nieman, DrPH

Reference

1. Calle EE, Kaaks R. Overweight, obesity and cancer: epidemiological evidence and proposed mechanisms. *Nat Rev Cancer.* 2004;4:579-591.

Lifetime Physical Activity and Risk of Endometrial Cancer
John EM, Koo J, Horn-Ross PL (Cancer Prevention Inst of California, Fremont)
Cancer Epidemiol Biomarkers Prev 19:1276-1283, 2010

Background.—The role of moderate physical activity and life patterns of activity in reducing endometrial cancer risk remains uncertain.

Methods.—We assessed lifetime histories of activity from recreation, transportation, chores, and occupation and other risk factors in a population-based case-control study of endometrial cancer conducted in the San Francisco Bay area. The analysis was based on 472 newly diagnosed cases ascertained by the regional cancer registry and 443 controls identified by random-digit dialing who completed an in-person interview.

Results.—Reduced risks associated with greater lifetime physical activity (highest versus lowest tertile) were found for both total activity [odds ratio (OR), 0.61; 95% confidence interval (95% CI), 0.43-0.87; $P_{trend} = 0.01$] and activity of moderate intensity (OR, 0.44; 95% CI, 0.30-0.64; $P_{trend} < 0.0001$). Compared with women with low lifetime physical activity (below median), those with greater activity throughout life had a higher reduction in risk (OR, 0.62; 95% CI, 0.44-0.88). Inverse associations were stronger in obese and overweight women, but differences were not statistically significantly different from those in normal-weight women.

Conclusion.—These findings suggest that physical activity in adulthood, even of moderate intensity, may be effective in lowering the risk of endometrial cancer, particularly among those at highest risk for this disease.

TABLE 2.—Lifetime Physical Activity and Risk of Endometrial Cancer, By Type of Activity and Intensity

	Cases ($n = 472$), n (%)	Controls ($n = 443$), n (%)	Age-, Race-, and BMI-Adjusted OR (95% CI)	Multivariate-Adjusted OR (95% CI)*
Total physical activity (h/wk)				
<13.4	204 (43)	149 (33)	1.0	1.0
13.4-27.1	147 (31)	145 (33)	0.78 (0.57-1.07)	0.89 (0.63-1.25)
≥27.2	121 (26)	149 (33)	0.62 (0.45-0.86)	0.67 (0.47-0.95)
			$P_{trend} = 0.004$	$P_{trend} = 0.03$
Total physical activity (MET-h/wk)				
<43.2	207 (44)	151 (34)	1.0	1.0
43.2-91.8	150 (32)	145 (33)	0.78 (0.57-1.06)	0.83 (0.59-1.17)
≥91.9	115 (24)	147 (33)	0.59 (0.43-0.83)	0.61 (0.43-0.87)
			$P_{trend} = 0.002$	$P_{trend} = 0.01$
Occupational activity				
Moderate or strenuous jobs (h/wk)				
0	276 (59)	223 (50)	1.0	1.0
<8.1	111 (24)	108 (24)	0.81 (0.59-1.12)	0.80 (0.56-1.13)
≥8.1	85 (18)	112 (25)	0.61 (0.43-0.86)	0.64 (0.44-0.92)
			$P_{trend} = 0.004$	$P_{trend} = 0.01$
Nonoccupational activity (h/wk)				
<6.3	196 (42)	149 (33)	1.0	1.0
6.3-12.3	147 (31)	149 (33)	0.78 (0.57-1.08)	0.79 (0.57-1.11)
≥12.4	128 (27)	149 (33)	0.70 (0.50-0.97)	0.77 (0.54-1.09)
			$P_{trend} = 0.03$	$P_{trend} = 0.13$
Exercise (h/wk)				
<0.75	150 (32)	146 (33)	1.0	1.0
0.75-2.57	166 (35)	147 (33)	1.09 (0.78-1.50)	1.07 (0.76-1.52)
≥2.58	156 (33)	150 (33)	1.02 (0.73-1.41)	0.93 (0.65-1.33)
			$P_{trend} = 0.93$	$P_{trend} = 0.67$
Walking/bicycling to school or work (h/wk)				
<0.23	174 (37)	147 (33)	1.0	1.0
0.23-0.47	164 (35)	144 (33)	0.92 (0.67-1.27)	0.99 (0.70-1.39)
≥0.48	134 (28)	152 (33)	0.79 (0.57-1.09)	0.80 (0.57-1.13)
			$P_{trend} = 0.16$	$P_{trend} = 0.22$
Strenuous household and outdoor chores (h/wk)				
<3.4	198 (42)	150 (34)	1.0	1.0
3.4-8.1	158 (33)	144 (33)	0.84 (0.62-1.16)	0.88 (0.63-1.24)
≥8.2	116 (25)	149 (33)	0.61 (0.44-0.85)	0.67 (0.46-0.96)
			$P_{trend} = 0.004$	$P_{trend} = 0.03$
Total moderate activity (h/wk)				
<6.9	229 (49)	150 (34)	1.0	1.0
6.9-15.5	151 (32)	148 (33)	0.67 (0.49-0.92)	0.68 (0.49-0.95)
≥15.6	92 (20)	145 (33)	0.41 (0.29-0.58)	0.44 (0.30-0.64)
			$P_{trend} < 0.0001$	$P_{trend} < 0.0001$

*OR and 95% CI were adjusted for age, race/ethnicity, education, family history of endometrial cancer, age at menarche, full-term pregnancies, duration of oral contraceptive use, duration of hormone therapy use, menopausal status, BMI, and height.

Impact.—The results emphasize the importance of evaluating lifetime histories of physical activity from multiple sources, including both recreational and nonrecreational activities of various intensities, to fully understand the relation between physical activity and disease risk (Table 2).

▶ There is growing evidence that physical activity protects against endometrial cancer.[1,2] However, many of the available studies have focused on recent physical activity, and given the slow development of cancer, a lifetime physical activity history is really required. This study used the case-control approach to explore the relationship between lifetime activity patterns and the risk of endometrial cancer, looking also at possible interactions between physical activity and obesity. It is quite difficult to obtain an accurate account of a person's lifetime activity patterns. However, the interviewers in this study seem to have been relatively successful, as judged by the substantial increase in the risk of cancer among those who reported little activity (Table 2). There are a number of surprises in the data, particularly the apparent lack of benefit from exercise and active transportation; the main protection appears to have been derived from occupational physical activity. Possibly, this may reflect the statistical adjustment of the data for the effects of obesity. The effects of body mass index were apparently relatively small, but much of the benefits of physical activity is generally thought to come through a reduction of body fat content and thus a lesser synthesis of estrogens[3]; moreover, it could be argued that exercise is helpful in controlling this obesity. At least 1 article has suggested that estrogen availability can be decreased by exercise even in the absence of fat loss.[4] This issue merits further exploration in a larger sample of subjects. Physical activity seems to have had the greatest beneficial impact if incurred between the ages of 20 and 30 years. There was apparently no significant benefit from greater physical activity between 10 and 19 years of age, although this might possibly reflect difficulties in the recall of such distant events.

R. J. Shephard, MD (Lond), PhD, DPE

References

1. Voskuil DW, Monninkhof EM, Elias SG, Vlems FA, van Leeuwen FE. Physical activity and endometrial cancer risk, a systematic review of current evidence. *Cancer Epidemiol Biomarkers Prev.* 2007;16:639-648.
2. Cust AE, Armstrong BK, Friedenreich CM, Slimani N, Bauman A. Physical activity and endometrial cancer risk: a review of the current evidence, biologic mechanisms and the quality of physical activity assessment methods. *Cancer Causes Control.* 2007;18:243-258.
3. McTiernan A, Tworoger SS, Ulrich CM, et al. Effect of exercise on serum estrogens in postmenopausal women: a 12-month randomized clinical trial. *Cancer Res.* 2004;64:2923-2928.
4. Patel AV, Feigelson HS, Talbot JT, et al. The role of body weight in the relationship between physical activity and endometrial cancer: results from a large cohort of U.S. women. *Int J Cancer.* 2008;123:1877-1882.

Effect of Active Resistive Exercise on Breast Cancer—Related Lymphedema: A Randomized Controlled Trial

Kim DS, Sim Y-J, Jeong HJ, et al (Kosin Univ College of Medicine, Busan, Republic of Korea)

Arch Phys Med Rehabil 91:1844-1848, 2010

Objective.—To investigate the differences between the effects of complex decongestive physiotherapy with and without active resistive exercise for the treatment of patients with breast cancer—related lymphedema (BCRL).

Design.—Randomized control-group study.

Setting.—An outpatient rehabilitation clinic.

Participants.—Patients (N = 40) with diagnosed BCRL.

Interventions.—Patients were randomly assigned to either the active resistive exercise group or the nonactive resistive exercise group. In the active resistive exercise group, after complex decongestive physiotherapy, active resistive exercise was performed for 15min/d, 5 days a week for 8 weeks. The nonactive resistive exercise group performed only complex decongestive physiotherapy.

Main Outcome Measures.—The circumferences of the upper limbs (proximal, distal, and total) for the volume changes, and the Short Form-36 version 2 questionnaire for the quality of life (QOL) at pretreatment and 8 weeks posttreatment for each patient.

Results.—The volume of the proximal part of the arm was significantly more reduced in the active resistive exercise group than that of the nonactive resistive exercise group (*P*<.05). In the active resistive exercise group, there was significantly more improvement in physical health and general health, as compared with that of the nonactive resistive exercise group (*P*<.05).

Conclusions.—For the treatment of patients with BCRL, active resistive exercise with complex decongestive physiotherapy did not cause additional swelling, and it significantly reduced proximal arm volume and helped improve QOL.

▶ Lymphedema is a significant problem in patients who have undergone treatment for breast cancer. Traditionally, physical therapy consisted of patient education, manual lymphatic drainage technique, nonelastic bandage compression therapy, and exercise. This study focuses on the effect of active resistive exercise in addition to the usual complex decongestive physical therapy regime. Although the sample size is small (40 in total: 20 in each group), the investigators conducted a well-designed randomized controlled trial with blind assessment and found that the resistive exercise component appears to be beneficial. Specifically, those who were in the experimental group had reduced proximal arm volume and greater improvement in physical health and general health. The importance of this study is that it suggests that resistive exercise should be added to the physical therapy regimen for breast cancer—related lymphedema. I also appreciated that the authors described the intervention in adequate detail in terms of the specific exercises that were performed.

D. E. Feldman, PT, PhD

Comparison of physiological response to cardiopulmonary exercise testing among cancer survivors and healthy controls

Klika RJ, Golik KS, Drum SN, et al (Cancer Survivor Ctr for Health and Wellbeing, Aspen, CO; Western State College of Colorado, Gunnison; et al)
Eur J Appl Physiol 2010 [Epub ahead of print]

Selected physiological responses, including lactate kinetics, to cardiopulmonary exercise testing (CPET) were evaluated among a group of cancer survivors (CS, $n = 55$) and healthy controls (HC, $n = 213$). It was uncertain if lactate testing in a group of cancer survivors could provide useful information about training intensity. It was hypothesized that chemotherapy, radiation, surgery, physical inactivity or some combination thereof would alter the normal lactate kinetics (curvilinearity) in the relationship of lactate concentration versus power. Physiologic responses of CS (heart rate, blood pressure, O_2 saturation, RPE, lactate, VO_{2peak}, and peak power) during cycle ergometry were compared to HC. Comparisons (*t* tests and Chi-square) were made between the groups and shape of lactate plots were analyzed for determination of a breakpoint. Multiple logistic regressions were then utilized to identify factors related to the inability to determine lactate breakpoints. Lactate breakpoints were common to all but one HC whereas among the CS there was a small subset of subjects ($n = 5$) who did not show a lactate breakpoint. Group differences indicated that female CS were significantly older, had greater BMI's, and lower work capacity than HC. Males CS had significantly lower work capacity than HC. Multiple logistical regression analyses, in all instances, yielded no statistically significant models predictive of the inability to determine a lactate breakpoint. In this sample of CS and HC, physiological responses and lactate kinetics during CPET were similar while work capacity among the CS was lower. Because lactate breakpoints were found, lactate threshold could be determined for all but a few individuals. For those working with CS, CPET with ECG monitoring and lactate threshold measures should be considered for those wishing for precise and safe training intensities.

▶ Prescribing exercise for enhanced athletic performance, amateur and elite, often includes measurement of lactate threshold by repeated blood sampling during graded exercise. The normal lactate response is a curvilinear relationship of blood lactate versus work, which typically presents a rapid increase in blood lactate at 40% to 80% of maximum work capacity. Lactate responses to work can be abnormal in persons with chronic disease states because of numerous physiological (eg, substrate utilization) and behavioral (eg, reduced physical activity) factors. In cancer survivors, the effects of cancer and treatments affect multiple physiological systems that could contribute to exercise intolerance and diminished performance. Whether cancer changes lactate kinetics was the focus of this investigation by Klika and colleagues. The 55 cancer survivors they studied had a range of cancer types, treatments, drug therapies, and time since diagnosis. Blood lactate was measured by fingerstick samples collected during a graded bicycle ergometer test. The identification of a lactate threshold was standardized, and the lactate responses were subjected to curve fitting. In comparison to the control subjects with no history of cancer, the survivors had significantly lower power at lactate threshold, lower maximal heart rate and maximal power, and lower VO_{2peak}. However, the relation of blood lactate to power output was curvilinear in 50 of the cancer survivors. The lactate to power curve was linear in 5 survivors (4 females) who were older and had lower work capacity compared with the other cancer survivors. The authors suggested that in relatively deconditioned individuals, the lactate threshold test may need to be adjusted to a lower starting load. One caveat of the study is that the cancer survivors were more fit compared with those in cohorts from other studies and lived in a resort community with a strong emphasis on physical activity. Nonetheless, because the lactate response retained the curvilinear relationship seen in controls, it is reasonable to use the lactate threshold approach to develop aerobic exercise prescriptions for cancer survivors.

C. M. Jankowski, PhD

Bone Status in Professional Cyclists
Campion F, Nevill AM, Karlsson MK, et al (Lund Univ, Malmö, Sweden; Univ of Wolverhampton, Walsall, West Midlands, UK; et al)
Int J Sports Med 31:511-515, 2010

Professional cycling combines extensive endurance training with non weight-bearing exercise, two factors often associated with lower bone mineral density (BMD). Therefore BMD was measured with dual-energy x-ray absorptiometry in 30 professional road cyclists (mean (SD) age: 29.1 (3.4) years; height: 178.5 (6.7) cm; weight: 71.3 (6.1) kg; % fat mass: 9.7 (3.2) % ; VO_2max: 70.5 (5.5) ml · kg^{-1} · min^{-1}) and in 30 young healthy males used as reference (28.6 (4.5) years; 176.5 (6.3) cm; 73.4 (7.3) kg; 20.7 (5.8) %). Adjusting for differences in age, height, fat mass, lean body mass, and calcium intake by ANCOVA, professional cyclists had similar head BMD (p = 0.383) but lower total body (1.135 (0.071) vs. 1.248 (0.104) g · cm^{-2} ; p < 0.001), arms (0.903 (0.075) vs. 0.950 (0.085), p = 0.028), legs (1.290 (0.112) vs. 1.479 (0.138); p < 0.001), spine (0.948 (0.100) vs. 1.117 (0.147) g · cm^{-2} ; p < 0.001), pelvis (1.054 (0.084) vs. 1.244 (0.142), p < 0.001), lumbar spine (1.046 (0.103) vs. 1.244 (0.167), P < 0.001), and femoral neck BMD (0.900 (0.115) vs. 1.093 (0.137), p < 0.001) compared to reference subjects. Professional cycling appears to negatively affect BMD in young healthy and highly active males, the femoral neck being the most affected site (−18%) in spite of the elevated muscle contractions inherent to the activity (Table 2).

▶ Surely exercise helps to prevent osteoporosis. This is not always the case, particularly if the high-energy expenditure of an endurance athlete is combined with an inadequate energy intake, a scenario long recognized in the "athletic triad."[1] Some previous studies of competitive road cyclists have found normal

TABLE 2.—BMD Values for PRO and REF

BMD (gcm^{-2})	PRO (n = 30) Mean	SD	REF (n = 30) Mean	SD	Difference Mean	95% CI		p
total	1.135	0.071	1.248	0.104	−0.119	−0.171	−0.067	< 0.001
head	2.041	0.228	2.085	0.226	−0.043	−0.142	0.056	0.383
arms	0.903	0.075	0.950	0.085	−0.077	−0.141	−0.014	0.018
legs	1.290	0.112	1.479	0.138	−0.160	−0.228	−0.092	< 0.001
ribs	0.655	0.052	0.720	0.060	−0.104	−0.163	−0.044	< 0.001
pelvis	1.054	0.084	1.244	0.142	−0.188	−0.254	−0.123	< 0.001
spine	0.948	0.100	1.117	0.147	−0.199	−0.283	−0.116	< 0.001
L1-L4	1.046	0.103	1.244	0.167	−0.197	−0.285	−0.108	< 0.001
femoral neck	0.900	0.115	1.093	0.137	−0.253	−0.348	−0.158	< 0.001
trochanter	0.787	0.097	0.927	0.147	−0.273	−0.372	−0.175	< 0.001
radius UD	0.394	0.057	0.434	0.052	−0.074	−0.182	0.033	0.171
radius 33 %	0.745	0.059	0.751	0.072	0.004	−0.071	0.078	0.919

Values as mean and SD. Mean difference between PRO and REF with 95 % confidence interval (95 % CI), and p-values calculated with repeated measures ANCOVA on log transformed data with age, log-height, log-LBM, log-FAT, and calcium as covariates.

bone densities.[2,3] However, it is important to underline that cycling events vary greatly in the total distance covered. In this report, the experimental subjects were all participants in 1 of 3 grueling 3-week mountain events (Tour de France, Giro d'Italia, or Vuelta a Espana), with a correspondingly stiff training schedule throughout most of the year; these particular events call for a daily energy expenditure of almost 30 MJ, with little opportunity for the cyclist to replace lost energy. An earlier study of Tour de France participants also noted that bone density was 10% lower than in controls, although perhaps because of a small sample size, the difference was not statistically significant in the previous report.[4] This study showed that relative to hospital staff controls, bone mineral density as estimated by dual X-ray absorptiometry was low in the body as a whole, arms, legs, pelvis, and spine, with particularly low values for the femoral neck and trochanter (Table 2). The deficiency of bone mineralization is important for cyclists because of their risk of falls. Calcium intake was adequate by European standards (800 mg/d) although lower than current North American recommendations. The practical lesson seems that every effort should be made to give distance cyclists adequate amounts of protein, calcium, and vitamin D.

R. J. Shephard, MD (Lond), PhD, DPE

References

1. Burrows M, Nevill AM, Bird SA, Simpson D. Physiological factors associated with low bone mineral density in female endurance runners. *Br J Sports Med.* 2003;37: 67-71.
2. Maïmoun L, Lumbrosa S, Manetta J, Paris F, Leroiux JL, Sultan C. Testosterone is significantly reduced in endurance athletes without impact on bone mineral density. *Horm Res.* 2003;59:285-292.
3. Warner SE, Shaw JM, Dalsky GP. Bone mineral density of competitive male mountain and road cyclists. *Bone.* 2002;30:281-286.
4. Sabo D, Bernd L, Pfeil J, Reiter A. Bone quality in lumbar spine in high performance athletes. *Eur Spine J.* 1996;5:258-263.

2010 clinical practice guidelines for the diagnosis and management of osteoporosis in Canada: summary

Papaioannou A, for the Scientific Advisory Council of Osteoporosis Canada
(McMaster Univ, Hamilton, Ontario, Canada; et al)
CMAJ 182:1864-1873, 2010

Since the publication of the Osteoporosis Canada guidelines in 2002, there has been a paradigm shift in the prevention and treatment of osteoporosis and fractures. The focus now is on preventing fragility fractures and their negative consequences, rather than on treating low bone mineral density, which is viewed as only one of several risk factors for fracture. Given that certain clinical factors increase the risk of fracture independent of bone mineral density, it is important to take an integrated approach and to base treatment decisions on the absolute risk of fracture. Current data suggest that many patients with fractures do not undergo appropriate assessment or treatment. To address this care gap for high-risk patients, the 2010 guidelines concentrate on the assessment and management of women and men over age 50 who are at high risk of fragility fractures and the integration of new tools for assessing the 10-year risk of fracture into overall management (Table 1).

▶ This is an extremely valuable review of current clinical practice guidelines used in Canada. Recent knowledge has been systematically reviewed based on priorities identified by surveys of primary care physicians, patients, osteoporosis specialists from various disciplines, radiologists, allied health professionals, and health policymakers. The authors used the Appraisal of Guidelines, Research and Evaluation framework to develop guidelines for assessment and management of osteoporosis in the target population of women and men older than

TABLE 1.—Indications for Measuring Bone Mineral Density

Older Adults (age ≥ 50 yr)	Younger Adults (age < 50 yr)
Age ≥ 65 yr (both women and men)	Fragility fracture
Clinical risk factors for fracture (menopausal women, men age 50–64 yr)	Prolonged use of glucocorticoids*
Fragility fracture after age 40 yr	Use of other high-risk medications†
Prolonged use of glucocorticoids*	Hypogonadism or premature menopause (age < 45 yr)
Use of other high-risk medications†	Malabsorption syndrome
Parental hip fracture	Primary hyperparathyroidism
Vertebral fracture or osteopenia identified on radiography	Other disorders strongly associated with rapid bone loss and/or fracture
Current smoking	
High alcohol intake	
Low body weight (< 60 kg) or major weight loss (> 10% of body weight at age 25 yr)	
Rheumatoid arthritis	
Other disorders strongly associated with osteoporosis	

*At least three months cumulative therapy in the previous year at a prednisone-equivalent dose ≥ 7.5 mg daily.
†For example, aromatase inhibitors or androgen deprivation therapy.

50 years. An expert panel developed the guidelines, which were then reviewed by the Guidelines Committee and the Executive Committee of the Osteoporosis Canada Scientific Advisory Council.

These clinical recommendations include who and how to assess for osteoporosis and fracture risk, initial investigations (including bone mineral density), and therapeutic options (including increasing exercise and prevention falls, calcium and vitamin D, pharmacological therapy, adverse effects, and special groups). Table 1 lists the indications for measuring bone mineral density in women of different ages, and Box 1 in the original article lists the recommended biochemical tests. Fig 2 in the original article shows a useful algorithm for an integrated approach to management of patients who are at risk for fracture. For assessing a 10-year fracture risk, 2 closely related tools are recommended for use in Canada: the updated tool of the Canadian Association of Radiologists and Osteoporosis Canada and a fracture risk assessment tool of the World Health Organization. Guidelines from 2 other organizations, the US National Osteoporosis Foundation and the UK National Osteoporosis Guideline groups, are compared and contrasted.

This article is a very compact assessment of management of osteoporosis, and the guidelines are ranked on the grade of evidence. It is very useful for practicing primary care physicians or specialists, such as orthopedic surgeons.

This writing group has developed a toolkit and a dissemination strategy. In addition, more than 10 professional organizations have endorsed these guidelines. Tools and resources can be found at www.osteoporosis.ca.

C. Lebrun, MD

Confounders in the Association between Exercise and Femur Bone in Postmenopausal Women

Beck TJ, Kohlmeier LA, Petit MA, et al (The Johns Hopkins Univ School of Medicine, Baltimore, MD; Spokane Osteoporosis Ctr, WA; Univ of Minnesota School of Kinesiology, Minneapolis; et al)
Med Sci Sports Exerc 43:80-89, 2011

Introduction.—Abundant animal and human evidence demonstrates that loading stimuli generate positive adaptive changes in bone, but effects of activity on bone mineral density (BMD) are often modest and frequently equivocal.

Hypothesis.—Physical activity effects on the femur would be better reflected in measurements of geometry than BMD.

Study Design.—Cross-sectional cohort study.

Methods.—We used data from 6032 women of mixed ethnicity aged 50−79 yr who had dual-energy x-ray absorptiometry (DXA) scans of the total body and hip from the Women's Health Initiative observational study. Subjects were distributed in three ways: self-report categories included 1) tertiles of MET and 2) reported minutes per week walking for exercise. A third, more objective, category was based on tertile of lean body mass fraction (LMF) from DXA scans. Femur outcomes included conventional femoral neck and total hip BMD, bone mineral content and region area, and geometry measurements using the Hip Structure Analysis software. Outcomes were compared between activity groups using models adjusted for common confounders.

Results.—Adjusted bone measurements showed similar activity effects with all three grouping variables, but these were greater and more significant when evaluated by LMF tertile. Women in the highest LMF tertile had the widest femurs. Differences in section modulus between highest and lowest tertile of LMF were 50%—80% greater than the association with bone mineral content and two to three times that on BMD.

Conclusions.—More active women in the Women's Health Initiative observational study had geometrically stronger femurs, although effects are underestimated, not apparent, or sometimes negative when using BMD as an outcome.

Clinical Relevance.—Exercise improves the strength of the femur largely by adding bone to the outer cortical surface; this improves resistance to bending, but because of the way DXA measurements are made, this may paradoxically reduce BMD.

▶ Most sports physicians assume that regular physical activity will increase bone mineral density and protect against osteoporosis, and this is supported by a reduced risk of fractures.[1] However, other factors such as a greater volume of muscle or improved balance could also be protecting the active subjects against fractures. Moreover, some reports have shown either little benefit or even on occasion a lower bone mineral density among physically active individuals.[2,3] Part of the problem may arise from studying athletes who are in negative energy balance, whether from participation in ultraendurance sport or a desire to develop a lean figure. However, a second factor seems that bone mineral density as measured by dual-energy X-ray absorptiometry is commonly expressed as g/cm^2 (bone mass per regional area), so that tends to be discounted in athletes who have a substantial increase in the regional area. The study of Beck and associates is based on a large sample of older postmenopausal women who were participating in the Women's Health Initiative. The most active women strengthened their femurs by adding tissue to the outer surface of the bone, and this tended to discount dual-energy absorptiometry estimates. Three estimates of habitual physical activity were adopted, the lean mass fraction being preferred to questionnaire indices. The positive effect of this measure of habitual physical activity became clear when the data were adjusted for total body mass and other variables (Fig 3 in the original article). A second possibility seems to adopt alternative indices of bone strength; thus, we have demonstrated a clear association between bone health and habitual physical activity using an osteosonic index (based on the transmission of sound waves through the bone under evaluation).[4]

R. J. Shephard, MD (Lond), PhD, DPE

References

1. Moayyeri A. The association between physical activity and osteoporotic fractures: a review of the evidence and implications for future research. *Ann Epidemiol.* 2008;18:827-835.
2. Barry DW, Kohrt WM. Exercise and the preservation of bone health. *J Cardiopulm Rehabil Prev.* 2008;28:153-162.
3. Barry DW, Kohrt WM. BMD decreases over the course of a year in competitive male cyclists. *J Bone Miner Res.* 2008;23:484-491.
4. Park H, Togo F, Watanabe E, et al. Relationship of bone health to yearlong physical activity in older Japanese adults: cross-sectional data from the Nakanojo Study. *Osteoporos Int.* 2007;18:285-293.

Minimal Detectable Change in Quadriceps Strength and Voluntary Muscle Activation in Patients With Knee Osteoarthritis

Kean CO, Birmingham TB, Garland SJ, et al (Univ of Western Ontario, London; Univ of British Columbia, Vancouver, Canada)
Arch Phys Med Rehabil 91:1447-1451, 2010

Objective.—To examine the test-retest reliability and quantify the minimal detectable change (MDC) in quadriceps strength and voluntary activation in patients with knee osteoarthritis (OA).

Design.—Repeated measures over a 1-week interval.

Setting.—Tertiary care center.

Participants.—A convenience sample of patients (N = 20) diagnosed with knee OA.

Intervention.—Isokinetic and isometric quadriceps strength testing and voluntary quadriceps activation testing using interpolated twitch technique.

Main Outcome Measures.—Peak isokinetic and isometric knee extension torque (Nm) and percentage of voluntary quadriceps activation (%).

Results.—The mean differences with 95% confidence intervals between the 2 test sessions for quadriceps isokinetic strength, isometric strength, and percent of voluntary activation were −4.34Nm (−14.01 to 5.34Nm), 1.56Nm (−5.56 to 8.68Nm), and 1.34% (−.53 to 3.22%), respectively. The intraclass correlation coefficients for all measures ranged from .93 to .98. The standard errors of measurement (SEMs) for quadriceps isokinetic and isometric strength were 14.57Nm and 10.76Nm, respectively. The SEM for percentage of voluntary activation was 2.84%. Based on these values, the MDCs were 33.90Nm, 25.02Nm, and 6.60% for quadriceps isokinetic strength, isometric strength, and percentage of voluntary activation, respectively.

Conclusions.—Maximal quadriceps isokinetic strength, isometric strength, and percentage of voluntary activation measures demonstrate excellent test-retest reliability in patients with knee OA. In addition to research applications, the present findings suggest these measures are appropriate for use when evaluating change in neuromuscular function of the quadriceps in individual patients.

▶ The ability of the quadriceps muscle group to hold or extend the knee is a requirement of many functional activities. Rehabilitation therapists frequently use specialized equipment to measure the isometric and isokinetic torque (2 measures of muscle strength, measured in Nm) of the quadriceps. The comparison of these torque measures before, during, and after rehabilitation intervention provides the rehabilitation therapist with evidence of intervention effectiveness. However, it is also important to know the minimal level of change that is needed to confidently detect a true change. In this article, Kean et al recruited 20 patients with radiographically confirmed severe knee osteoarthritis to determine the 90% confidence minimal detectable change (MDC) of peak isometric (knee at 90 degrees) and peak isokinetic (knee extension of 60 degrees/s) torques during 2 test sessions separated by at least 24 hours within a 1-week interval. They report that the isometric and isokinetic MDCs were 25.0 and 33.9 Nm, respectively. The clinical significance of this article is that it informs the rehabilitation therapist of the minimal change in quadriceps torque required to be confident that their intervention is effective.

M. R. Pierrynowski, PhD

Effects of a supervised exercise program on the physical fitness and immunological function of HIV-infected patients

Farinatti PTV, Borges JP, Gomes RD, et al (Laboratory of Physical Activity and Health Promotion/State Univ of Rio de Janeiro, Rio de Janeiro, Brazil)
J Sports Med Phys Fitness 50:511-518, 2010

Exercise effects in subjects with HIV/AIDS are not entirely understood. The study aimed to investigate the effects of a supervised exercise program on the physical fitness and immunological function of HIV-infected subjects. Twenty-seven highly active antiretroviral therapy treated HIV-infected patients (age: 45 ± 2 years; CD4-T: $21.3 \pm 2.2\%$) were assigned to a control (CG, n=8) or experimental (EG, n=19) group. The EG participated in a 12-week exercise program, consisting of aerobic training, strength, and flexibility exercises (3 times/wk; aerobic-30min: PWC 150; strength-50min: 3 sets of 12 reps of 5 exercises at 60-80% 12 RM; flexibility-10min: 2 sets of 30 s at maximal range of motion of 8 exercises). Prior to training there was no significant difference in any variable between the EG and the CG. Flexibility (23%, P<0.05), 12 repetition maximum in the leg press and seated bilateral row exercises (54% and 65% respectively, P<0.05) increased, while the heart rate at a given cycle ergometer workload declined (19% for slope and 12% for intercept, P<0.05) in the EG, but not in the CG. No significant differences were found for the relative and absolute CD4 T-cell counts between groups prior to or after training, but there was a slight enhancement trend in the EG (16%, P=0.19). Overall training can improve the muscle and aerobic fitness of HIV-infected patients with no negative effect on their immunological function.

▶ Although antiretroviral therapy has dramatically increased the lifespan of patients with human immunodeficiency virus (HIV) infections, muscle wasting and osteoporosis (in part, side effects of medication) are a continuing concern.[1,2] The logical remedy might be to develop an appropriate exercise prescription, but there has been surprisingly little research on this issue.[3-6] Many of the existing studies are compromised by a small sample size, poor adherence to exercise programs, and lack of a control group. The study of Farinatti et al is somewhat larger than most, with a randomized allocation of subjects, although there were some significant exclusion criteria, including smoking and medical contraindications to exercise. Also, a larger number of subjects were assigned to the experimental group because of fears of poor program compliance, although in fact 87% adherence to exercise sessions was achieved over the 12-week investigation. A combined aerobic, strength, and flexibility program (90 minutes, 3 times per week) yielded substantial improvements in strength, aerobic performance, and flexibility relative to control subjects. One danger of exercise for those with HIV/AIDS is that the potential immunosuppressive effect of vigorous physical activity might further compromise an already weakened immune system, and some authors have even advised a restriction of physical activity because of this. However, in this study, the T-cell count of the experimental group (initially at or below the lower limit of normality, at an average of 504 cells/mm^2) remained unchanged over the program. The authors make no comment on possible use of protein supplements or hormone therapy to increase lean tissue mass, but the effects of any such parallel treatments would presumably also have been reflected in scores for the control subjects, where fitness levels remained unchanged over the 12-week period. The present data set seems to suggest that good results can be obtained safely by exercise, without the use of such adjuvants.

R. J. Shephard, MD (Lond), PhD, DPE

References

1. Safrin S, Grunfeld C. Fat distribution and metabolic change in patients with HIV infection. *AIDS*. 1999;13:2493-2505.
2. Serrano S, Mariñoso ML, Soriano JC, et al. Bone remodelling in human immunodeficiency virus-1-infected patients. A histomorphometric study. *Bone*. 1995;16:185-191.
3. Shephard RJ, Shek PN. Exercise and CD4+/CD8+ cell counts: Influence of various contributing factors in health and HIV infection. *Exerc Immunol Rev*. 1996;2:65-83.
4. Shephard RJ. *Physical Activity, Training and the Immune System*. Carmel, IN: Cooper Publications; 1997.
5. O'Brien K, Nixon S, Tynan AM, Glazier RH. Effectiveness of aerobic exercise in adults living with HIV/AIDS: systematic review. *Med Sci Sports Exerc*. 2004;36:1659-1666.
6. Ciccolo JT, Jowers EM, Bartholomew JB. The benefits of exercise training for quality of life in HIV/AIDS in the post-HAART era. *Sports Med*. 2004;34:487-499.

How Much Physical Activity Is Needed To Maintain Erectile Function? Results of the Androx Vienna Municipality Study

Kratzik CW, Lackner JE, Märk I, et al (Med Univ of Vienna, Austria)
Eur Urol 55:509-517, 2009

Objective.—To assess the correlation of erectile function (EF) and physical activity (PhA) by using standardized, validated instruments in healthy men.

Methods.—A urologist examined 674 men aged 45—60 yr at their place of work. That included a urological physical examination, medical history, and assessment of testosterone (T) and sex hormone—binding globulin; all men completed the 5-item International Index of Erectile Function (IIEF-5) as well as the Paffenbarger score. PhA was assessed in kilojoules per week (4.2 kJ = 1 kcal).

Results.—A positive correlation between the IIEF-5 and the Paffenbarger score ($r = 0.164$, $p < 0.001$) was found. The IIEF-5 score increased with an increasing Paffenbarger score up to a level of 4000 kcal/wk. T revealed a trend to a significant impact on the IIEF-5 score, but showed no association with the Paffenbarger score. The risk of severe erectile dysfunction (ED) was decreased by 82.9% for males with PhA of at least 3000 kcal/wk compared with males with PhA under 3000 kcal/wk ($OR = 0.171$, $p = 0.018$).

Conclusion.—Increasing PhA from 1000 to 4000 kcal/wk may reduce the risk of ED (Fig 1).

▶ Given current sales of Viagra, the suggestion that regular physical activity enhances erectile function (previously reported[1,2] and apparently accepted by Kratzik and associates) might be thought a powerful factor encouraging many middle-aged and older men to engage in regular exercise. But before too much hope is invested in this concept, it is important to underline a number of limitations to the Androx Vienna Municipality Study. Firstly, the authors have only demonstrated a correlation, so there is no guarantee that exercise is the causal factor. Physical activity could be beneficial by reducing the risk of diabetes and/or hypertension or increasing the release of vasodilating nitric oxide. However, individuals who choose to exercise are not typical of the general population; they are generally younger, more health conscious, likely to avoid smoking and an excessive consumption of alcohol, and unlikely to be suffering from anxiety or depression (both of which tend to reduce habitual physical activity). Unfortunately, these authors did not consider all of these variables in their multivariate analysis; however, their data suggest that some of the variance in erectile function was explained by age, body mass index, and hypertension, and no association was seen with their measures of smoking and alcohol consumption. Secondly, the observed correlation between physical activity score and erectile dysfunction was quite weak ($r = 0.16$, Fig 1), so many factors are probably having a much larger influence on erectile function than cumulative weekly energy expenditure. Finally, although some advantage is seen in those with an expenditure of 4 MJ per week, the total amount of

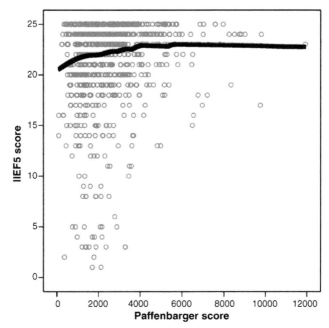

FIGURE 1.—Correlation between Paffenbarger score and IIEF-5. Since data were not normal distributed and not suitable for a linear regression this association is illustrated by a curve calculated with a local linear regression. The local linear regression curve revealed a non-linear association between PhA and EF. (Reprinted from Kratzik CW, Lackner JE, Märk I, et al. How much physical activity is needed to maintain erectile function? Results of the Androx Vienna Municipality Study. *Eur Urol.* 2009;55:509-517. Copyright 2009, with permission from the European Association of Urology.)

physical activity associated with substantial benefit (12 MJ/wk) is much greater than that accepted by the majority of the population who consider themselves physically active.

R. J. Shephard, MD (Lond), PhD, DPE

References

1. Bacon CG, Mittleman MA, Kawachi I, Giovannucci E, Glasser DB, Rimm EB. A prospective study of risk factors for erectile dysfunction. *J Urol.* 2006;176:217-221.
2. Ponholzer A, Temml C, Mock K, Marszalek M, Obermayr R, Madersbacher S. Prevalence and risk factors for erectile dysfunction in 2869 men using a validated questionnaire. *Eur Urol.* 2005;47:80-85 (discussion 85–86).

Physical activities and future risk of Parkinson disease

Xu Q, Park Y, Huang X, et al (Natl Inst of Environmental Health Sciences, Res Triangle Park, NC; Natl Cancer Inst, Rockville, MD; Pennsylvania State Univ—Milton S. Hershey Med Ctr, Hershey; et al)
Neurology 75:341-348, 2010

Objective.—To prospectively investigate the relationship between physical activity and Parkinson disease (PD).

Methods.—We evaluated physical activity in relation to PD among 213,701 participants of the NIH-AARP Diet and Health Study cohort. Physical activities over 4 periods (ages 15—18, 19—29, and 35—39, and in the past 10 years) were noted in 1996—1997, and physician-diagnosed PD was reported on the 2004—2006 follow-up questionnaire. Only cases diagnosed after 2000 (n = 767) were included in the analyses.

Results.—Higher levels of moderate to vigorous activities at ages 35—39 or in the past 10 years as reported in 1996—1997 were associated with lower PD occurrence after 2000 with significant dose-response relationships. The multivariate odds ratios (OR) between the highest vs the lowest levels were 0.62 (95% CI confidence interval [CI] 0.48—0.81, *p* for trend 0.005) for ages 35—39 and 0.65 (95% CI 0.51—0.83, p for trend 0.0001) for in the past 10 years. Further analyses showed that individuals with consistent and frequent participation in moderate to vigorous activities in both periods had approximately a 40% lower risk than those who were inactive in both periods. Moderate to vigorous activities at earlier ages or light activities were not associated with PD. Finally, the association between higher moderate to vigorous physical activities and lower PD risk was demonstrated in a metaanalysis of prospective studies.

Conclusions.—Although we cannot exclude the possibility that less participation in physical activity is an early marker of PD, epidemiologic evidence suggests that moderate to vigorous exercise may protect against PD (Fig 1).

▶ Large-scale epidemiological studies continue to find new benefits from regular physical activity. Parkinson disease (PD) is a particularly unpleasant condition to develop, in part because of the physical limitations that it imposes and in part because of its relatively prolonged clinical course. Previous analyses of protection against PD through regular physical activity have yielded inconsistent results.[1-3] However, animal experiments suggest that enforced exercise can protect the function of neurons in the nigrostriatal dopaminergic system that is critical to PD. The 40% reduction of PD risk here associated with moderate or vigorous physical activity during middle age (Fig 1) seems fairly convincing, although it is a little surprising that no benefit is associated with activity in the period of 19-29 years. Subjects reported relatively stable physical activity histories, diminishing the likelihood that early precursors of clinical PD were responsible for associations between inadequate physical activity and development of the disease. The underlying mechanisms remain a matter of debate. Possibly, modulation of cerebral vascular disease may be a factor.

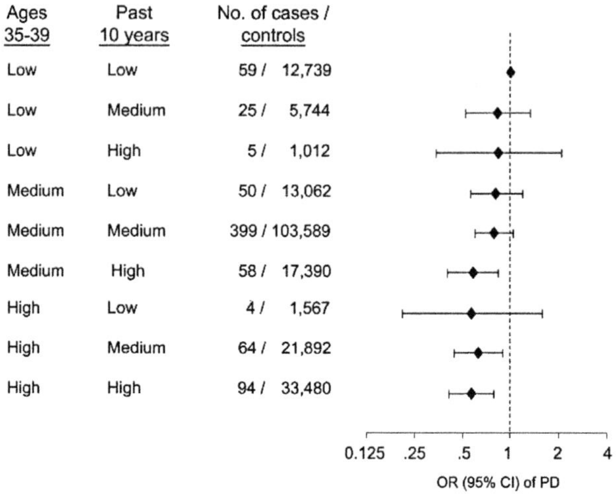

Ages 35-39	Past 10 years	No. of cases / controls
Low	Low	59 / 12,739
Low	Medium	25 / 5,744
Low	High	5 / 1,012
Medium	Low	50 / 13,062
Medium	Medium	399 / 103,589
Medium	High	58 / 17,390
High	Low	4 / 1,567
High	Medium	64 / 21,892
High	High	94 / 33,480

FIGURE 1.—Changes of physical activities in relation to risk of Parkinson disease (PD). Odds ratios (OR) and 95% confidence intervals (CI) of PD after 2000 according to changes of moderate to vigorous physical activities between ages 35–39 and in the past 10 years as reported at the risk factor survey in 1996–1997. The analysis adjusted for age at risk factors survey, gender, race, education levels, smoking status, and coffee consumption. (Reprinted from Xu Q, Park Y, Huang X, et al. Physical activities and future risk of Parkinson disease. *Neurology* 2010;75:341-348.)

Other suggested benefits of regular physical activity include greater neural plasticity, downregulation of dopamine transporter, and increased levels of plasma urate.

R. J. Shephard, MD (Lond), PhD, DPE

References

1. Chen H, Zhang SM, Schwarzschild MA, Hernán MA, Ascherio A. Physical activity and the risk of Parkinson disease. *Neurology.* 2005;64:664-669.
2. Logroscino G, Sesso HD, Paffenbarger RS Jr, Lee I-M. Physical activity and risk of Parkinson's disease: a prospective cohort study. *J Neurol Neurosurg Psychiatry.* 2006;77:1318-1322.
3. Thacker EL, Chen H, Patel AV, et al. Recreational physical activity and risk of Parkinson's disease. *Mov Disord.* 2008;23:69-74.

Predicting Exercise Capacity Through Submaximal Fitness Tests in Persons With Multiple Sclerosis

Kuspinar A, Andersen RE, Teng SY, et al (McGill Univ, Montreal, QC, Canada)
Arch Phys Med Rehabil 91:1410-1417, 2010

Objective.—To estimate, for persons with multiple sclerosis (MS), the extent to which peak oxygen consumption (Vo_2peak) can be predicted by the results on submaximal tests.
Design.—Cross-sectional study.

Setting.—Three MS clinics in the Greater Montreal region, Canada.

Participants.—A center-stratified random sample of 135 women and 48 men was drawn (N = 183). A subgroup of 59 subjects with MS, who were able to perform the step test, was selected from this sample to complete the maximal exercise test.

Interventions.—Not applicable.

Main Outcome Measure.—Vo$_2$peak.

Results.—In this sample (mean age ± SD, 39 ± 9y; median Expanded Disability Status Scale = 1.5), the mean Vo$_2$peak ± SD was 27.6 ± 7.3 mL·kg^{-1}·min^{-1}. This value is considerably low when compared with healthy persons, ranking below the 25th percentile for both men and women. In a multivariate regression analysis, the step test and grip strength were identified as the only significant predictors of Vo$_2$peak. When combined with body weight, grip strength and the step test explained 74% of the variance in Vo$_2$peak.

Conclusions.—Patients with MS with a mild degree of disability exhibit marked reductions in exercise capacity. Also, in persons with MS, submaximal tests are good predictors of exercise capacity. These measures may be used in clinical settings to help assess and monitor maximum oxygen consumption and in research to evaluate the effect of exercise-related interventions. Furthermore, they will allow people with MS to self-monitor their exercise capacity and be more actively engaged in taking charge of their fitness level (Table 5).

▶ Physicians are often reluctant to make direct measurements of the peak exercise capacity of patients with chronic disease,[1] and reliance is often placed on the distance walked in 6 minutes.[2] However, this study suggests that if a submaximal method of exercise testing is desired, the best results are obtained from use of the Canadian Home Fitness Test[3,4]; the one proviso is whether the patient can perform the test (a quarter of the patients with multiple sclerosis could not). Although the correlation with direct measurement is less close than in healthy individuals, the step test score alone accounts for 66% of the variance in peak oxygen intake, and if information from a simple grip test and body mass is added, the proportion rises to 74% (Table 5). In contrast, the 6-minute walk accounts for only 6% of the variance in absolute peak oxygen

TABLE 5.—Multiple Linear Regression Model for Absolute VO$_2$peak

	Unstandardized Coefficients B	SE	Standardized Coefficients	Cumulative R^2 by Step	P
Step test (L/min)	1.091	.180	.31	.64	<.001
Grip strength (kg)	0.009	.003	.22	.72	.004
Body weight (kg)	0.009	.004	.14	.74	.02
Sex	0.067	.180	NA	NA	.71

NOTE. Outcome variable: VO$_2$peak in L/min. Total R^2 = .74; P<.001. Intercept is −1.176; SE = .589; P =.05. Standardized coefficient = ß × 1 SD; used to standardize the measurement scale of the different variables.
Abbreviation: NA, not applicable.

intake and 23% of the variance in relative peak oxygen intake. The Canadian Home Fitness Test thus provides a useful tool for both repeated outpatient assessment and self-monitoring of physical condition in multiple sclerosis, and it appears to be a substantially better approach than a 6-minute walk. Nevertheless, the Canadian Home Fitness Test data should be interpreted in a relative rather than an absolute sense because there is a substantial systematic error in the score (approaching 20%) relative to direct measurements.

R. J. Shephard, MD (Lond), PhD, DPE

References

1. Noonan V, Dean E. Submaximal exercise testing: clinical application and interpretation. *Phys Ther.* 2000;80:782-807.
2. ATS Committee on Proficiency Standards for Clinical Pulmonary Function Laboratories. ATS statement: guidelines for the six-minute walk test. *Am J Respir Crit Care Med.* 2002;166:111-117.
3. Weller IM, Thomas SG, Gledhill N, Paterson D, Quinney A. A study to validate the modified Canadian Aerobic Fitness Test. *Can J Appl Physiol.* 1995;20:211-221.
4. Weller IM, Thomas SG, Corey PN, Cox MH. Prediction of maximal oxygen uptake from a modified Canadian aerobic fitness test. *Can J Appl Physiol.* 1993; 18:175-188.

8 Environmental Factors

Aural Canal, Esophageal, and Rectal Temperatures During Exertional Heat Stress and the Subsequent Recovery Period
Gagnon D, Lemire BB, Jay O, et al (Univ of Ottawa, Ontario, Canada)
J Athl Train 45:157-163, 2010

Context.—The measurement of body temperature is crucial for the initial diagnosis of exertional heat injury and for monitoring purposes during a subsequent treatment strategy. However, little information is available about how different measurements of body temperature respond during and after exertional heat stress.

Objective.—To present the temporal responses of aural canal (T_{ac}), esophageal (T_{es}), and rectal (T_{re}) temperatures during 2 different scenarios (S1, S2) involving exertional heat stress and a subsequent recovery period.

Design.—Randomized controlled trial.

Setting.—University research laboratory.

Patients or Other Participants.—Twenty-four healthy volunteers, with 12 (5 men, 7 women) participating in S1 and 12 (7 men, 5 women) participating in S2.

Intervention(s).—The participants exercised in the heat (42°C, 30% relative humidity) until they reached a 39.5°C cutoff criterion, which was determined by T_{re} in S1 and by T_{es} in S2. As such, participants attained different levels of hyperthermia (as determined by T_{re}) at the end of exercise. Participants in S1 were subsequently immersed in cold water (2°C) until T_{re} reached 37.5°C, and participants in S2 recovered in a temperate environment (30°C, 30% relative humidity) for 60 minutes.

Main Outcome Measure(s).—We measured T_{ac}, T_{es}, and T_{re} throughout both scenarios.

Results.—The T_{es} (S1 = 40.19 ± 0.41°C, S2 = 39.50 ± 0.02°C) was higher at the end of exercise compared with both T_{ac} (S1 = 39.74 ± 0.42°C, S2 = 38.89 ± 0.32°C) and T_{re} (S1 = 39.41 ± 0.04°C, S2 = 38.74 ± 0.28°C) (for both comparisons in each scenario, $P < .001$). Conversely, T_{es} (S1 = 36.26 ± 0.74°C, S2 = 37.36 ± 0.34°C) and T_{ac} (S1 = 36.48 ± 1.07°C, S2 = 36.97 ± 0.38°C) were lower compared with T_{re} (S1 = 37.54 ± 0.04°C, S2 = 37.78 ± 0.31°C) at the end of both scenarios (for both comparisons in each scenario, $P < .001$).

Conclusions.—We found that T_{ac}, T_{es}, and T_{re} presented different temporal responses during and after both scenarios of exertional heat stress and a subsequent recovery period. Although these results may not have direct practical implications in the field monitoring and treatment of individuals with exertional heat injury, they do quantify the extent to which these body temperature measurements differ in such scenarios (Fig 1).

▶ Because of convenience, most sports physicians and exercise physiologists have used the rectal temperature as a measure of the thermal stress induced by a bout of exercise. In events such as a marathon run, a rectal temperature of 40°C is commonly used as a simple field test to distinguish cases of heat exhaustion from exertional heat stroke.[1,2] However, it has long been recognized that the rectal temperature differs substantially from that recorded elsewhere in the body[3-6] (Fig 1). Readings from the mouth are usually distorted by mouth breathing and resultant cooling of the tongue, but other sites, such as the esophagus or the tympanic membrane can be used in the laboratory, and indeed, it has been suggested that such data provide a better measure of the thermal hazards faced by an individual because they reflect more closely the temperature of blood perfusing the brain. Given that during running, most of the heat is generated in the leg muscles, it is at first inspection a little surprising that rectal temperature lags behind the other indicators; possible factors include a greater tissue mass surrounding the rectal probe and an exercise-induced reduction in visceral flow.[7] During the recovery phase, the rectal temperature remains higher than at alternative measuring sites in part because the tissue mass around the probe takes longer to cool and in part because heat is still being liberated from the leg muscles. The rectal temperature will remain the method of choice for monitoring thermal stress in the field, but one important

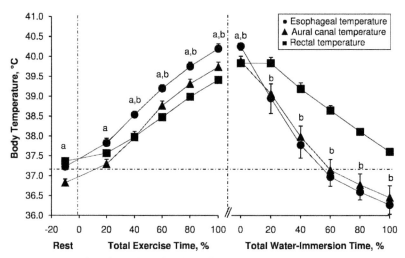

FIGURE 1.—Esophageal, aural canal, and rectal temperatures during exertional heat stress and throughout the subsequent period of coldwater immersion in scenario 1. Values are mean ± standard error for 12 participants. [a] Indicates different from aural canal temperature ($P < .05$). [b] Indicates different from rectal temperature ($P < .05$). The vertical dashed lines delimit each period. The horizonal dashed line represents the mean of all 3 resting core temperatures. (Reprinted from Gagnon D, Lemire BB, Jay O, et al. Aural canal, esophageal, and rectal temperatures during exertional heat stress and the subsequent recovery period. *J Athl Train*. 2010;45:157-163.)

practical lesson is that if one waits until rectal temperature has normalized, a patient may be cooled for too long.[8]

R. J. Shephard, MD (Lond), PhD, DPE

References

1. American College of Sports Medicine, Armstrong LE, Casa DJ, et al. American College of Sports Medicine position stand: Exertional heat illness during training and competition. *Med Sci Sports Exerc.* 2007;39:556-572.
2. Binkley HM, Beckett J, Casa DJ, Kleiner DM, Plummer PE. National Athletic Trainers'Association Position Statement: Exertional Heat Illnesses. *J Athl Train.* 2002;37:329-343.
3. Cranston WI, Gerbrandy J, Snell ES. Oral, rectal and oesophageal temperatures and some factors affecting them in man. *J Physiol.* 1954;126:347-358.
4. Minard D, Copman L, Dasler AR. Elevation of body temperature in health. *Ann N Y Acad Sci.* 1964;121:12-25.
5. Newsham KR, Saunders JE, Nordin ES. Comparison of rectal and tympanic thermometry during exercise. *South Med J.* 2002;95:804-810.
6. Casa DJ, Becker SM, Ganio MS, et al. Validity of devices that assess body temperature during outdoor exercise in the heat. *J Athl Train.* 2007;42:333-342.
7. Rowell LB. Human cardiovascular adjustments to exercise and thermal stress. *Physiol Rev.* 1974;54:75-159.
8. Proulx CI, Ducharme MB, Kenny GP. Safe cooling limits from exercise-induced hyperthermia. *Eur J Appl Physiol.* 2006;96:434-445.

Heat acclimation improves exercise performance

Lorenzo S, Halliwill JR, Sawka MN, et al (Univ of Oregon, Eugene; US Army Res Inst of Environmental Medicine, Natick, MA)

J Appl Physiol 109:1140-1147, 2010

This study examined the impact of heat acclimation on improving exercise performance in cool and hot environments. Twelve trained cyclists performed tests of maximal aerobic power ($\dot{V}_{O_{2max}}$), time-trial performance, and lactate threshold, in both cool [13°C, 30% relative humidity (RH)] and hot (38°C, 30% RH) environments before and after a 10-day heat acclimation ($\sim 50\%$ $\dot{V}_{O_{2max}}$ in 40°C) program. The hot and cool condition $\dot{V}_{O_{2max}}$ and lactate threshold tests were both preceded by either warm (41°C) water or thermoneutral (34°C) water immersion to induce hyperthermia (0.8−1.0°C) or sustain normothermia, respectively. Eight matched control subjects completed the same exercise tests in the same environments before and after 10 days of identical exercise in a cool (13°C) environment. Heat acclimation increased $\dot{V}_{O_{2max}}$ by 5% in cool (66.8 ± 2.1 vs. 70.2 ± 2.3 ml·kg^{-1}·min^{-1}, $P = 0.004$) and by 8% in hot (55.1 ± 2.5 vs. 59.6 ± 2.0 ml·kg^{-1}·min^{-1}, $P = 0.007$) conditions. Heat acclimation improved time-trial performance by 6% in cool (879.8 ± 48.5 vs. 934.7 ± 50.9 kJ, $P = 0.005$) and by 8% in hot (718.7 ± 42.3 vs. 776.2 ± 50.9 kJ, $P = 0.014$) conditions. Heat acclimation increased power output at lactate threshold by 5% in cool (3.88 ± 0.82 vs. 4.09 ± 0.76 W/kg, $P = 0.002$) and by 5% in hot (3.45 ± 0.80 vs. 3.60 ± 0.79 W/kg, $P < 0.001$)

conditions. Heat acclimation increased plasma volume ($6.5 \pm 1.5\%$) and maximal cardiac output in cool and hot conditions ($9.1 \pm 3.4\%$ and $4.5 \pm 4.6\%$, respectively). The control group had no changes in $\dot{V}_{O_{2max}}$, time-trial performance, lactate threshold, or any physiological parameters. These data demonstrate that heat acclimation improves aerobic exercise performance in temperate-cool conditions and provide the scientific basis for employing heat acclimation to augment physical training programs.

▶ This study was the first to show that 10 days of heat acclimation provided ergogenic benefits in both cool and hot conditions (Fig 2A-C in the original article). Multiple studies indicate that heat acclimation induces physiological adaptations including reduced oxygen uptake at a given power output, muscle glycogen sparing, reduced blood lactate at a given power output, plasma volume expansion, improved myocardial efficiency, increased ventricular compliance, and enhanced muscle force generation. These heat acclimation benefits may persist for 1 or 2 weeks and are analogous to those of the live high and train low system of training.[1] Heat acclimation training, however, requires less time and logistical support than living at high elevations and training near sea level. The authors concluded that "robust adaptations to environmental exposure can be leveraged to augment aerobic performance in highly trained athletes."

D. C. Nieman, DrPH

Reference

1. Levine BD, Stray-Gundersen J. "Living high-training low": effect of moderate-altitude acclimatization with low-altitude training on performance. *J Appl Physiol.* 1997;83:102-112.

Safety in the Heat: A Comprehensive Program for Prevention of Heat Illness Among Workers in Abu Dhabi, United Arab Emirates
Joubert D, Thomsen J, Harrison O (Dept of Public Health and Res, Abu Dhabi, United Arab Emirates; Division of Public Health and Policy, Abu Dhabi, United Arab Emirates)
Am J Public Health 101:395-398, 2011

The Safety in the Heat program was developed in response to the extreme heat stress conditions experienced by workers in the United Arab Emirates and other Middle Eastern countries each summer, where ambient air temperatures often reach 45°C (135°F) and higher with 90% humidity. A comprehensive, multimedia, economical education and awareness program targeting companies in the region was developed; 465 companies employing 814 996 heat-exposed workers across 6254 work and labor residence sites were reached. Feedback from program participants indicated a high level of support and satisfaction. Results indicated a marked reduction in heat related illness over a period of 2 years

(2008–2009) at 2 companies, one of which reported a combined 79.5% decrease in cases (15.3 vs 1.16 cases per 1000 workers) while the other experienced a 50% reduction in serious cases (0.08–0.04 cases per 100 000 work hours).

▶ This article reports on a successful public health intervention that was instituted to target workers in 465 companies in Abu Dhabi where temperatures in the summer are extremely hot. The interest for sport medicine practitioners is that a similar public health program could be instituted for sport activities. The program, called Safety in the Heat, refined and validated a novel heat stress index called the Thermal Work Limit. Program materials were distributed to companies in several languages, using posters, pamphlets, videos, banners, Web sites, etc. These addressed general awareness of heat hazards, symptoms, precautions, and emergency measures. Although there is not much information in this short article about the Thermal Work Limit, perhaps a similar measure could be implemented for sports activities and used to warn people against playing sport under certain conditions. Similarly, a program providing information on safety of sports in the heat could be developed for the general population within local community sport organizations.

D. E. Feldman, PT, PhD

Thermoregulation, pacing and fluid balance during mass participation distance running in a warm and humid environment

Lee JKW, Nio AQX, Lim CL, et al (Defence Med and Environmental Res Inst, Singapore; et al)
Eur J Appl Physiol 109:887-898, 2010

Deep body temperature (T_c), pacing strategy and fluid balance were investigated during a 21-km road race in a warm and humid environment. Thirty-one males (age 25.3 ± 3.2 years; maximal oxygen uptake 59.1 ± 4.2 ml kg^{-1} min^{-1}) volunteered for this study. Continuous T_c responses were obtained in 25 runners. Research stations at approximately 3-km intervals permitted accurate assessment of split times and fluid intake. Environmental conditions averaged 26.4°C dry bulb temperature and 81% relative humidity. Peak T_c was 39.8 ± 0.5 (38.5–40.7) °C with 24 runners achieving $T_c > 39.0$°C, 17 runners ≥39.5°C, and 10 runners ≥40.0°C. In 12 runners attaining peak $T_c \geq 39.8$°C, running speed did not differ significantly when T_c was below or above this threshold (208 ± 15 cf. 205 ± 24 m min^{-1}; $P = 0.532$). Running velocity was the main significant predictor variable of $\triangle T_c$ at 21 km ($R^2 = 0.42$, $P < 0.001$) and was the main discriminating variable between hyperthermic ($T_c \geq 39.8$°C) and normothermic runners ($T_c < 39.8$°C) up to 11.8 km. A reverse J-shaped pacing profile characterised by a marked reduction in running speed after 6.9 km and evidence of an end-spurt in 16 runners was observed. Variables relating to fluid balance were not associated with any T_c parameters or pacing. We conclude that hyperthermia,

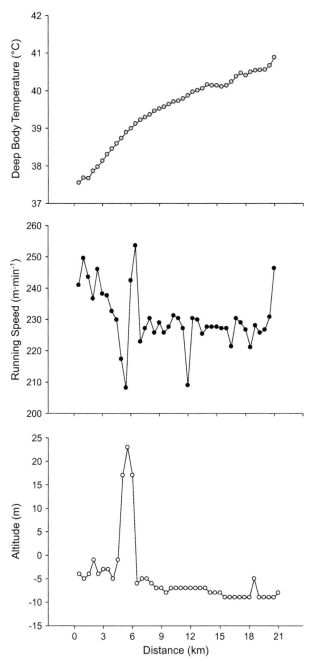

FIGURE 3.—Deep body temperature, running speed and elevation versus race distance for the fastest runner. (Reprinted from Lee JKW, Nio AQX, Lim CL, et al. Thermoregulation, pacing and fluid balance during mass participation distance running in a warm and humid environment. *Eur J Appl Physiol.* 2010;109:887-898. With kind permission of Springer Science+Business Media.)

defined by a deep body temperature greater than 39.5°C, is common in trained individuals undertaking outdoor distance running in environmental heat, without evidence of fatigue or heat illness (Fig 3).

▶ For a number of years, Noakes[1] has argued that the competitive pace of the distance runner is set by some hypothetical "Central Governor." This acts by feed-forward regulation, but functioning somewhat like the governor of an old-fashioned steam engine, limiting a runner's pace in such a way as to avert tissue damage, particularly problems arising from hyperthermia. There is little direct or indirect evidence for the existence of such a brain structure,[2] and even if it were to exist, it could not be regarded as a very effective control mechanism because dangerous levels of hyperthermia can develop during marathon running, unless competitors and their environment are monitored very carefully by a competent team of sports physicians. In the study of Lee and associates, 17 of 25 runners exceeded a "safe" gastrointestinal temperature of 39.5°C over a half marathon (21 km) under warm and humid conditions (26.4°C, 81% relative humidity), and in 10 of the runners, temperatures reached values of more than 40°C. Contrary to Noakes' hypothesis, there was no evidence that the pace of the runners slowed when their rectal temperature reached 39.8°C, and indeed many of the group showed a sharp increase of speed during the final kilometer of their run, when temperature was already 40.6°C (Fig 3). At least 2 other reports have shown sharp increases of running speed when the body temperature was already 40°C.[3,4] We must conclude that any regulation of speed in distance runners reflects a learned conservation of muscle glycogen for a final sprint, rather than the action of some nebulous "Central Governor."

R. J. Shephard, MD (Lond), PhD, DPE

References

1. Noakes TD. The central governor model of exercise regulation applied to the marathon. *Sports Med.* 2007;37:374-377.
2. Shephard RJ. Is it time to retire the 'central governor'? *Sports Med.* 2009;39: 709-721.
3. Ely BR, Ely MR, Cheuvront SN, Kenefick RW, DeGroot DW, Montain SJ. Evidence against a 40 °C core temperature threshold for fatigue in humans. *J Appl Physiol.* 2009;107:1519-1525.
4. Maron MB, Wagner JA, Horvarth SM. Thermoregulatory responses during competitive marathon running. *J Appl Physiol.* 1977;42:909-914.

Thermoregulatory Responses and Hydration Practices in Heat-Acclimatized Adolescents During Preseason High School Football

Yeargin SW, Casa DJ, Judelson DA, et al (Indiana State Univ, Terre Haute; Univ of Connecticut, Storrs; California State Univ, Fullerton; et al)
J Athl Train 45:136-146, 2010

Context.—Previous researchers have not investigated the thermoregulatory responses to multiple consecutive days of American football in adolescents.

Objective.—To examine the thermoregulatory and hydration responses of high school players during formal preseason football practices.

Design.—Observational study.

Setting.—Players practiced outdoors in late August once per day on days 1 through 5, twice per day on days and 7, and once per day on days 8 through 10. Maximum wet bulb globe temperature averaged 23 ± 4°C.

Patients or Other Participants.—Twenty-five heat-acclimatized adolescent boys (age = 15 ± 1 years, height = 180 ± 8 cm, mass = 81.4 ± 15.8 kg, body fat = 12 ± 5%, Tanner stage = 4 ± 1).

Main Outcome Measure(s).—We observed participants within and across preseason practices of football. Measures included gastrointestinal temperature (T_{GI}), urine osmolality, sweat rate, forearm sweat composition, fluid consumption, testosterone to cortisol ratio, perceptual measures of thirst, perceptual measures of thermal sensation, a modified Environmental Symptoms Questionnaire, and knowledge questionnaires assessing the participants' understanding of heat illnesses and hydration. Results were analyzed for differences across time and were compared between younger (14–15 years, n = 13) and older (16–17 years, n = 12) participants.

Results.—Maximum daily T_{GI} values remained less than 40°C and were correlated with maximum wet bulb globe temperature ($r = 0.59$, $P = .009$). Average urine osmolality indicated that participants generally experienced minimal to moderate hypohydration before (881 ± 285 mOsmol/kg) and after (856 ± 259 mOsmol/kg) each practice as a result of replacing approximately two-thirds of their sweat losses during exercise but inadequately rehydrating between practices. Age did not affect most variables; however, sweat rate was lower in younger participants (0.6 ± 0.2 L/h) than in older participants (0.8 ± 0.1 L/h) ($F_{1,18} = 8.774$, $P = .008$).

Conclusions.—Previously heat-acclimatized adolescent boys ($T_{GI} < 40°C$) can safely complete the initial days of preseason football practice in moderate environmental conditions using well-designed practice guidelines. Adolescent boys replaced most sweat lost during practice but remained mildly hypohydrated throughout data collection, indicating inadequate hydration habits when they were not at practice.

▶ We are in need of more studies like this one that provide information on hydration status of athletes in real-world situations. Adequate hydration is critical for both optimizing sports performance and avoiding heat illness, which can be life threatening. But we don't have a great deal of information regarding what athletes actually drink and how their hydration status changes during periods of training and competition. The findings in this case provide an important, yet not perhaps unexpected, lesson. Focusing on adequate drinking practices during sports play is appropriate, but athletes shouldn't forget that even with the best drinking habits, they are seldom euhydrated when they finish training sessions or competitions. Increasing fluid intake between times is critical to prevent arriving at the beginning of the next session of play with a fluid deficit. The take-home message is that athletes need to drink adequately both during and between training sessions.

T. Rowland, MD

Ice Slurry Ingestion Increases Core Temperature Capacity and Running Time in the Heat

Siegel R, Maté J, Brearley MB, et al (Edith Cowan Univ, Joondalup, Western Australia, Australia; Northern Territory Inst of Sport, Australia)

Med Sci Sports Exerc 42:717-725, 2010

Purpose.—To investigate the effect of ice slurry ingestion on thermoregulatory responses and submaximal running time in the heat.

Methods.—On two separate occasions, in a counterbalanced order, 10 males ingested 7.5 g·kg^{-1} of either ice slurry ($-1°C$) or cold water (4°C) before running to exhaustion at their first ventilatory threshold in a hot environment (34.0°C ± 0.2°C, 54.9% ± 5.9% relative humidity). Rectal and skin temperatures, HR, sweating rate, and ratings of thermal sensation and perceived exertion were measured.

Results.—Running time was longer ($P = 0.001$) after ice slurry (50.2 ± 8.5 min) versus cold water (40.7 ± 7.2 min) ingestion. Before running, rectal temperature dropped 0.66°C ± 0.14°C after ice slurry ingestion compared with 0.25°C ± 0.09°C ($P = 0.001$) with cold water and remained lower for the first 30 min of exercise. At exhaustion, however, rectal temperature was higher ($P = 0.001$) with ice slurry (39.36°C ± 0.41°C) versus cold water ingestion (39.05°C ± 0.37°C). During exercise, mean skin temperature was similar between conditions ($P = 0.992$), as was HR ($P = 0.122$) and sweat rate ($P = 0.242$). After ice slurry ingestion, subjects stored more heat during exercise (100.10 ± 25.00 vs 78.93 ± 20.52 W·m^{-2}, $P = 0.005$), and mean ratings of thermal sensation ($P = 0.001$) and perceived exertion ($P = 0.022$) were lower.

Conclusions.—Compared with cold water, ice slurry ingestion lowered preexercise rectal temperature, increased submaximal endurance running time in the heat (+19% ± 6%), and allowed rectal temperature to become higher at exhaustion. As such, ice slurry ingestion may be an effective and practical precooling maneuver for athletes competing in hot environments.

▶ This study discusses precooling strategies for athletes to enhance performance times and reduce core body temperature prior to exercising. The goal is to find the most practical and effective strategy. In this study, the investigators compare 2 strategies: ingestion of ice slurry (slushie) versus ingestion of cold water. Although the sample size was small (10 males), there was adequate power in this random crossover design to demonstrate that the ice slurry strategy lowered rectal temperature before running, increased running time in the heat, and increased rectal temperature afterward (at exhaustion). Furthermore, mean ratings of thermal sensation and perceived exertion were lower after ingestion of the ice slurry as compared with drinking of cold water (Fig 4 in the original article). There are other types of precooling strategies such as ice vests or jackets and external immersion in cold water, but these are less practical for use on the field. The ice slurry represents a practical precooling strategy that can be used in the field and appears to be superior to simply drinking cold water prior to exercising.

D. E. Feldman, PT, PhD

Thermoregulatory responses to ice-slush beverage ingestion and exercise in the heat
Stanley J, Leveritt M, Peake JM (Queensland Academy of Sport, Brisbane, Australia; Griffith Univ, Gold Coast, Australia)
Eur J Appl Physiol 110:1163-1173, 2010

We compared the effects of an ice-slush beverage (ISB) and a cool liquid beverage (CLB) on cycling performance, changes in rectal temperature (T_{re}) and stress responses in hot, humid conditions. Ten trained male cyclists/triathletes completed two exercise trials (75 min cycling at ~60% peak power output + 50 min seated recovery + 75% peak power output × 30 min performance trial) on separate occasions in 34°C, 60% relative humidity. During the recovery phase before the performance trial, the athletes consumed either the ISB (mean ± SD −0.8 ± 0.1°C) or the CLB (18.4 ± 0.5°C). Performance time was not significantly different after consuming the ISB compared with the CLB (29.42 ± 2.07 min for ISB vs. 29.98 ± 3.07 min for CLB, $P = 0.263$). T_{re} (37.0 ± 0.3°C for ISB vs. 37.4 ± 0.2°C for CLB, $P = 0.001$) and physiological strain index (0.2 ± 0.6 for ISB vs. 1.1 ± 0.9 for CLB, $P = 0.009$) were lower at the end of recovery and before the performance trial after ingestion of the ISB compared with the CLB. Mean thermal sensation was lower ($P < 0.001$) during recovery with the ISB compared with the CLB. Changes in plasma volume and the concentrations of blood variables (i.e., glucose, lactate, electrolytes, cortisol and catecholamines) were similar between the two trials. In conclusion, ingestion of ISB did not significantly alter exercise performance even though it significantly reduced pre-exercise T_{re} compared with CLB. Irrespective of exercise performance outcomes, ingestion of ISB during recovery from exercise in hot humid environments is a practical and effective method for cooling athletes following exercise in hot environments (Fig 2).

▶ Several reports have previously suggested that when exercising in hot and humid conditions, a reduction of core temperatures is achieved by ingesting cold (4°C-10°C) beverages.[1-4] This small-scale controlled trial compared the effects of administering 1 L of ice-slush (14 g/kg of slush) versus 1 L of a standard 18°C beverage during recovery from a 75-minute bout of cycle ergometer exercise (75% of peak power output) in the heat (33.7°C, 60% relative humidity). The findings confirmed an earlier study[5] that showed substantial thermal benefit

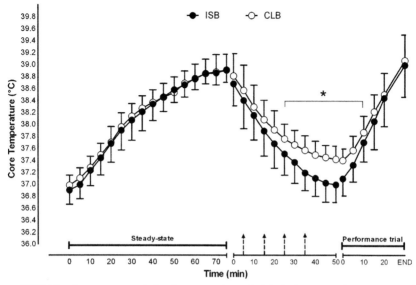

FIGURE 2.—Core temperature during the two experimental trials. *Broken arrows* denote ingestion of experimental beverage. Recovery phase is the 50-min period between steady-state and performance trial. Data are presented as mean ± SD. *Significantly different between conditions, $P < 0.05$. (Reprinted from Stanley J, Leveritt M, Peake JM. Thermoregulatory responses to ice-slush beverage ingestion and exercise in the heat. *Eur J Appl Physiol.* 2010;110:1163-1173. With kind permission of Springer Science+Business Media.)

from drinking ice-slush relative to a standard cold beverage (Fig 2). The thermal benefit is hardly surprising, given the substantial latent heat of fusion (333 kJ/kg) associated with the transition from ice to water. More importantly, the physiological strain index was reduced relative to the control condition, and the subsequent time trial performance was not adversely affected by drinking the ice-slush. It remains to be examined how far slush ingestion would reduce fluid absorption and thus more long-term performance in the heat.

R. J. Shephard, MD (Lond), PhD, DPE

References

1. Lee JKW, Shirreffs SM. The influence of drink temperature on thermoregulatory responses during prolonged exercise in a moderate environment. *J Sports Sci.* 2007;25:975-985.
2. Lee JKW, Maughan RJ, Shirreffs SM. The influence of serial feeding of drinks at different temperatures on thermoregulatory responses during cycling. *J Sports Sci.* 2008;26:583-590.
3. Lee JKW, Shirreffs SM, Maughan RJ. Cold drink ingestion improves exercise endurance capacity in heat. *Med Sci Sports Exerc.* 2008;40:1637-1644.
4. Mündel T, King J, Collacott E, Jones DA. Drink temperature influences fluid intake and endurance capacity in men during exercise in a hot, dry environment. *Exp Physiol.* 2006;91:925-933.
5. Siegel R, Maté J, Brearley MB, Watson G, Nosaka K, Laursen PB. Ice slurry ingestion increases core temperature capacity and running time in the heat. *Med Sci Sports Exerc.* 2010;42:717-725.

Can Changes in Body Mass and Total Body Water Accurately Predict Hyponatremia After a 161-km Running Race?

Lebus DK, Casazza GA, Hoffman MD, et al (Univ of California Davis Med Ctr, Sacramento; et al)

Clin J Sport Med 20:193-199, 2010

Objective.—To relate changes in body mass, total body water (TBW), extracellular fluid (ECF), and serum sodium concentration ([Na$^+$]) from a 161-km ultramarathon to finish time and incidence of hyponatremia.

Design.—Observational.

Setting.—The 2008 Rio Del Lago 100-Mile (161-km) Endurance Run in Granite Bay, California.

Participants.—Forty-five runners.

Main Outcome Measurements.—Pre-race and post-race body mass, TBW, ECF, and serum [Na$^+$].

Results.—Body mass and serum [Na$^+$] significantly decreased 2% to 3% ($P < 0.001$) from pre-race to post-race, but TBW and ECF were unchanged. Significant relationships were observed between finish time and percentage change in body mass ($r = 0.36$; $P = 0.01$), TBW ($r = 0.50$; $P = 0.007$), and ECF ($r = 0.61$; $P = 0.003$). No associations were found between post-race serum [Na$^+$] and percentage change in body mass ($r = -0.04$; $P = 0.94$) or finish time ($r = 0.5$; $P = 0.77$). Hyponatremia (serum [Na$^+$] < 135 mmol/L) was present among 51.2% of finishers. Logistic regression prediction equation including pre-race TBW and percentage changes in TBW and ECF had an 87.5% concordance with the classification of hyponatremia.

Conclusions.—Hyponatremia occurred in over half of the 161-km ultramarathon finishers but was not predicted by change in body mass. The combination of pre-race TBW and percentage changes in TBW and ECF explained 87.5% of the variation in the incidence of hyponatremia (Fig 4).

▶ An introductory article in the 2007 *Year Book of Sports Medicine*[1] queried how far hyponatremia was a problem in well-managed athletic competition. The study by Lebus and associates provides pre- and postrace sodium ion concentrations for 41 runners completing an ultramarathon event. The time to cover 161 km averaged almost 26 hours. Environmental temperatures during this period ranged widely from 12.2° to 37.6°C, but no other details on weather conditions are given. Twenty-four aid stations provided various foods, including salty snacks, water, and sports drinks, but the nutritional advice given to the runners is not detailed, but probably followed the Western States Endurance Run Participants Guide.[2] None of the group required medical treatment for hyponatremia, although 16 of 41 athletes had what some have termed a biochemical hyponatremia (Na+ concentration of 130-135 mM/L), and 5 athletes were in the clinically hyponatremic zone (Na+ concentration < 130 mM/L).[3] The study makes several interesting observations. Firstly, the average prerace sodium ion concentration (138 mM/L) was a little low, suggesting that some runners had hyperhydrated prior to the event. Secondly,

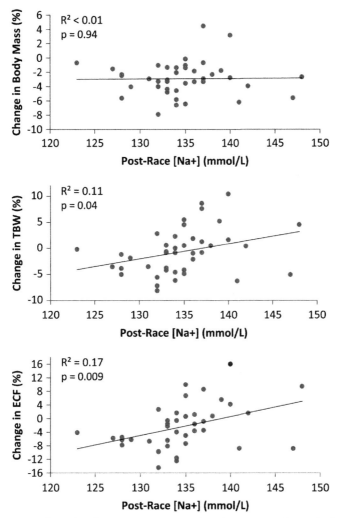

FIGURE 4.—Relationships for post-race serum [Na$^+$] with percentage changes in body mass ($r = -0.04$; $P = 0.94$; $n = 41$), TBW ($r = 0.33$; $P = 0.04$; $n = 41$), and ECF ($r = 0.41$; $P = 0.009$; $n = 40$). (Reprinted from Lebus DK, Casazza GA, Hoffman MD, et al. Can changes in body mass and total body water accurately predict hyponatremia after a 161-km running race? *Clin J Sport Med.* 2010;20:193-199, with permission from Lippincott Williams & Wilkins.)

although the average decrease in body mass was around 2 kg or 2.9% of body mass, there was no change in total body water or extracellular fluids. In the fastest 3 competitors, there was a 5.6% to 6.6% decrease in body mass, without deterioration of performance. This casts doubt on the practice of insisting on fluid ingestion when weight loss reaches 5%[2] and makes untenable the current ACSM recommendation of limiting weight loss to 2%; some of these individuals had sodium concentrations below 135 mM/L, and further fluid intake would have been inappropriate (Fig 4). Weight-based recommendations for the rehydration of ultramarathon runners too frequently neglect weight loss resulting from the metabolism of fat and water liberated as glycogen is metabolized.[4] The latter is likely to be exaggerated in ultramarathoners as a consequence of carbohydrate loading prior to an event.

R. J. Shephard, MD (Lond), PhD, DPE

References

1. Shephard RJ. Hype or hyponatremia?. In: Shephard RJ, ed. *Yearbook of Sports Medicine.* Philadelphia, PA: Elsevier; 2007.
2. Western States Endurance Run Participant's Guide, http://www.ws100.com/PGuide09.pdf; August 19, 2009. Accessed.
3. Noakes TD, Sharwood K, Speedy D, et al. Three independent biological mechanisms cause exercise-associated hyponatremia: evidence from 2,135 weighed competitive athletic performances. *Proc Natl Acad Sci U S A.* 2005;102:18550-18555.
4. Olsson KE, Saltin B. Variation in total body water with muscle glycogen changes in man. *Acta Physiol Scand.* 1970;80:11-18.

The incidence of exercise-associated hyponatraemia in the London marathon
Kipps C, Sharma S, Pedoe DT (Univ of London, UK; Kings College Hosp, London, UK; Homerton Hosp, London, UK)
Br J Sports Med 45:14-19, 2011

Background.—Exercise-associated hyponatraemia (EAH) is a potentially fatal cause of collapse in endurance exercise. It is understood to be a dilutional hyponatraemia caused by an increase of total body water relative to the amount of exchangeable sodium stores. Fourteen runners presented to one London hospital with symptomatic EAH several hours after finishing the 2003 London Marathon, and more recently, a young male runner died from the complications of severe EAH after crossing the finish line of the London Marathon.

Objectives.—To determine the incidence of EAH in runners in the London Marathon.

Methods.—Volunteers were recruited at race registration where they were weighed, had blood tests and completed a demographic and experience questionnaire. Weights, blood tests and a fluid intake questionnaire were repeated after the finish. Blood was analysed on-site using handheld i-STAT blood analysers.

Results.—Of the 88 volunteers, 11 (12.5%) developed asymptomatic hyponatraemia (serum sodium 128–134 mmol/l). They consumed more fluid (p<0.001) and gained more weight (p<0.001) than did those without hyponatraemia.

Conclusions.—A significant proportion (12.5%) of healthy volunteers developed asymptomatic hyponatraemia running a marathon in cool conditions. On average, these runners consumed more fluid and gained more weight than did non-hyponatraemic runners, although fluid intake

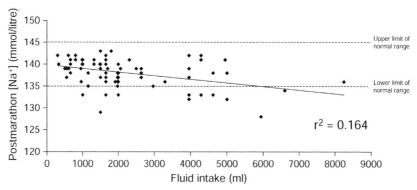

FIGURE 3.—Postmarathon [Na⁺] against fluid intake. (Reprinted from Kipps C, Sharma S, Pedoe DT. The incidence of exercise-associated hyponatraemia in the London marathon. *Br J Sports Med.* 2011;45:14-19 and reproduced with permission from the BMJ Publishing Group.)

was not related to weight gain in this study. Four of the 11 hyponatraemic runners lost weight over the course of the marathon, strengthening the case for an additional factor, such as inappropriate antidiuretic hormone release during exercise, in the development of EAH (Fig 3).

▶ There has been much speculation as to the likelihood of developing hyponatremia during long-distance events.[1] Previous electrolyte-based estimates from Europe and the United States have ranged from 3% to 22%,[2,3] with 5 possible deaths from this problem in recent years. Hyponatremia is commonly diagnosed whenever serum sodium (Na^+) concentrations fall below the lower normal limit of 135 mmol/L during or within 24 hours following a race[4]; however, blood electrolyte levels are not always a reliable indicator of the clinical severity of the condition. Early clinical signs (including bloating, nausea, vomiting, and headache) are rare until the serum Na^+ concentrations fall below 130 mmol/L. In this sample of runners from the London marathon, 12.5% of 88 runners had a serum Na^+ concentration of less than 135 mmol/L (some as low as 128 mmol/L) (Fig. 3), but none developed any symptoms that were attributable to hyponatremia. The race was held under cool (9°C-12°C) and rainy conditions. In general, the cause of low Na^+ concentrations appears to have been an excessive intake of fluid (and this was reflected in changes of the individual's body mass over the event). But there were a few exceptions where inappropriate arginine vasopressin secretion may have been a contributing factor.[5] In general, Na^+ balance was well maintained in those individuals whose body mass decreased by 0% to 2.5% over the run. One weakness in this study that should be emphasized is that blood electrolytes were determined at registration rather than at the start of the event; thus, some runners may have begun the race in a hyperhydrated state.

R. J. Shephard, MD (Lond), PhD, DPE

References

1. Shephard RJ. Hype or hyponatremia?. In: Shephard RJ, ed. *Year Book of Sports Medicine 2007.* Philadelphia, PA: Elsevier Mosby; 2008:xix-xxviii.

2. Mettler S, Rusch C, Frey WO, Bestmann L, Wenk C, Colombani PC. Hyponatremia among runners in the Zurich Marathon. *Clin J Sport Med.* 2008;18:344-349.

3. Chorley J, Cianca J, Divine J. Risk factors for exercise-associated hyponatremia in non-elite marathon runners. *Clin J Sport Med.* 2007;17:471-477.

4. Hew-Butler T, Ayus JC, Kipps C, et al. Statement of the Second International Exercise-Associated Hyponatremia Consensus Development Conference, New Zealand, 2007. *Clin J Sport Med.* 2008;18:111-121.

5. Siegel AJ, Verbalis JG, Clement S, et al. Hyponatremia in marathon runners due to inappropriate arginine vasopressin secretion. *Am J Med.* 2007;120:461.e11-461.e17.

Protective Effect of Erythropoietin on Renal Injury Induced by Acute Exhaustive Exercise in the Rat

Lin X, Qu S, Hu M, et al (Med College of Hunan Normal Univ, Changsha, China; Public Health College of Central South Univ, Changsha, China)
Int J Sports Med 31:847-853, 2010

We investigated the protective effect of Erythropoietin (EPO) analogue rHuEPO on renal injury induced by acute exhaustive exercise in the rat. Rats were randomly allocated to one of 3 groups: normal control (C), exhaustive exercise test (ET) and EPO pre-treatment (rHuEPO 2000 U/kg) plus ET (EPO + ET). Compared with controls, animals in the ET group had increased serum urea nitrogen, serum creatinine, urine protein, and renal tissue malondialdehyde (MDA) and decreased renal tissue nitric oxide (NO), nitric oxide synthase (NOS) and superoxide dismutase (SOD) activities. There was severe damage in renal tubular epithelial cells with a lot of cell apoptosis, and TUNEL assay revealed a remarkably high apoptotic index ($p < 0.01$). Changes in renal function and kidney tissue were much less in the EPO + ET group ($p < 0.05$) and the apoptotic index was much lower than in the ET group (18.45 ± 0.32 vs. 27.55 ± 0.49, $p < 0.05$). EPO pretreatment thus significantly prevented renal cell apoptosis, and counteracted high MDA and low NO and NOS renal contents induced by exhaustive exercise. The data point to a potential value of EPO in preventing the acute renal injury after exhaustive exercise (Table 3).

▶ It has long been recognized that the blood flow to the viscera is greatly reduced during vigorous endurance exercise, particularly if an athlete is

TABLE 3.—Apoptosis Rate and Apoptosis Index in the Renal Cortex of the Different Groups (mean ± SD, n = 8)

Group	Apoptosis Rate (%)	Apoptosis Index (%)
Control	20[a]	5.49 ± 0.46[a]
ET	100[b**]	27.55 ± 0.49[b**]
ET + EPO	100[b**]	18.45 ± 0.32[c*]

Statistical differences between groups in each column were indicated by different alphabetic superscripts: (b) differs from (a) ** $P < 0.01$; (b) differs from (c) $P < 0.05$; (c) differs from (a) $P < 0.05$, ANOVA test.

competing under hot conditions.[1,2] One consequence is an increase of renal protein loss,[3] and under severe conditions, local hypoxia may be sufficient to cause renal failure,[4] with increases in serum lactate dehydrogenase fractions 1 and 2. There is also a risk that further injury may occur during the period of reperfusion.[5] Sports physicians naturally try to avoid pushing competitors to the point of renal failure, and human experimentation is correspondingly sparse. There is thus interest in studying the reactions of experimental animals such as laboratory rats to prolonged endurance exercise in the heat. The studies of Lin and associates suggest that rats are quite vulnerable to this type of renal injury. Their laboratory was warm (25°C ; 3°C), and under these conditions, a run of 3 hours to exhaustion was enough to cause marked pathological damage to the kidneys, including a degeneration of the tubular cells and an accumulation of red cells and casts in the lumina. Recombinant human erythropoietin has recently been shown to protect against ischemic injury in various tissues, including the kidneys.[6] This study shows that the administration of 2000 U/kg of erythropoietin (EPO) intraperitoneally 30 minutes before exhausting exercise countered the increase in renal malondialdehyde and decrease in renal nitric oxide, nitric oxide synthase, and superoxide dismutase and perhaps more importantly reduced the apoptotic index (Table 3). The mechanisms of protection are as yet unclear; EPO may activate tubular enzymes that initiate the gene transcription of antiapoptotic factors, or it may act on any one of several mechanisms that conserve renal nitric oxide. If the present findings are confirmed, there may be demands for the prophylactic administration of EPO to endurance athletes, further complicating the already difficult task of controlling blood doping.

R. J. Shephard, MD (Lond), PhD, DPE

References

1. Rowell LB. Visceral blood flow and metabolism during exercise. In: Shephard RJ, ed. *Frontiers of Fitness*. Springfield, IL: C.C. Thomas; 1971:210-232.
2. Rowell LB. Human cardiovascular adjustments to exercise and thermal stress. *Physiol Rev.* 1974;54:75-159.
3. Poortmans JR. The level of plasma proteins in normal human urine. In: Peeters H, ed. *Protides of the Biological Fluids*. London: Academic Press; 1969:503-609.
4. Rose LI, Bosser JE, Cooper KH. Serum enzymes after marathon running. *J Appl Physiol.* 1970;29:355-357.
5. Singbartl K, Green SA, Ley K. Blocking P-selectin protects from ischemia/reperfusion-induced acute renal failure. *FASEB J.* 2000;14:48-54.
6. Chatterjee PK. Pleiotropic renal actions of erythropoietin. *Lancet.* 2005;365:1890-1892.

Effects of athletes' muscle mass on urinary markers of hydration status
Hamouti N, Del Coso J, Ávila A, et al (Univ of Castilla-La Mancha, Avda, Spain; Univ El Bosque, Bogotá, Colombia)
Eur J Appl Physiol 109:213-219, 2010

To determine if athletes' muscle mass affects the usefulness of urine specific gravity (U_{sg}) as a hydration index. Nine rugby players and nine endurance runners differing in the amount of muscle mass (42 ± 6 vs. 32 ± 3 kg, respectively; $P = 0.0002$) were recruited. At waking during six consecutive days, urine was collected for U_{sg} analysis, urine osmolality (U_{osm}), electrolytes ($U_{[Na^+]}$, $U_{[K^+]}$ and $U_{[Cl^-]}$) and protein metabolites ($U_{[Creatinine]}$, $U_{[Urea]}$ and $U_{[Uric\ acid]}$) concentrations. In addition, fasting blood serum osmolality (S_{osm}) was measured on the sixth day. As averaged during 6 days, U_{sg} (1.021 ± 0.002 vs. 1.016 ± 0.001), U_{osm} (702 ± 56 vs. 554 ± 41 mOsmol kg^{-1} H$_2$O), $U_{[Urea]}$ (405 ± 36 vs. 302 ± 23 mmol L^{-1}) and $U_{[Uric\ acid]}$ (2.7 ± 0.3 vs. 1.7 ± 0.2 mmol L^{-1}) were higher in rugby players than runners ($P < 0.05$). However, urine electrolyte concentrations were not different between groups. A higher percentage of rugby players than runners (56 vs. 11%; $P = 0.03$) could be cataloged as hypohydrated by U_{sg} (i.e., >1.020) despite S_{osm} being below 290 mOsmol kg^{-1} H$_2$O in all participants. A positive correlation was found between muscle mass and urine protein metabolites ($r = 0.47$; $P = 0.04$) and between urine protein metabolites and U_{sg} ($r = 0.92$; $P < 0.0001$). In summary, U_{sg} specificity to detect hypohydration was reduced in athletes with large muscle mass. Our data suggest that athletes with large muscle mass (i.e., rugby players) are prone to be incorrectly classified as hypohydrated based on U_{sg} (Fig 1).

▶ Two simple methods of detecting dehydration are to look for a change in body mass relative to pre-event levels (taking due account of any release of 1.5-2.0 L of water associated with glycogen molecules) and to measure the specific gravity (sg) of the urine. The latter approach has the advantage that it can be used to assess cumulative dehydration, even if the normal body mass is not known,[1,2] and it is not affected by changes in body fat content. However, as with so many physiological variables, the data for athletes do not always coincide with what one expects to see in sedentary individuals (an upper sg limit of 1.020 as a marker of euhydration). One study of wrestlers found that 69% of tests using this limit gave false-positive indications of

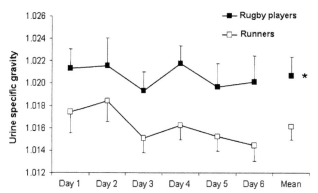

FIGURE 1.—First morning urine specific gravity of rugby players and runners during six consecutive days. Data are mean ± SEM. *Different from runners, $P < 0.05$. (Reprinted from Hamouti N, Del Coso J, Ávila A, et al. Effects of athletes' muscle mass on urinary markers of hydration status. *Eur J Appl Physiol.* 2010;109:213-219. With kind permission of Springer Science+Business Media.)

dehydration,[3] although in endurance runners, the same criterion yielded only 8% of false-positive results.[4] Problems arise because the sg of the urine reflects not only the individual's hydration status but also the urinary solute content of around 4%. More than a half of total solutes reflects protein metabolites from muscle catabolism and protein digestion. Athletes with a large muscle mass have increased creatinine excretion, and if they opt for a high protein diet, their urea excretion is also increased. The sg is thus increased by about 0.004 units relative to athletes with a low muscle mass (Fig 1). The urinary sg is closely correlated with the urinary concentration of protein metabolites ($r = 0.92$). Thus, it seems that if sg is to be used as a test of dehydration, sport-specific limits are required.

R. J. Shephard, MD (Lond), PhD, DPE

References

1. Godek SF, Bartolozzi AR, Godek JJ. Sweat rate and fluid turnover in American football players compared with runners in a hot and humid environment. *Br J Sports Med.* 2005;39:205-211.
2. Shirreffs SM, Maughan RJ. Urine osmolality and conductivity as indices of hydration status in athletes in the heat. *Med Sci Sports Exerc.* 1998;30:1598-1602.
3. Oppliger RA, Magnes SA, Popowski LA, et al. Accuracy of urine specific gravity and osmolality as indicators of hydration status. *Int J Sport Nutr Exerc Metab.* 2005;15:236-251.
4. Popowski LA, Oppliger RA, Patrick Lambert G, Johnson RF, Kim Johnson A, Gisolf CV. Blood and urinary measures of hydration status during progressive acute dehydration. *Med Sci Sports Exerc.* 2001;33:747-753.

Human Phase Response Curves to Three days of Daily Melatonin: 0.5 mg *Versus* 3.0 mg

Burgess HJ, Revell VL, Molina TA, et al (Rush Univ Med Ctr, Chicago, IL; Univ of Surrey, UK)
J Clin Endocrinol Metab 95:3325-3331, 2010

Context.—Phase response curves (PRCs) to melatonin exist, but none compare different doses of melatonin using the same protocol.

Objective.—The aim was to generate a PRC to 0.5 mg of oral melatonin and compare it to our previously published 3.0 mg PRC generated using the same protocol.

Design and Setting.—The study included two 5-d sessions in the laboratory, each preceded by 7—9 d of fixed sleep times. Each session started and ended with a phase assessment to measure the dim light melatonin onset (DLMO). In between were 3 d in an ultradian dim light (<150 lux)/dark cycle (light:dark, 2.5:1.5).

Participants.—Healthy adults (16 men, 18 women) between the ages of 18 and 42 yr participated in the study.

Interventions.—During the ultradian days of the laboratory sessions, each participant took one pill per day at the same clock time (0.5 mg melatonin or placebo, double blind, counterbalanced).

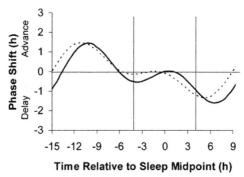

Time Relative to Sleep Midpoint (h)

FIGURE 5.—The three-pulse PRC to 0.5 mg (*solid curve*) and 3.0 mg (*dashed curve*) of exogenous oral melatonin generated from subjects free-running during 3 d of an ultradian light/dark cycle (LD 2.5:1.5). Phase shifts of the circadian clock, measured by the DLMO, are plotted against the time of administration of the melatonin pill relative to the midpoint of each individual's assigned baseline sleep schedule at home before the laboratory sessions. The *vertical lines* show the average assigned baseline bedtime and wake time. (Reprinted from Burgess HJ, Revell VL, Molina TA, et al. Human phase response curves to three days of daily melatonin: 0.5 mg *versus* 3.0 mg. *J Clin Endocrinol Metab*. 2010;95:3325-3331, with permission from The Endocrine Society.)

Main Outcome Measure.—Phase shifts to melatonin were derived by subtracting the phase shift to placebo. A PRC with time of pill administration relative to baseline DLMO and a PRC relative to midpoint of home sleep were generated.

Results.—Maximum advances occurred when 0.5 mg melatonin was taken in the afternoon, 2–4 h before the DLMO, or 9–11 h before sleep midpoint. The time for maximum phase delays was not as distinct, but a fitted curve peaked soon after wake time.

Conclusions.—The optimal administration time for advances and delays is later for the lower dose of melatonin. When each dose of melatonin is given at its optimal time, both yield similarly sized advances and delays (Fig 5).

▶ Melatonin treatment to assist in the adjustment of athletes to a differing time zone is a controversial practice, in part because of individual differences in intrinsic melatonin cycles and in part because of substantial differences in the biological availability of melatonin contained in over the counter preparations. This article describes the phase shifts induced by 2 doses of melatonin (0.5 and 3.0 mg), each administered once per day at varying points over the sleep/waking cycle (Fig 5). Advances of the cycle were achieved more readily than retardation. Differences between the 2 doses, although statistically significant, were not of great practical importance. The publishing of these curves may provide some guidance to athletes who wish to include this treatment as a part of their adaptation to a new time zone.

R. J. Shephard, MD (Lond), PhD, DPE

Effect of Air Pollution on Marathon Running Performance

Marr LC, Ely MR (Virginia Tech, Blacksburg; US Army Res Inst of Environmental Medicine, Natick, MA)
Med Sci Sports Exerc 42:585-591, 2010

Before the 2008 Olympic Games, there was concern that air pollution in Beijing would affect the performance of marathon runners. Air pollutant concentrations during marathon running and their effect on performance have not been reported. Evidence suggests that the lung function of females may be more susceptible than that of males to air pollution, but it is uncertain if this translates to decreased marathon performance.

Purpose.—The purposes of this study were to 1) describe ambient air pollutant concentrations present during major US marathons, 2) quantify performance decrements associated with air pollutants, and 3) examine potential sex difference in performance related to air pollutants.

Methods.—Marathon race results, weather data, and air pollutant concentrations were obtained for seven marathons for 8–28 yr. The top three male and female finishing times were compared with the course record and contrasted with air pollutant levels and wet bulb globe temperature (WBGT). A WBGT-adjusted performance decrement was calculated, and regression analysis was used to quantify performance decrements associated with pollutants.

Results.—The air pollutant concentrations of carbon monoxide, ozone, particulate matter smaller than 10 μm (PM_{10}), $PM_{2.5}$, nitrogen dioxide, and sulfur dioxide ranged from 0 to 5.9 ppm, from 0 to 0.07 ppm, from 4.5 to 41.0 $\mu g \cdot m^{-3}$, from 2.8 to 42.0 $\mu g \cdot m^{-3}$, from 0 to 0.06 ppm, and from 0 to 0.05 ppm, respectively. After adjusting for WBGT-associated performance decrements, only PM_{10} was associated with decrements in performance of women. For every 10-$\mu g \cdot m^{-3}$ increase in PM_{10}, performance can be expected to decrease by 1.4%.

Conclusions.—The concentrations of air pollution present during marathons rarely exceed health-based national standards and levels known to affect lung function in laboratory situations. Regardless, PM_{10} was significantly correlated with performance of women marathon runners (Table 2).

▶ In the 1950s, cities such as London experienced thousands of excess deaths that were attributed to air pollution; subsequently, a combination of more rigorous legislation and deindustrialization has greatly improved air quality over many large cities in Europe and North America. Unfortunately, China has not shared in this decrease of atmospheric pollutants; indeed, a combination of rapid industrialization and coal-fired electricity generation has led to very severe levels of pollution for much of the year. Nevertheless, fears of major interference with the Beijing Olympic Games proved unfounded because of drastic measures to curb both vehicle traffic and industrial production during the games.[1,2] There are still occasional thermal inversions that cause air quality standards to be exceeded in large North American cities, and questions remain

TABLE 2.—Correlation Matrix and Significance Level (*<0.05) Between Marathon Performance (Percent off the Course Record) for Women and Men with Air Pollutants and WBGT

	Men % off Course Record	CO	O_3	PM_{10}	$PM_{2.5}$	NO_2	SO_2	WBGT
Women % off course record	0.65*	−0.09	0.06	0.55*	0.12	−0.05	0.14	0.16*
Men % off course record		−0.07	0.07	0.34*	−0.03	−0.11	−0.05	0.27*
CO			0.06	0.37*	0.50*	0.23*	0.35*	0.13
O_3				−0.05	−0.65*	0.13	0.16	0.33*
PM_{10}					0.69*	0.57*	0.58*	0.22
$PM_{2.5}$						0.29	0.11	−0.02
NO_2							0.41*	0.34*
SO_2								0.23*

about the effects of such pollution on various categories of athlete. Marathon runners are a particularly vulnerable group on 2 counts. During the course of a 3-hour run, they inhale as large a volume of air as a sedentary person would in several days; moreover, a switch from nasal to mouth breathing carries pollutants further into their airways.[3-6] The attention of environmental monitoring agencies has focused recently on harm from ozone and fine particulate matter. It is thus particularly interesting to note that in this study, the negative effect on the race performance of female competitors was associated with the concentrations of larger particulate matter (Table 2), even though levels remained below currently accepted limits. In a sedentary person, large particles are deposited in the turbinates, and the main health concern arises from fine particulates, but once mouth breathing begins, large particulates can also become a problem. The main acute effect of large particles is probably to induce some bronchospasm, and the increased work of breathing would be enough to account for a 1% to 2% decrease in performance. Women may have more responsive airways than men because of a greater fractional deposition of large particulates.[7] As a final comment, none of the races studied in this report were held at very high temperatures, and there is some evidence that the effects of air pollutants on the marathoner may be exacerbated under hot conditions.[8]

R. J. Shephard, MD (Lond), PhD, DPE

References

1. Hao J, Wang L. Improving urban air quality in China: Beijing case study. *J Air Waste Manag Assoc.* 2005;55:1298-1305.
2. Sun Y, Zhuang G, Wang Y, et al. The air-borne particulate pollution in Beijing—concentration, composition, distribution and sources. *Atmos Environ.* 2004;38:5991-6004.
3. Niinimaa V, Cole P, Mintz S, Shephard RJ. The switching point from nasal to oronasal breathing. *Resp Physiol.* 1980;42:61-71.
4. Kabel JR, Ben-Jebria A, Ultman JS. Longitudinal distribution of ozone absorption in the lung: comparison of nasal and oral quiet breathing. *J Appl Physiol.* 1994;77:2584-2592.
5. Bowes SM, Francis M, Laube BL, Frank R. Acute exposure to acid fog: influence of breathing pattern on effective dose. *Am Ind Hyg Assoc J.* 1995;56:143-150.

6. McDonnell WF, Smith MV. Description of acute ozone response as a function of exposure rate and total inhaled dose. *J Appl Physiol.* 1994;76:2778-2784.
7. Kim CS, Hu SC. Regional deposition of inhaled particles in human lungs: comparison between men and women. *J Appl Physiol.* 1998;84:1834-1844.
8. Folinsbee LJ, Horvath SM, Raven PB, et al. Influence of exercise and heat stress on pulmonary function during ozone exposure. *J Appl Physiol.* 1977;43:409-413.

Investigating performance and lung function in a hot, humid and ozone-polluted environment

Gomes EC, Stone V, Florida-James G (Edinburgh Napier Univ, UK)
Eur J Appl Physiol 110:199-205, 2010

Large urbanized areas, where sports events take place, have a polluted environment and can also reach high temperatures and humidity levels. The aim of this study was to investigate the impact of a hot, humid and ozone-polluted (O_3) environment on (1) performance of an 8 km time trial run, (2) pulmonary function, and (3) subjective respiratory symptoms in endurance-trained runners. Using crossover randomized design, 10 male participants (mean $\dot{V} O_{2\ max} = 64.4$ mlO$_2$ kg^{-1} min^{-1}, SD = 4.4) took part in a time trial run under four different conditions: 20°C + 50% relative humidity (rh) (Control), 20°C + 50% rh + 0.10 ppm O_3 (Control + O_3), 31°C + 70% rh (Heat), 31°C + 70% rh + 0.10 ppm O_3 (Heat + O_3). Heart rate, ratings of perceived exertion and minute ventilation were collected during the run. Lung function was measured pre and post-exercise. The runners completed a respiratory symptoms questionnaire after each trial. The completion time of both the Heat (32 min 35 s) and Heat + O_3 (33 min 09 s) trials were significantly higher ($P < 0.0001$) when compared to the Control + O_3 (30 min 27 s) and Control (30 min 15 s) trials. There were no significant changes between pre/post lung function measures or between trials. The effective dose of ozone simulated in the present study did not affect the performance and therefore, ozone-pollution, at an environmentally relevant concentration, did not compound the impairment in performance beyond that induced by a hot, humid environment (Table 1).

▶ Previous reports, well summarized by Folinsbee and Schelegle,[1] have noted an adverse effect upon physical performance from exposure to ozone concentrations of 0.2 ppm and greater. This seems in keeping with the ceiling of 0.15 ppm recommended for the general population in the World Health Organization air quality guidelines. With 60 minutes of ozone exposure, athletes have shown small decreases in maximal oxygen intake and endurance time, and these changes have been linked to the combined impact of decrements in 1-second forced expiratory volume and respiratory discomfort. If the total dose of ozone is increased by prolonging vigorous effort to > 60 minutes, respiratory symptoms and a small decrement in respiratory function have been described even at concentrations < 0.09 ppm.[2,3] However, most of the available data have been collected in environmental chambers, and in some instances,

TABLE 1.—Effect of Exercise Trial on Heart Rate, RPE, Speed, Expired Air and Oxygen Consumption

	Control	Control + O_3	Heat	Heat + O_3
Average speed (km h^{-1})	16.1 ± 0.9	15.9 ± 1.6	$14.9 \pm 1.2^{\dagger}$	$14.6 \pm 1.2^{\dagger}$
Mean heart rate (beats min^{-1})	168 ± 3	170 ± 6	172 ± 3	170 ± 6
Peak heart rate (beats min^{-1})	187 ± 6	190 ± 6	192 ± 3	190 ± 6
Mean RPE	14 ± 0.9	15 ± 0.9	15 ± 0.9	$16 \pm 0.9^{*}$
Peak RPE	17 ± 0.9	17 ± 0.9	18 ± 0.9	$19 \pm 0.9^{\dagger}$
Expired volume (l min^{-1})	134 ± 16.7	124 ± 21.1	109 ± 17.4	$106 \pm 19.2^{*}$
$\dot{V}$ O_2 consumption (mlO$_2$ kg^{-1} min^{-1})	58.1 ± 4.3	56.4 ± 7.4	$49.4 \pm 7.4^{*}$	$48.4 \pm 5.3^{*,\,\S}$
O_3 effective dose (ED)	0	383.9 ± 86.8	0	366.5 ± 68.5

Values are mean ± SD.
*Significantly different from control trial, $P < 0.05$.
†Significantly different from both control and control + O3 trial, $P < 0.01$.
§Borderline significance, $P = 0.056$ compared with Control + O3.

the air in these chambers has been cool and at a fairly low relative humidity. This may be an important issue when testing the effects of a pollutant that is a respiratory irritant, and it could explain the somewhat disparate findings of Gomes et al.

R. J. Shephard, MD (Lond), PhD, DPE

References

1. Folinsbee LJ, Schelegle ES. Air pollutants and human performance. In: Shepard, RJ, Åstrand, P-O, eds. *Endurance in Sport*. Oxford, UK: Blackwell Scientific; 2000:628-638.
2. Brunekreef B, Hoek G, Breugelmans O, Leentvaar M. Respiratory effects of low-level photochemical air pollution in amateur cyclists. *Am J Respir Crit Care Med*. 1994;150:962-966.
3. Grievink L, Jansen SMA, van't Veer P, Brunekreef B. Acute effects of ozone on pulmonary function of cyclists. *Occup Environ Med*. 1998;55:13-17.

Cardiorespiratory and immune response to physical activity following exposure to a typical smoking environment

Flouris AD, Metsios GS, Jamurtas AZ, et al (Inst of Human Performance and Rehabilitation, Thessaly, Trikala, Greece; Univ of Thessaly, Trikala, Greece)
Heart 96:860-864, 2010

Objective.—Millions of non-smokers suffer daily passive smoking (PS) at home or at work, many of whom then have to walk fast for several minutes or climb a few sets of stairs. We conducted a randomised single-blind crossover experiment to assess the cardiorespiratory and immune response to physical activity following PS.

Design.—Data were obtained from 17 (eight women) nonsmoking adults during and following 30 minutes of moderate cycling administered at baseline and at 0 hour, 1 hour and 3 hours following a 1-hour PS exposure set at bar/restaurant PS levels.

Results.—We found that PS was associated with a 36% and 38.7% decrease in mean power output in men and women, respectively, and that this effect persisted up to 3 hours (p<0.05). Moreover, at 0 hour almost all cardiorespiratory and immune variables measured were markedly reduced (p<0.05). For instance, FEV_1 values at 0 hour dropped by 10.2% in men and 10.8% in women, while IL-5 increased by 59.2% in men and 44% in women, respectively (p<0.05). At 3-hour mean values of respiratory quotient, mean power, perceived exertion, cotinine, FEV_1, IL-5, IL-6 and INFγ in both sexes, recovery diastolic and mean arterial pressure, IL-4 and TNFα in men, as well as percentage predicted FEV_1 in women remained different compared to baseline (p<0.05). Also, some of the PS effects were exacerbated in less fit individuals.

Conclusion.—It is concluded that 1hour of PS at bar/restaurant levels adversely affects the response to moderate physical activity in healthy non-smokers for at least 3 hours following PS.

▶ The topic of human responses to passive smoking at rest and during exercise was examined by our laboratory many years ago under carefully controlled environmental conditions[1]; this was before the current interest in immune responses, but otherwise, the contention of Flouris et al that the article is severely outdated seems both unsubstantiated and unwarranted. The study of Flouris and associates was in fact different from and less satisfactory than ours, in that they apparently accumulated smoke simply by leaving cigarettes to smolder in an ash tray, whereas we used a smoking machine that accurately simulated the breathing pattern of a typical smoker. Carbon monoxide concentrations provide a reasonable estimate of passive exposure to cigarette smoke, but the value selected for the present experiment (23 ppm) reflects a well-ventilated tavern. If poorly ventilated, carbon monoxide levels can rise as high as 38 ppm.[2] The exposure was for 1 hour, compared with 2 hours in our earlier experiments. The substantial drop of forced expiratory volume that is reported here was not seen in our earlier trial; possibly, it is an effect of exposure to smoldering cigarettes rather than normal smoking. We also observed only small effects of passive smoking upon exercise performance at a fixed external loading. The large decrease in power output here reported for a fixed rate of oxygen consumption seems bizarre and possibly has a psychological rather than a physiological basis. There are many good reasons to avoid passive exposure to cigarette smoke, but if this health hazard is to be controlled, it is important that assaults on cigarette manufacturers be based on well-conceived and carefully performed science.

R. J. Shephard, MD (Lond), PhD, DPE

References

1. Pimm PE, Shephard RJ, Silverman F. Physiological effects of acute passive exposure to cigarette smoke. *Arch Environ Health.* 1978;33:201-213.
2. Sebben J, Pimm P, Shephard RJ. Cigarette smoke in enclosed public facilities. *Arch Environ Health.* 1977;32:53-58.

Volatile organic compounds in runners near a roadway: increased blood levels after short-duration exercise

Blair C, Walls J, Davies NW, et al (Univ of Tasmania, Australia)
Br J Sports Med 44:731-735, 2010

Objective.—To determine if non-elite athletes undertaking short duration running exercise adjacent to a busy roadway experience increased blood levels of common pollutant volatile organic compounds (benzene, toluene, ethylbenzene and xylene (BTEX)).

Design and Setting.—The study was observational in design. Participants (nine males/one female non-elite athletes) ran for 20 min, near a busy roadway along a 100 m defined course at their own pace. Blood levels of BTEX were determined both pre- and post-exercise by SPME-GC-MS. Environmental BTEX levels were determined by passive adsorption samplers.

Results.—Subjects completed a mean (range) distance of 4.4 (3.4 to 5.2) km over 20 min (4.5 (3.8 to 5.9) min/km pace), with a mean (SD) exercise intensity of 93 (2.3)% HR_{max}, and mean (SD) ventilation significantly elevated compared with resting levels (86.2 (2.3) vs 8.7 (0.9) l/min; $p<0.001$). The mean (SD) environmental levels (time weighted average) were determined as 53.1 (4.2), 428 (83), and 80.0 (3.7) $\mu g/m^3$ for toluene, ethylbenzene and xylenes, respectively, while benzene was below the detectable limit due to the short exposure period. Significant increases in blood BTEX levels were observed in runners between pre- and postexercise for toluene (mean increase of 1.4 ng/ml; $p = 0.002$), ethylbenzene (0.7 ng/ml; $p = 0.0003$), *m/p*-xylene (2.0 ng/ml; $p = 0.004$) and *o*-xylene (1.1 ng/ml; $p = 0.002$), but no change was observed for benzene.

Conclusions.—Blood BTEX levels are increased during high-intensity exercise such as running undertaken in areas with BTEX pollution, even with a short duration of exercise. This may have health implications for runners who regularly exercise near roadways (Table 2).

▶ The risks to urban runners from exposure to carbon monoxide and ozone have been well documented. Less is known of the risk from the volatile organic compounds found in petroleum products, although studies of cyclists have

TABLE 2.—Mean (SD) Blood Benzene, Toluene, Ethylbenzene and Xylene Concentrations (ng/ml) in Runners Pre- and Postexercise

		Subjects	
	Pre-exercise	Postexercise	Concentration Change
Benzene	1.4 (0.3)	1.5 (0.5)	+0.1
Toluene	1.4 (0.7)	2.8 (0.9)	+1.4*
Ethylbenzene	1.2 (0.4)	1.9 (0.4)	+0.7*
m/p-Xylene	3.5 (1.1)	5.5 (1.6)	+2.0*
o-Xylene	1.6 (0.6)	2.7 (0.7)	+1.1*

*p<0.05.

found increased blood levels postexercise.[1,2] In this study, 20 minutes of running along a busy roadway were sufficient to increase blood levels of toluene, ethylbenzene, *m/p* xylene, and *o*-xylene (Table 2). These substances are plainly bad for respiratory health,[3] but with the possible exception of ethylbenzene,[4,5] they are not normally carcinogenic. The atmosphere contained no detectable benzene, and blood levels of benzene remained unchanged; the risk of lung cancer is thus unlikely to have been changed by this exposure. Nevertheless, the data point to a need for further study of the effects of vehicle exhaust and underline the need for pedestrian walkways that are away from exhaust fumes.

R. J. Shephard, MD (Lond), PhD, DPE

References

1. Andreoli R, Manini P, Bergamaschi E, Brustolin A, Mutti A. Solid-phase microextraction and gas chromatography-mass spectrometry for determination of monoaromatic hydrocarbons in blood and urine: application to people exposed to air pollutants. *Chromatographia.* 1999;50:167-172.
2. Bergamaschi E, Brustolin A, De Palma G, et al. Biomarkers of dose and susceptibility in cyclists exposed to monoaromatic hydrocarbons. *Toxicol Lett.* 1999;108:241-247.
3. ACGIH. *Threshold Limit Values for Chemical Substances and Physical Agents and Biological Exposure Indices.* Cincinnati, OH: American Conference of Governmental Industrial Hygienists; 2001.
4. NTP. *United States Department of Health and Human Services, Public Health Service, National Toxicology Program.* Research Triangle Park, NC: National Institute of Environmental Health Sciences; 2001.
5. IARC. Ethylbenzene. *IARC Monogr Eval Carcinog Risks Hum.* 2000;77:227-266.

Changes in total body and limb composition and muscle strength after a 6–8 weeks sojourn at extreme altitude (5000–8000 m)
Sergi G, Imoscopi A, Sarti S, et al (Univ of Padua, Italy)
J Sports Med Phys Fitness 50:450-455, 2010

Weight loss at extreme altitudes affects quantitative changes in fat-free mass (FFM), muscle mass and fat mass. No studies to date have focused on regional body composition and physical performance using reference methods after stays at extreme altitudes. The aim of this study was to investigate the changes in total and regional body composition, and muscle strength induced by the extreme altitudes. Eight men aged 38.8 ± 5.8 who took part in two different Italian expeditions on Mt. Everest (group A) and on Gasherbrum II (group B). Before and after the expedition all participants underwent anthropometric measurements, total and regional body composition assessment by DEXA, and handgrip and knee extensor strength measurements by dynamometry. The variations in body composition mainly involved FFM, with a similar loss in group A (-2.4 ± 1.9 kg; $P<0.05$) and group B (-2.4 ± 1.2 kg; $P<0.05$). Most of the FFM loss involved the limbs (-2.1 ± 1.4 kg; $P<0.01$), and especially the upper limbs (-1.6 ± 1.1 kg; $P<0.01$). The isotonic knee extensor strength declined in 6 of the 8 study participants, with a mean drop of -4.4 ± 6.1 kg. In conclusion, our study evidence that extreme altitudes induce weight loss due mainly to a loss of fat-free mass in the limb.

▶ Several previous reports have noted a negative energy balance during the later phases of expeditions to high altitude,[1-3] particularly on venturing above 5000-m altitude.[4] Problems arise from a combination of the heavy physical demands of the climb, additional metabolism stimulated by cold, difficulties in cooking palatable food at very high altitudes, a depressant effect of hypoxia upon protein synthesis, and decreased insulin levels.[5] In this uncontrolled study, 2 small parties of middle-aged men spent relatively long periods of preparation at a base camp (40, 53 days) and at a high camp (16, 40 days), and the source of muscle loss (as seen in dual energy X-ray absorptiometry performed before and 6 days after return from the base camp) seems to have been too little rather than too much physical activity. A dietician kept note of the food intake, and this also dropped from about 12.5 MJ/d at the base camp to a rather inadequate intake of around 8.3 MJ/d at the high camp. The use of muscle protein rather than body fat is in contrast with earlier studies such as the study by Reynolds et al,[3] and it probably reflects in part low initial body fat stores (only about 12% of body mass). Losses of both isotonic knee extensor strength and handgrip force were substantial (> 20%), suggesting the need for greater attention to both diet and possible limitation of exercise during sojourn at high altitude camps.

R. J. Shephard, MD (Lond), PhD, DPE

References

1. Kayser B. Nutrition and high altitude exposure. *Int J Sports Med.* 1992;13: S129-132.
2. Hamad N, Travis SPL. Weight loss at high altitude: pathophysiology and practical implications. *Eur J Gastroenterol Hepatol.* 2006;18:5-10.
3. Reynolds RD, Lickteig JA, Deuster PA, et al. Energy metabolism increases and regional body fat decreases while regional muscle mass is spared in humans climbing Mt. Everest. *J Nutr.* 1999;129:1307-1314.
4. Westerterp KR. Limits to sustainable metabolic rate. *J Exp Biol.* 2001;204: 3183-3187.
5. Kayser B. Nutrition and energetics of exercise at altitude. Theory and possible practical implications. *Sports Med.* 1994;17:309-323.

Continuous positive airway pressure increases haemoglobin O_2 saturation after acute but not prolonged altitude exposure

Agostoni P, on behalf of the HIGHCARE Investigators (Università di Milano, Italy; et al)
Eur Heart J 31:457-463, 2010

Aims.—It is unknown whether subclinical high-altitude pulmonary oedema reduces spontaneously after prolonged altitude exposure. Continuous positive airway pressure (CPAP) removes extravascular lung fluids and improves haemoglobin oxygen saturation in acute cardiogenic

TABLE 3.—Cardiorespiratory Parameters Pre-Continuous Positive Airway Pressure and During Continuous Positive Airway Pressure (30 min) at Capanna Regina Margherita and Mount Everest South Base Camp

	Capanna Regina Margherita			Mount Everest South Base Camp			Δ Pre-CPAP at CM vs. Δ pre-CPAP at MEBC (P-value)
	Pre-CPAP	30′ CPAP	P-value	Pre-CPAP	30′ CPAP	P-value	
HbO$_2$-sat (%)	80 (78–81)	91 (84–97)	<0.001	81 (78–85)	80 (78–85)	0.80	<0.001
HR (b.p.m.)	88 (77–101)	84 (77–86)	<0.001	76 (68–91)*	73 (63–85)	0.01	0.24
RR (b.p.m.)	17 (14–21)	16 (14–18)	0.79	13 (11–17)	13 (10–17)	0.52	0.62
SBP (mmHg)	126 (122–134)	130 (122–136)	0.89	131 (119–144)	132 (111–140)	0.23	0.61
DBP (mmHg)	87 (81–90)	90 (83–96)	0.57	80 (71–88)	84 (74–92)	0.26	0.51
PAPs (mmHg)	35 (31–40)	33 (24–35)	0.005	32 (27–40)	37 (33–38)	0.60	0.03

Data are reported as median and inter-quartile range (first and third quartiles). CPAP, continuous positive airway pressure; HbO$_2$-sat, arterial haemoglobin saturation for oxygen; HR, heart rate; RR, respiratory rate; SBP, systolic blood pressure; DBP, diastolic blood pressure; PAPs, pulmonary artery systolic pressure. *P*-values represent significance vs. the same parameter pre-continuous positive airway pressure in the same conditions.

*$P < 0.05$ vs. HR pre-continuous positive airway pressure at Capanna Regina Margherita.

oedema. We evaluated the presence of pulmonary extravascular fluid increase by assessing CPAP effects on haemoglobin oxygen saturation under acute and prolonged altitude exposure.

Methods and Results.—We applied 7 cm H_2O CPAP for 30 min to healthy individuals after acute (Capanna Margherita, CM, 4559 m, 2 days permanence, and <36 h hike) and prolonged altitude exposure (Mount Everest South Base Camp, MEBC, 5350 m, 10 days permanence, and 9 days hike). At CM, CPAP reduced heart rate and systolic pulmonary artery pressure while haemoglobin oxygen saturation increased from 80% (median), 78—81 (first to third quartiles), to 91%, 84—97 ($P < 0.001$). After 10 days at MEBC, haemoglobin oxygen saturation spontaneously increased from 77% (74—82) to 86% (82—89) ($P < 0.001$) while heart rate (from 79, 64—92, to 70, 54—81; $P < 0.001$) and respiratory rate (from 15, 13—17, to 13, 13—15; $P < 0.001$) decreased. Under such conditions, these parameters were not influenced by CPAP.

Conclusion.—After ascent excessive lung fluids accumulate affecting haemoglobin oxygen saturation and, in these circumstances, CPAP is effective. Acclimatization implies spontaneous haemoglobin oxygen saturation increase and, after prolonged altitude exposure, CPAP is not associated with HbO_2-sat increase suggesting a reduction in alveolar fluids (Table 3).

▶ Although only 1% to 2% of patients develop severe high-altitude pulmonary edema, there is increasing evidence that some fluid accumulation occurs in the lungs of most climbers, and this contributes to the decrease in arterial oxygen saturation that they experience in the first few days after ascent.[1,2] Positive pulmonary pressure is commonly used to treat pulmonary edema at sea level,[3-5] and it is thus a logical option for those with the acute pulmonary edema of high-altitude sickness. Under acute conditions (a 36-hour hike followed by 2 days in a comfortable heated hut on Mt Rosa at 4559 meters, Table 3), all of the climbers who were tested showed a substantial gain of trans-cutaneously estimated arterial oxygen saturation in response to the wearing of a positive pressure mask. The authors of the present report attribute this gain to a forcing of edema fluid from the alveoli into the pulmonary interstitial tissue. However, no significant benefit was seen after climbers spent a longer period in a less comfortable environment (10 days at 5350 meters on Mount Everest). The authors suggest that there may be a decrease of alveolar fluid accumulation with the longer period of residence at high altitude and in support of this view the arterial oxygen saturations were certainly higher at 10 days than on first arrival at 5350 meters, even without the application of positive pressure. The practical implication of this research is that a pressure-breathing mask might be helpful to individuals who are particularly vulnerable to mountain sickness during their first few days at altitude.

R. J. Shephard, MD (Lond), PhD, DPE

References

1. Grocott M, Martin D, Levett D, McMorrow R, Windsor J, Montgomery HE. Arterial blood gases and oxygen content in climbers on Mount Everest. *N Engl J Med.* 2009;360:140-148.

2. Cremona G, Asnaghi R, Baderna P, et al. Pulmonary extravascular fluid accumulation in recreational climbers: a prospective study. *Lancet.* 2002;359:303-309.
3. Masip J, Roque M, Sánchez B, Fernández R, Subirana M, Expósito JA. Non invasive ventilation in acute cardiogenic pulmonary edema: systematic review and meta-analysis. *JAMA.* 2005;294:3124-3130.
4. Bersten AD, Holt AW, Vedig AE, Skowronski GA, Baggoley CJ. Treatment of severe cardiogenic pulmonary edema with continuous positive airway pressure delivered by face mask. *N Engl J Med.* 1991;325:1825-1830.
5. Gray A, Goodacre S, Newby D, Masson M, Sampson F, Nicholl J. Non-invasive ventilation in acute cardiogenic pulmonary edema. *N Engl J Med.* 2008;359: 142-151.

Effectiveness of intermittent training in hypoxia combined with live high/train low

Robertson EY, Saunders PU, Pyne DB, et al (Australian Inst of Sport, Canberra, Australia; et al)
Eur J Appl Physiol 110:379-387, 2010

Elite athletes often undertake altitude training to improve sea-level athletic performance, yet the optimal methodology has not been established. A combined approach of live high/train low plus train high (LH/TL+TH) may provide an additional training stimulus to enhance performance gains. Seventeen male and female middle-distance runners with maximal aerobic power ($\dot{V}O_{2max}$) of 65.5 ± 7.3 mL kg^{-1} min^{-1} (mean $\pm$ SD) trained on a treadmill in normobaric hypoxia for 3 weeks (2,200 m, 4 week^{-1}). During this period, the train high (TH) group ($n = 9$) resided near sea-level (~ 600 m) while the LH/ TL+TH group ($n = 8$) stayed in normobaric hypoxia (3,000 m) for 14 hours day^{-1}. Changes in 3-km time trial performance and physiological measures including $\dot{V}O_{2max}$; running economy and haemoglobin mass (Hb$_{mass}$) were assessed. The LH/TL+TH group substantially improved $\dot{V}O_{2max}$ (4.8%; ± 2.8%, mean; ± 90% CL), Hb$_{mass}$ (3.6%; ± 2.4%) and 3-km time trial performance (-1.1%; ± 1.0%) immediately post-altitude. There was no substantial improvement in time trial performance 2 weeks later. The TH group substantially improved $\dot{V}O_{2max}$ (2.2%; ± 1.8%), but had only trivial changes in Hb$_{mass}$ and 3-km time-trial performance. Compared with TH, combined LH/TL+TH substantially improved $\dot{V}O_{2max}$ (2.6%; ± 3.2%), Hb$_{mass}$ (4.3%; ± 3.2%), and time trial performance (-0.9%; ± 1.4%) immediately post-altitude. LH/TL+TH elicited greater enhancements in physiological capacities compared with TH, however, the transfer of benefits to time-trial performance was more variable (Table 4).

▶ For those athletes who wish to boost their hemoglobin levels by a permitted process, the current approach is to spend a period living at high altitude (real or simulated) but to continue training at sea level (live high/train low [LH/TL]).[1-5] Such a regimen not only boosts maximal oxygen intake and hemoglobin concentration but also induces at least a temporary increase in the endurance performance of elite athletes.[6] However, not all athletes are able to spend as

TABLE 4.—Absolute and Percent Change (mean ± SD) Within Each Altitude Group (LH/TL+TH, LH/TL and TH) and the Control Group Following 3 Weeks of Simulated Altitude Exposure/Training or Sea-Level Training

	Δ Time Trial[a]		Δ $\dot{V}O_{2max}$		Δ Hb_{mass}	
	s	%	mL kg^{-1} min^{-1}	%	g	%
LH/TL+TH ($n=8$)	-5.8 ± 8.3	-1.1 ± 1.6	3.1 ± 2.6	$4.8 \pm 4.2^*$	28 ± 28	$3.6 \pm 3.3^*$
LH/TL ($n=8$)	-11.8 ± 13.8	$-1.4 \pm 1.7^*$	1.5 ± 2.3	$2.1 \pm 3.2^*$	25 ± 28	2.8 ± 3.2
TH ($n=9$)	0.8 ± 9.2	-0.1 ± 1.6	1.5 ± 1.9	$2.2 \pm 2.9^*$	-8 ± 41	-0.7 ± 3.9
Control ($n=8$)	4.1 ± 19.2	0.5 ± 2.2	0.6 ± 2.8	0.9 ± 4.2	12 ± 39	1.4 ± 4.0

[a]Time trial: LH/TL + TH and TH (3-km); LH/TL and Control (4.5-km)
*Substantially different from pre-test.

long as 3 weeks living in a hypoxic environment, and there have been suggestions that even among those who can spare this much time, skeletal muscle physiology may be enhanced by undertaking at least some of the training under hypoxic conditions.[7] This article compares control athletes with those training for 4 to 5 hours per week at a moderate altitude (600 meters), those living at the equivalent of a higher altitude (2000 meters) but training at sea level, and those in whom the last regimen was supplemented by some training at an altitude of 600 meters (Table 4). One of the 4 data sets was obtained 2 weeks later on—mainly the same group of individuals. At least with this less-than-optimal test design, the effect of the combined regimen (a gain of 4.8%) was more than twice than yielded by the currently accepted protocol. The apparent benefit from the new approach is sufficient to warrant testing with a statistically balanced comparison between the conventional LH/TL and the new approach.

R. J. Shephard, MD (Lond), PhD, DPE

References

1. Hahn AG, Gore CJ, Martin DT, Ashenden MJ, Roberts AD, Logan PA. An evaluation of the concept of living at moderate altitude and training at sea level. *Comp Biochem Physiol.* 2001;128:777-789.
2. Nummela A, Rusko H. Acclimatization to altitude and normoxic training improve 400-m running performance at sea-level. *J Sports Sci..* 2000;18:411-419.
3. Robertson EY, Saunders PU, Pyne DB, Aughey RJ, Anson J, Gore CJ. Reproducibility of performance changes to simulated live high/train low altitude. *Med Sci Sports Exerc.* 2010;42:394-401.
4. Stray-Gundersen J, Chapman RF, Levine BD. "Living high-training low" altitude training improves sea level performance in male and female elite runners. *J Appl Physiol.* 2001;91:1113-1120.
5. Wehrlin JP, Zuest P, Hallen J, Marti B. Live High-Train Low for 24 days increases hemoglobin mass and red cell volume in elite endurance athletes. *J Appl Physiol.* 2006;100:1938-1945.
6. Bonetti DL, Hopkins WG. Sea-level exercise performance following adaptation to hypoxia: a meta-analysis. *Sports Med.* 2009;39:107-127.
7. Hoppeler H, Klossner S, Vogt M. Training in hypoxia and its effects on skeletal muscle tissue. *Scand J Med Sci Sports.* 2008;18:38-49.

Assessment of Extravascular Lung Water and Cardiac Function in Trimix SCUBA Diving

Marinovic J, Ljubkovic M, Obad A, et al (Univ of Split School of Medicine, Croatia; et al)
Med Sci Sports Exerc 42:1054-1061, 2010

An increasing number of recreational self-contained underwater breathing apparatus (SCUBA) divers use trimix of oxygen, helium, and nitrogen for dives deeper than 60 m of sea water. Although it was seldom linked to the development of pulmonary edema, whether SCUBA diving affects the extravascular lung water (EVLW) accumulation is largely unexplored.

Methods.—Seven divers performed six dives on consecutive days using compressed gas mixture of oxygen, helium, and nitrogen (trimix), with diving depths ranging from 55 to 80 m. The echocardiographic parameters (bubble grade, lung comets, mean pulmonary arterial pressure (PAP), and left ventricular function) and the blood levels of the N-terminal part of pro-brain natriuretic peptide (NT-proBNP) were assessed before and after each dive.

Results.—Venous gas bubbling was detected after each dive with mean probability of decompression sickness ranging from 1.77% to 3.12%. After each dive, several ultrasonographically detected lung comets rose significantly, which was paralleled by increased pulmonary artery pressure (PAP) and decreased left ventricular contractility (reduced ejection fraction at higher end-systolic and end-diastolic volumes) as well as the elevated NT-proBNP. The number of ultrasound lung comets and mean PAP did not return to baseline values after each dive.

Conclusions.—This is the first report that asymptomatic SCUBA dives are associated with accumulation of EVLW with concomitant increase in PAP, diminished left ventricular contractility, and increased release of NT-proBNP, suggesting a significant cardiopulmonary strain. EVLW and PAP did not return to baseline during repetitive dives, indicating possible cumulative effect with increasing the risk for pulmonary edema (Fig 3).

▶ Many factors potentially contribute to pulmonary edema in the self-contained underwater breathing apparatus diver, including an increase of gas density at depth, central blood pooling caused by body cooling, and the delivery of gas at pressures less than those applied to the chest by the water,[1,2] vigorous exercise, hyperoxia, a rise of pulmonary arterial pressure, and damage to the pulmonary endothelium by gas bubbles during decompression. These various issues are exacerbated by the use of heliox mixtures that allow the diver to explore greater depths, with the potential for a progressive development of pulmonary edema over the course of repeated dives. This small-scale study on 7 healthy and experienced middle-aged divers demonstrated that despite an absence of symptoms, there was a progressive increase in the number of ultrasound comets[3] indicative of pulmonary edema (Fig 3) as dives were repeated over a period of several days. Moreover, this was sufficient

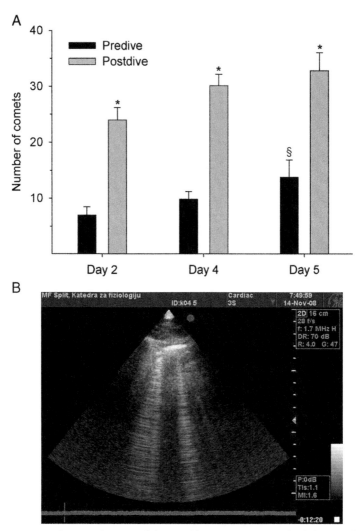

FIGURE 3.—A. Shown are the means of ultrasound lung comets (ULC) number before and after dives on days 2, 4, and 5. *$P < 0.05$ vs predive value on the same day; §$P < 0.05$ vs predive on days 2 and 4. B. An example of the chest ultrasound recording in a single IC space showing several ULC. (Reprinted from Marinovic J, Ljubkovic M, Obad A, et al. Assessment of extravascular lung water and cardiac function in trimix SCUBA diving. *Med Sci Sports Exerc.* 2010;42:1054-1061.)

to increase pulmonary arterial pressure, impair left ventricular contractility, and release N-terminal probrain natriuretic protein. However, perhaps because of the small sample size, the development of edema was unrelated to gas bubble counts. The findings suggest the need for caution, particularly if less healthy individuals are contemplating multiple dives using heliox gas mixtures.

R. J. Shephard, MD (Lond), PhD, DPE

References

1. Pons M, Blickenstorfer D, Oechslin E, et al. Pulmonary oedema in healthy persons during scuba-diving and swimming. *Eur Respir J.* 1995;8:762-767.
2. Slade JB Jr, Hattori T, Ray CS, Bove AA, Cianci P. Pulmonary edema associated with scuba diving: case reports and review. *Chest.* 2001;120:1686-1694.
3. Agricola E, Bove T, Oppizzi M, et al. "Ultrasound comet-tail images": a marker of pulmonary edema: a comparative study with wedge pressure and extravascular lung water. *Chest.* 2005;127:1690-1695.

9 Special Considerations: Children, Women, the Elderly, and Special Populations

Adults Born at Very Low Birth Weight Exercise Less than Their Peers Born at Term
Kajantie E, Strang-Karlsson S, Hovi P, et al (Natl Inst for Health and Welfare, Helsinki, Finland; et al)
J Pediatr 157:610-616, 2010

Objective.—To study the effects of very low birth weight (VLBW, <1500 g) birth on physical activity, an important protective and modifiable factor.

Study Design.—VLBW participants (n = 163) with no major disability and 188 individuals born at term (mean age, 22.3 years; range, 18.5–27.1) completed a standardized questionnaire of physical activity.

Results.—VLBW participants reported less leisure-time conditioning physical activity. They were 1.61-fold more likely to "not exercise much," 1.61-fold more likely to exercise infrequently (once a week or less), 2.75-fold more likely to exercise with low intensity (walking), and 3.11-fold more likely to have short exercise sessions (<30 minutes). The differences were present even in subjects with no history of bronchopulmonary dysplasia or asthma and were only slightly attenuated when adjusted for height, parental education, lean body mass, and percent body fat.

Conclusions.—Unimpaired adults who were VLBW exercise less during their leisure time than adults born at term. Promoting physical activity may be particularly important in the VLBW population to counteract the risks of chronic disease in adult life (Table 2).

▶ Kajantie and associates have demonstrated here a dramatic difference in habitual physical activity between adults with a normal birth weight and those born with a body mass of less than 1.5 kg (Table 2). Given the well-recognized association between physical activity and social class,[1] the first

TABLE 2.—Odds Ratios (95% CIs) for Low Levels Leisure-Time Conditioning Physical Activity in Very Low Birth Weight Adults Compared with Participants Born at Term

	Physically Inactive	Low Frequency (<1/Week)	Low Intensity (Walking)	Short Session Duration (<30 min)
Model 1	1.61 (1.01-2.55)	1.61 (1.05-2.46)	2.75 (1.63-4.65)	3.11 (1.44-6.75)
Model 2	1.38 (0.84-2.37)	1.54 (0.98-2.41)	2.41 (1.38-4.20)	3.22 (1.42-7.32)
Model 3	1.47 (0.88-2.45)	1.73 (1.07-2.78)	2.59 (1.43-4.68)	3.37 (1.45-7.85)
Model 4	1.66 (0.90-3.08)	1.30 (0.74-2.27)	2.81 (1.35-5.84)	3.07 (1.14-8.24)

Model 1 adjusted for sex and age.
Model 2, Model 1 + height; Model 3, Model 2 + parental education, maternal smoking during pregnancy, and current daily smoking of the subject; Model 4, Model 3 + lean body mass + percent body fat (data available for 134 VLBW and 135 term subjects).

explanation that comes to mind is that premature and low-birth-weight infants are seen more frequently in lower socioeconomic segments of the population. Kajantie and associates endeavored to adjust their data for this factor, with little resulting change in the handicap shown by those with a low body mass at birth; however, such statistical adjustments are often less than complete. There may also be physical and psychomotor effects of the premature birth that last through much of childhood, including poorer lung function,[2,3] a lower lean tissue mass,[4] delays in motor development,[5] and a smaller overall body size, all of which could reduce self-confidence and inhibit participation in some forms of sport and vigorous physical activity. Given the ever-increasing survival rate of premature infants, the issue seems of some importance for policy makers. There are 2 immediate practical lessons. Firstly, efforts to promote regular physical activity should be directed particularly to this subgroup of the adult population, and secondly, the focus for all of the population should be upon encouraging forms of physical activity that are accessible to all, rather than on sports where physical size and the ability to intimidate opponents seem prerequisites.[6]

R. J. Shephard, MD (Lond), PhD, DPE

References

1. Shephard RJ, Bouchard C. Principal components of fitness: relationship to physical activity and lifestyle. *Can J Appl Physiol.* 1994;19:200-214.
2. Kilbride HW, Gelatt MC, Sabath RJ. Pulmonary function and exercise capacity for ELBW survivors in preadolescence: effect of neonatal chronic lung disease. *J Pediatr.* 2003;143:488-493.
3. Vrijlandt EJ, Gerritsen J, Boezen HM, Grevink RG, Duiverman EJ. Lung function and exercise capacity in young adults born prematurely. *Am J Respir Crit Care Med.* 2006;173:890-896.
4. Keller H, Bar-Or O, Kriemler S, Ayub BV, Saigal S. Anaerobic performance in 5- to 7-yr-old children of low birthweight. *Med Sci Sports Exerc.* 2000;32:278-283.
5. Marlow N, Hennessy EM, Bracewell MA, Wolke D. Motor and executive function at 6 years of age after extremely preterm birth. *Pediatrics.* 2007;120:793-804.
6. Shephard RJ, Lavallée H, Larivière G. Competitive selection among age-class ice-hockey players. *Br J Sports Med.* 1978;12:11-13.

Six-minute walk test in children with chronic conditions

Hassan J, van der Net J, Helders PJM, et al (Univ Med Centre Utrecht, The Netherlands)
Br J Sports Med 44:270-274, 2010

Objectives.—The 6-minute walk test (6MWT) is a frequently used indicator of functional exercise capacity. The goals of this study were to compare the 6-minute walk performance of three paediatric patient groups with that of healthy peers, to assess differences between published reference values and to investigate which anthropometric characteristics best predict 6-minute walk performance.

Methods.—47 children with haemophilia (mean (SD) age 12.5 (2.9) years), 44 with juvenile idiopathic arthritis (JIA) (mean age 9.3 (2.2) years) and 22 with spina bifida (SB) (mean age 10.3 (3.1) years) were included. Subjects performed a 6MWT, and the distance walked (6MWD) was compared with published reference values.

Results.—The haemophilia, JIA and SB patients achieved 90%–92%, 72%–75% and 60%–62% of predicted walking distances, respectively. There were significant associations between 6MWD and age, height and weight in the haemophilia group and 6MWD and height in the JIA group. None of the anthropometric variables was significantly related to 6MWD in the SB group. All anthropometric variables were strongly correlated with walking distance—body weight product (6Mwork) in all groups. Height explained 24% (haemophilia) and 11% (JIA) of the variance in 6MWD and 84% (haemophilia), 78% (JIA) and 73% (SB) of the variance in 6Mwork.

Conclusions.—Walking distances of children with haemophilia, JIA and SB are significantly reduced compared with healthy references. Walking distance—body weight product seems to be a better outcome measure of the 6MWT compared with distance walked alone. Height is the best predictor of 6MWD and 6Mwork (Fig 2).

▶ It is quite feasible to measure the maximal oxygen intake of children directly in the laboratory by using a progressive treadmill test,[1] and in the field, reliable estimates of physical work capacity can be made on a cycle ergometer.[2] Nevertheless, the field testing of aerobic power in children has often been based on walk-run tests carried out over distances of 274 to 549 meters (300-600 yards). These are unsatisfactory in part because scores depend on motivation and knowledge of pacing, and in part because the primary determinants of performance in the growing child are height and body mass rather than aerobic ability.[3] The 6-minute walk test has proven to be a useful tool in the field assessment of elderly patients, and there have been suggestions that this test can also be used to evaluate the aerobic power of clinical pediatric populations.[3-6] Unfortunately, as the present data show, in children, height and body mass are the principal predictors of the distance walked in 6 minutes. Although mean scores may differ between healthy children and those with various diseases, the test is indicating more about body build than aerobic

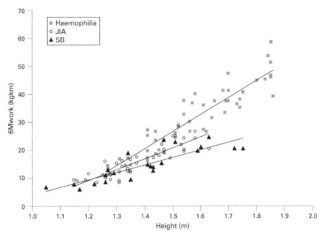

FIGURE 2.—Association between 6Mwork and height. 6Mwork, product of 6-minute walking distance (km) and weight (kg). (Reprinted from Hassan J, van der Net J, Helders PJM, et al. Six-minute walk test in children with chronic conditions. *Br J Sports Med.* 2010;44:270-274, and reproduced with permission from the BMJ Publishing Group.)

power (Fig 2). Aerobic inferences can be increased if a child's score is related to norms that include standing height, age,[7,8] and preferably, body mass.[9]

R. J. Shephard, MD (Lond), PhD, DPE

References

1. Shephard RJ, Allen C, Benade AJS, et al. The working capacity of Toronto schoolchildren. *Can Med Assoc J.* 1968;100:560-566. 705-714.
2. Howell M, MacNab R. *The Physical Working Capacity of Canadian Children 7-17 Years.* Ottawa: Canadian Association for Health, Physical Education & Recreation; 1968.
3. Cumming GR. Body size and the assessment of physical performance. In: Shephard RJ, Lavallé H, eds. *Physical Fitness Assessment: Principles, Practice and Application.* Springfield IL: C.C. Thomas; 1978:18-31.
4. Nixon PA, Joswiak ML, Fricker FJ. A six-minute walk test for assessing exercise tolerance in severely ill children. *J Pediatr.* 1996;129:362-366.
5. Gulmans VA, van Veldhoven NH, de Meer K, Helders PJ. The six-minute walking test in children with cystic fibrosis: reliability and validity. *Pediatr Pulmonol.* 1996;22:85-89.
6. Lelieveld OT, Takken T, van der Net J, van Weert E. Validity of the 6-minute walking test in juvenile idiopathic arthritis. *Arthritis Rheum.* 2005;53:304-307.
7. Geiger R, Strasak A, Treml B, et al. Six-minute walk test in children and adolescents. *J Pediatr.* 2007;150:395-399.
8. Li AM, Yin J, Au JT, et al. Standard reference for the six-minute-walk test in healthy children aged 7 to 16 years. *Am J Respir Crit Care Med.* 2007;176: 174-180.
9. Lammers AE, Hislop AA, Flynn Y, Haworth SG. The 6-minute walk test: normal values for children of 4–11 years of age [published online ahead of print August 3 2007]. *Arch Dis Child.* 2008;93:464-468. 10.1136/adc.2007.123653.

Youth Marathon Runners and Race Day Medical Risk Over 26 years

Roberts WO, Nicholson WG (Univ of Minnesota Med School, Minneapolis; HealthEast St Johns Hosp, Maplewood, MN)
Clin J Sport Med 20:318-321, 2010

Objective.—To report the number of marathon finishers younger than 18 years and race day medical encounters at the same site and to compare them with adult finishers.

Design.—Retrospective cohort study.

Setting.—Urban 42-km road race.

Participants.—Twin Cities Marathon finishers.

Assessment of Risk Factors.—The race records from 1982 to 2007 were assessed for finishers younger than 18 years to determine the number of finishers and medical encounters, incidence of race-related medical encounters, and type and severity of medical problems.

Main Outcome Measures.—Age group marathon finishers and medical encounters.

Results.—Three hundred ten marathon (225 boys and 85 girls) aged 7 to 17 years finished the race with times ranging from 2:53:22 to 6:10:00. There were 4 medical encounters (minor in nature and required no intervention beyond a short period of rest) for an incidence of 12.9 per 1000 finishers. The odds ratio for youth compared with adult finish line medical encounters was 0.52 (*P* = 0.2658; 95% confidence interval, 0.19-1.39).

Conclusions.—Three hundred ten youth marathon successfully finished Twin Cities Marathon over 26 years with only 4 requiring post-race medical evaluations. The relative risk of requiring acute race day medical

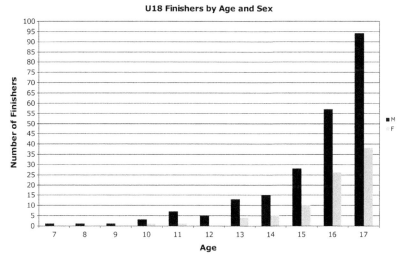

FIGURE 2.—Number of marathon finishers who are younger than 18 years by age and sex. (Reprinted from Roberts WO, Nicholson WG. Youth marathon runners and race day medical risk over 26 years. *Clin J Sport Med.* 2010;20:318-321.)

attention was less than, but not statistically different from, adult finishers (Fig 2).

▶ Conventional wisdom has been that a marathon race is too demanding for children to participate.[1] However, there have been a growing number of competitors under the age of 18; data from the Twin Cities (Minneapolis) marathon show some competitors as young as 7 years of age (Fig 2). It is thus useful to inquire what the medical experience is with this age group. The data of Roberts and Nicholson, accumulated from 310 finishers over 25 years, show only 4 cases of mild exhaustion, compared with 24.6 medical encounters per 1000 adult contestants. Nevertheless, those aged 7 to 12 years ran relatively slowly (completion times of 3:21 to 6:10). Fears of poorer heat tolerance in children have now been largely disproved,[2-4] and this article supports the conclusion of Brenner[5]: there seems "no reason to disallow participation in a properly run marathon as long as the athlete enjoys the activity and is asymptomatic." The conclusion merits confirmation on a larger sample of young runners.

R. J. Shephard, MD (Lond), PhD, DPE

References

1. Rice SG, Waniewski S. Children and marathoning: how young is too young? *Clin J Sport Med.* 2003;13:369-373.
2. Inbar O, Morris N, Epstien Y, Gass G. Comparison of thermoregulatory responses to exercise in dry heat among prepubertal boys, young adults and older males. *Exp Physiol.* 2004;89:691-700.
3. Rowland T, Garrison A, Prober D. Determinants of endurance exercise capacity in the heat in prepubertal boys. *Int J Sports Med.* 2007;28:26-32.
4. Rivera Brown AM, Rowland TW, Ramirez Marrero FA, Santacana G, Vann A. Exercise tolerance in a hot and humid climate in heat acclimatized girls and women. *Int J Sports Med.* 2006;27:943-950.
5. Brenner JS, American Academy of Pediatrics Council on Sports Medicine and Fitness. Overuse injuries, overtraining, and burnout in child and adolescent athletes. *Pediatrics.* 2007;119:1242-1245.

Secular trends and distributional changes in health and fitness performance variables of 10–14-year-old children in New Zealand between 1991 and 2003
Albon HM, Hamlin MJ, Ross JJ (Lincoln Univ, Canterbury, New Zealand)
Br J Sports Med 44:263-269, 2010

Background.—New Zealand children's health and fitness performance is declining over time, but whether this change is because of deterioration in all children's health and fitness performance or can be attributed to just a certain portion of the population, is unknown.

Objectives.—In this study, secular trends and distributional changes in health-related and performance-related fitness components among New Zealand primary school children aged 10 to 14 years between 1991 and 2003 were tracked.

Methods.—Health-and performance-related fitness parameters including height, weight, body mass index (BMI), flexibility, standing broad jump, 4×9-m agility run, abdominal curl-ups, and 550-m run were collected up to twice a year from 3306 children (10—14 years old) from a New Zealand school between 1991 and 2003.

Results.—Over the 12-year period, the boys' weight increased by 4.5 kg (95% CL 2.7 to 6.2, or 0.8% per year) and girls' by 3.9 kg (95% CL 2.0 to 5.9, or 0.7% per year). Mean BMI increased by 0.12 kg m^{-2} (0.6%) and 0.11 kg m^{-2} (0.5%) per year for boys and girls, respectively. Children's 550-m run performance declined by 1.5% and 1.7% per year for boys and girls, respectively. Little difference existed between children located in the highest performing and leanest percentiles in 1991 and 2003, but for children in the poorest performing and fattest percentiles, their results were substantially worse in 2003.

Conclusion.—These results suggest that the deterioration in the health-related and performance-related fitness components of New Zealand 10—14-year-olds is not homogeneous but skewed towards those children who are the heaviest and perform worst in fitness tests. Previous research on health-related fitness parameters among children in New Zealand is limited but shows secular trends of increasing body mass in conjunction with deteriorating aerobic fitness performance, muscular endurance and explosive muscular power. Internationally, similar increases in body mass have been observed in children since the 1980s. Secular trends of deteriorating health-related fitness performance have also been reported among children around the world, with the most significant decreases observed in aerobic performance. However, trends in health-related variables reported as changes in mean body mass index (BMI) and mean aerobic fitness performance do not reveal possible changes in the distribution of BMI or aerobic performance within the population. Changes in such measures may come about because of a shift in the entire population under investigation or a change in a portion of the population. It is not clear whether New Zealand's entire childhood population is becoming heavier and less aerobically fit or whether only a portion of the children are becoming even heavier and more unfit, with the remaining children showing little secular change. The aim of this study was to track secular trends and distributional changes in body weight and physical fitness parameters among New Zealand primary school children aged 10 to 14 years.

▶ This study is important because it underscores the importance of looking beyond oversimplified assumptions when examining changes in fitness in populations. Yes, as expected, performance on motor tasks deteriorated in New Zealand over time, and at first glance this seems to parallel (and is probably causally related to) trends in increasing obesity. But on closer analysis, the authors found that such trends weren't quite that simple. The decline in performance occurred most prominently in those who were most unfit and most fat. This resembles the profile one sees in examining the trends for increasing obesity in the population; it is the fattest who are getting fatter. The implications are obvious. We need to look carefully at subgroups when trying to decipher trends in fitness and activity in the population. Failure to do so may lead to spurious conclusions.

T. Rowland, MD

Physical Activity, Fitness, Weight Status, and Cognitive Performance in Adolescents

Ruiz JR, on behalf of the AVENA Study Group (Univ of Granada, Spain; et al)
J Pediatr 157:917-922, 2010

Objective.—To examine the association of participation in physical sports activity during leisure time, sedentary behaviors, cardiorespiratory and muscular fitness, and weight status with cognitive performance in Spanish adolescents.

Study Design.—This cross-sectional study comprised a total of 1820 adolescents (958 female) aged 13.0 to 18.5 years. Cognitive performance (verbal, numeric and reasoning abilities, and an overall score) was measured with the "SRA-Test of Educational Ability." Participation in physical sports activity during leisure time (yes/no) and time devoted to study, television viewing, and playing video games were self-reported and categorized as ≤3 hours/day and >3 hours/day. We assessed cardiorespiratory and muscular fitness with field-based tests. Adolescents were classified as underweight, normal weight, overweight, and obese.

Results.—Participation in physical sports activities during leisure time was associated with better cognitive performance study variables (all $P < .001$), independent of potential confounders including cardiorespiratory fitness and body mass index. We did not observe an association of time devoted to study, television viewing, or playing video-games with cognitive performance. Likewise, cognitive performance was similar across cardiorespiratory and muscular fitness levels and body weight categories.

Conclusion.—Participation in physical sports activity during leisure time may positively influence cognitive performance in adolescents.

▶ The ancient Greeks maintained that a physically fit and strong body leads to a sound mind. Evidence, however, on the chronic benefits of exercise training on mental cognition for young and middle-aged adults is lacking. This linkage is much stronger for older adults whose cognitive function is below peak levels.[1,2] Interestingly, adults who adopt physically active lifestyles experience a delay in the onset of cognitive decline and Alzheimer disease as they age.[3] Among the elderly, regular physical activity improves or maintains cognitive function, with the specific improvements seen in speed of cognition and attention. Less is known in this area among children and youth. Studies indicate a positive association between physical activity and academic performance in children and a negative relationship to sedentary behaviors, such as television viewing.[4] In this study, adolescents engaged in physical sports activities during leisure time had significantly better cognitive performance than those who were not. The authors reason that physical activity during the pubertal period offers high possibilities of stimulating cognitive function because this is a period of life when the brain has profound plasticity.

D. C. Nieman, DrPH

References

1. Hillman CH, Erickson KI, Kramer AF. Be smart, exercise your heart: exercise effects on brain and cognition. *Nat Rev Neurosci.* 2008;9:58-65.
2. Klusmann V, Evers A, Schwartzer R, et al. Complex mental and physical activity in older women and cognitive performance: a 6-month randomized controlled trial. *J Gerontol A Biol Sci Med Sci.* 2010;65:680-688.
3. Scarmeas N, Luchsinger JA, Schupf N, et al. Physical activity, diet, and risk of Alzheimer disease. *JAMA.* 2009;302:627-637.
4. Trudeau F, Shephard RJ. Physical education, school physical activity, school sports and academic performance. *Int J Behav Nutr Phys Act.* 2008;5:10.

Aerobic Fitness and Executive Control of Relational Memory in Preadolescent Children
Chaddock L, Hillman CH, Buck SM, et al (Univ of Illinois at Urbana-Champaign; Chicago State Univ, IL)
Med Sci Sports Exerc 43:344-349, 2011

Purpose.—The neurocognitive benefits of an active lifestyle in childhood have public health and educational implications, especially as children in today's technological society are becoming increasingly overweight, unhealthy, and unfit. Human and animal studies show that aerobic exercise affects both prefrontal executive control and hippocampal function. This investigation attempts to bridge these research threads by using a cognitive task to examine the relationship between aerobic fitness and executive control of relational memory in preadolescent 9- and 10-yr-old children.

Method.—Higher-fit and lower-fit children studied faces and houses under individual item (i.e., nonrelational) and relational encoding conditions, and the children were subsequently tested with recognition memory trials consisting of previously studied pairs and pairs of completely new items. With each subject participating in both item and relational encoding conditions, and with recognition test trials amenable to the use of both item and relational memory cues, this task afforded a challenge to the flexible use of memory, specifically in the use of appropriate encoding and retrieval strategies. Hence, the task provided a test of both executive control and memory processes.

Results.—Lower-fit children showed poorer recognition memory performance than higher-fit children, selectively in the relational encoding condition. No association between aerobic fitness and recognition performance was found for faces and houses studied as individual items (i.e., nonrelationally).

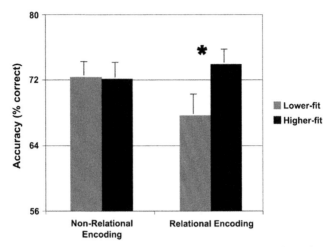

FIGURE 2.—Recognition memory performance (percent correct) for nonrelational and relational encoding conditions as a function of aerobic fitness group. Error bars, SEM. *Significant difference between higher-fit and lower-fit groups at $P < 0.05$. (Reprinted from Chaddock L, Hillman CH, Buck SM, et al. Aerobic fitness and executive control of relational memory in preadolescent children. *Med Sci Sports Exerc.* 2011;43:344-349, with permission from the American College of Sports Medicine.)

Conclusions.—The findings implicate childhood aerobic fitness as a factor in the ability to use effective encoding and retrieval executive control processes for relational memory material and, possibly, in the strategic engagement of prefrontal- and hippocampal-dependent systems (Fig 2).

▶ There has been a long debate about the effects of regular physical activity upon the academic attainments of young children.[1,2] Some parent groups and teachers have been opposed to increasing the time allocated to physical education programs, fearing that the consequent devotion of less time to academic subjects would impair such learning. We studied this question in French Canada, using a quasi-experimental design, where preceding and succeeding classes at the same primary school served as controls. An hour of physical education per day reduced academic time by some 14%, but the academic success of the experimental students was certainly no poorer than that of the controls. Indeed, on both teacher assessments and province-wide examinations, there was a suggestion that the experimental students performed better on both language and mathematical skills. The article of Chaddock and associates offers an interesting and novel approach to this controversial issue. The children in their study were not randomly selected students but were rather a fairly small sample of boys who were attending a sports camp, and the comparison of physical activity was based on attained fitness as measured by a treadmill test of maximal oxygen intake rather than by documented allocation of class time. Nevertheless, the fitter students performed better than the less fit on a relational encoding task (Fig 2). The weakness in this particular proof is that it is correlational, and the less fit boys were also of lower socioeconomic status (median score 2.5 vs 2.9), and this may have influenced their success with the encoding task.

R. J. Shephard, MD (Lond), PhD, DPE

References

1. Trudeau F, Shephard RJ. Physical education, school physical activity, school sports and academic performance. *Int J Behav Nutr Phys Act.* 2008;5:10.
2. Trudeau F, Shephard RJ. Relationships of physical activity to brain health and the academic performance of schoolchildren. *Am J Lifestyle Med.* 2010;4:138-150.

Aerobic Fitness and Executive Control of Relational Memory in Preadolescent Children
Chaddock L, Hillman CH, Buck SM, et al (Univ of Illinois at Urbana-Champaign, IL; Chicago State Univ, IL)
Med Sci Sports Exerc 43:344-349, 2011

Purpose.—The neurocognitive benefits of an active lifestyle in childhood have public health and educational implications, especially as children in today's technological society are becoming increasingly overweight, unhealthy, and unfit. Human and animal studies show that aerobic exercise affects both prefrontal executive control and hippocampal function. This investigation attempts to bridge these research threads by using a cognitive task to examine the relationship between aerobic fitness and executive control of relational memory in preadolescent 9- and 10-yr-old children.

Method.—Higher-fit and lower-fit children studied faces and houses under individual item (i.e., nonrelational) and relational encoding conditions, and the children were subsequently tested with recognition memory trials consisting of previously studied pairs and pairs of completely new items. With each subject participating in both item and relational encoding conditions, and with recognition test trials amenable to the use of both item and relational memory cues, this task afforded a challenge to the flexible use of memory, specifically in the use of appropriate encoding and retrieval strategies. Hence, the task provided a test of both executive control and memory processes.

Results.—Lower-fit children showed poorer recognition memory performance than higher-fit children, selectively in the relational encoding condition. No association between aerobic fitness and recognition performance was found for faces and houses studied as individual items (i.e., nonrelationally).

Conclusions.—The findings implicate childhood aerobic fitness as a factor in the ability to use effective encoding and retrieval executive control processes for relational memory material and, possibly, in the strategic engagement of prefrontal- and hippocampal-dependent systems (Fig 2).

▶ The chronic benefit of exercise training on mental cognition for children, adolescents, young- and middle-aged adults, and the elderly is controversial.

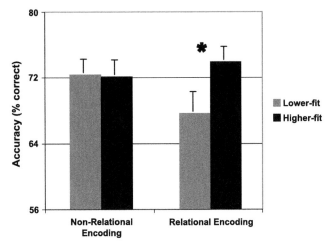

FIGURE 2.—Recognition memory performance (percent correct) for nonrelational and relational encoding conditions as a function of aerobic fitness group. Error bars, SEM. *Significant difference between higher-fit and lower-fit groups at $P < 0.05$. (Reprinted from Chaddock L, Hillman CH, Buck SM, et al. Aerobic fitness and executive control of relational memory in preadolescent children. *Med Sci Sports Exerc*. 2011;43:344-349, with permission from the American College of Sports Medicine.)

Data from this cross-sectional study of 9- and 10-year-old children are interesting, but the statistical model only included socioeconomic status as a potential confounder (Fig 2). The linkage is strongest for older adults whose cognitive function is below peak levels.[1,2] Among the elderly, regular physical activity improves or maintains cognitive function, with specific improvements seen in speed of cognition and attention. Potential mechanisms are still being debated but may include reduced inflammation, enhanced brain perfusion with blood through a buildup of extra brain capillaries, improved neural connections between brain regions, and an enhanced caffeine-like arousal.[3]

D. C. Nieman, DrPH

References

1. Angevaren M, Aufdemkampe G, Verhaar HJ, Aleman A, Vanhees L. Physical activity and enhanced fitness to improve cognitive function in older people without known cognitive impairment. *Cochrane Database Syst Rev*. 2008;(3). CD005381.
2. Hillman CH, Motl RW, Pontifex MB, et al. Physical activity and cognitive function in a cross-section of younger and older community-dwelling individuals. *Health Psychol*. 2006;25:678-687.
3. Lambourne K, Tomporowski P. The effect of exercise-induced arousal on cognitive task performance: a meta-regression analysis. *Brain Res*. 2010;1341:12-24.

A neuroimaging investigation of the association between aerobic fitness, hippocampal volume, and memory performance in preadolescent children
Chaddock L, Erickson KI, Prakash RS, et al (Univ of Illinois at Urbana-Champaign; Univ of Pittsburgh, PA; The Ohio State Univ, Columbus)
Brain Res 1358:172-183, 2010

Because children are becoming overweight, unhealthy, and unfit, understanding the neurocognitive benefits of an active lifestyle in childhood has important public health and educational implications. Animal research has indicated that aerobic exercise is related to increased cell proliferation and survival in the hippocampus as well as enhanced hippocampal-dependent learning and memory. Recent evidence extends this relationship to elderly humans by suggesting that high aerobic fitness levels in older adults are associated with increased hippocampal volume and superior memory performance. The present study aimed to further extend the link between fitness, hippocampal volume, and memory to a sample of preadolescent children. To this end, magnetic resonance imaging was employed to investigate whether higher- and lower-fit 9- and 10-year-old children showed differences in hippocampal volume and if the differences were related to performance on an item and relational memory task. Relational but not item memory is primarily supported by the hippocampus. Consistent with predictions, higher-fit children showed greater bilateral hippocampal volumes and superior relational memory task performance compared to lower-fit children. Hippocampal volume was also positively associated with performance on the relational but not the item memory task. Furthermore, bilateral hippocampal volume was found to mediate the relationship between fitness level (VO_2 max) and relational memory. No relationship between aerobic fitness, nucleus accumbens volume, and memory was reported, which strengthens the hypothesized specific effect of fitness on the hippocampus. The findings are the first to indicate that aerobic fitness may relate to the structure and function of the preadolescent human brain (Fig 1).

▶ Our semilongitudinal study of primary school students in the Trois Rivières region of Québec[1-5] demonstrated a positive relationship between additional required physical education (five 1-hour periods per week taught by a physical education specialist) and academic performance. Unlike a number of other reports that had advanced similar claims, our study was controlled, with students in the immediately preceding and succeeding classes at the same schools receiving only the standard allocation of one 40-minute period of physical education per week, taught by the homeroom teacher. Nevertheless, a causal physiological relationship between physical activity and enhanced academic performance was far from proven. Possibly the normal classroom teachers may have been able to teach more effectively when given a 1-hour break per day, and the students may also have been better behaved and more attentive after release of their surplus energy in an hour of vigorous physical education. Particularly in older children, involvement in sports may also have

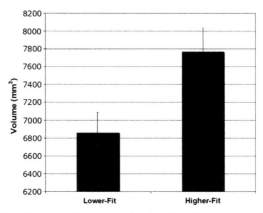

FIGURE 1.—Bilateral hippocampal volume as a function of aerobic fitness group. Error bars represent standard error. (Reprinted from Brain Research, Chaddock L, Erickson KI, Prakash RS, et al. A neuro-imaging investigation of the association between aerobic fitness, hippocampal volume, and memory performance in preadolescent children. *Brain Res.* 2010;1358:172-183. Copyright 2010, with permission from Elsevier.)

increased their self-esteem, with a positive effect on learning. Finally, our experimental design made it impossible to blind the community as to subject grouping, and since most teachers favored the introduction of more physical education, this may have biased the marks that they awarded to experimental classes (although their assessment of superior academic performance was generally supported by the better achievements of the experimental students in province-wide examinations). Studies of seniors have suggested a causal relationship, a reduction of memory loss in fit and active old people being linked to an increased secretion of neurotrophins[6] and thus repair of damaged neuronal links. It has been less clear that this explains the benefit observed in children and adolescents. However, the present cross-sectional report shows that students who are more fit have a substantial advantage of hippocampal volume relative to those who are unfit (Fig 1), much as previously has been demonstrated in the elderly,[7] and that this is linked in turn to a better relational memory. From the practical viewpoint, the important conclusion for educators is that a substantial amount of academic time can be allocated to physical education, with an improvement rather than a deterioration in a child's academic performance.

R. J. Shephard, MD (Lond), PhD, DPE

References

1. Shephard RJ, Lavallée H, Volle M, LaBarre R, Beaucage C. Academic skills and required physical education: The Trois Rivières experience. *CAHPER Research Supplement.* 1994;1:1-12.
2. Shephard RJ. Habitual physical activity and academic performance. *Nutr Rev.* 1996;54:S32-S36.
3. Shephard RJ. Curricular physical activity and academic performance. *Pediatr Ex Sci.* 1997;9:113-126.
4. Trudeau F, Shephard RJ. Physical education, school physical activity and school sports and academic performance. *Int J Behav Nutr Phys Activ.* 2008;5:10.

5. Trudeau F, Shephard RJ. Relationships of physical activity to brain health and the academic performance of school children. *Am J Lifestyle Med.* 2009;4:138-150.
6. Cotman CW, Berchthold NC. Exercise: a behavioral intervention to enhance brain health and plasticity. *Trends Neurosci.* 2002;25:295-301.
7. Erickson KL, Prakash RS, Voss MW, et al. Aerobic fitness is associated with hippocampus volume in elderly humans. *Hippocampus.* 2009;19:1030-1039.

Cardiovascular fitness is associated with cognition in young adulthood

Åberg MAI, Pedersen NL, Torén K, et al (Univ of Gothenburg, Sweden; Univ of Southern California, Los Angeles; et al)
Proc Natl Acad Sci U S A 106:20906-20911, 2009

During early adulthood, a phase in which the central nervous system displays considerable plasticity and in which important cognitive traits are shaped, the effects of exercise on cognition remain poorly understood. We performed a cohort study of all Swedish men born in 1950 through 1976 who were enlisted for military service at age 18 ($N = 1,221,727$). Of these, 268,496 were full-sibling pairs, 3,147 twin pairs, and 1,432 monozygotic twin pairs. Physical fitness and intelligence performance data were collected during conscription examinations and linked with other national databases for information on school achievement, socioeconomic status, and sibship. Relationships between cardiovascular fitness and intelligence at age 18 were evaluated by linear models in the total cohort and in subgroups of full-sibling pairs and twin pairs. Cardiovascular fitness, as measured by ergometer cycling, positively associated with intelligence after adjusting for relevant confounders (regression coefficient $b = 0.172$; 95% CI, 0.168–0.176). Similar results were obtained within monozygotic twin pairs. In contrast, muscle strength was not associated with cognitive performance. Cross-twin cross-trait analyses showed that the associations were primarily explained by individual specific, non-shared environmental influences ($\geq 80\%$), whereas heritability explained <15% of covariation. Cardiovascular fitness changes between age 15 and 18 y predicted cognitive performance at 18 y. Cox proportional-hazards models showed that cardiovascular fitness at age 18 y predicted educational achievements later in life. These data substantiate that physical exercise could be an important instrument for public health initiatives to optimize educational achievements, cognitive performance, as well as disease prevention at the society level.

▶ Evidence continues to accumulate that regular physical activity, participation in sports, and physical fitness are related to cognitive function and intellectual performance. Initially such evidence was entirely cross-sectional, but studies like this one begin to give us a longitudinal perspective. Such data provide a more convincing argument for a cause-effect relationship compared with the earlier cross-sectional information. However, there is still much to be learned. Which direction might the causal arrow go? Are intelligent people more likely to play sports or be physically fit? Or does regular exercise influence brain electrical patterns that enhance cognitive abilities? If the latter is true, what are the mechanisms for this? This whole question has significant bearing on a number of important issues. For instance, those who create school curricula might be convinced that sacrificing physical education classes for academic subject matter may not be justified. Or, at the other end of the life span, we might have evidence to support the idea that exercise would be an effective means of inhibiting the decline in mental functioning in the aged. There is already evidence in animals to support this idea. Future investigations should focus on both longitudinal and interventional designs that will give us better insight on this exercise-brain function relationship.

T. Rowland, MD

Clinical Report—Identification and Management of Eating Disorders in Children and Adolescents
Rosen DS, the Committee on Adolescence
Pediatrics 126:1240-1253, 2010

The incidence and prevalence of eating disorders in children and adolescents has increased significantly in recent decades, making it essential for pediatricians to consider these disorders in appropriate clinical settings, to evaluate patients suspected of having these disorders, and to manage (or refer) patients in whom eating disorders are diagnosed. This clinical report includes a discussion of diagnostic criteria and outlines the initial evaluation of the patient with disordered eating. Medical complications of eating disorders may affect any organ system, and careful monitoring for these complications is required. The range of treatment options, including pharmacotherapy, is described in this report. Pediatricians are encouraged to advocate for legislation and policies that ensure appropriate services for patients with eating disorders, including medical care, nutritional intervention, mental health treatment, and care coordination (Table 1).

▶ The female athlete triad is a constellation of 3 separate yet potentially intertwined clinical disorders, with significant short-term and long-term health implications for active females. Previously, one of the entities was disordered eating, including the frank eating disorders of anorexia nervosa (AN) and

---

TABLE 1.—The SCOFF Questionnaire[56]

---

1. Do you make yourself **sick** because you feel uncomfortably full?
2. Do you worry you have lost **control** over how much you eat?
3. Have you recently lost **>1 stone** (6.3 kg or 14 lb) in a 3-mo period?
4. Do you believe yourself to be **fat** when others say you are too thin?
5. Would you say that **food** dominates your life?

One point should be given for every "yes" answer; a score of ≥2 indicates a likelihood of AN or BN.
Editor's Note: Please refer to original journal article for full references.

---

bulimia nervosa (BN). The other 2 were amenorrhea and osteoporosis. When any of the triad disorders were diagnosed in a patient, clinicians were advised to look for evidence of the other 2 conditions. For example, follow-up questions regarding menarche and the regularity of menstrual cycles as well as nutritional habits should be a natural part of the medical history of a young female athlete presenting with a stress fracture.

With the latest position stand on the female athlete triad of the American College of Sports Medicine,[1] the triad has been redefined to include low energy availability (with or without an eating disorder), functional hypothalamic amenorrhea, and osteoporosis. All 3 conditions exist on a spectrum from health to disease, and an athlete can move in different directions and at different speeds, along any of the axes of the spectrum.

Even though the energy imbalance is often inadvertent (ie, not enough energy taken in for the energy demands of training and competition), some female athletes will still have more pathological conditions. Therefore, early identification and management of eating disorders in children and adolescents is critical. If missed, and left untreated, there can be significant problems, such as growth retardation, short stature, and pubertal delay, in addition to low—bone mineral density, which may be irreversible. This updated clinical report from the Committee on Adolescence of the American Academy of Pediatrics thoroughly covers the diagnostic criteria, initial evaluation, medical complications, and treatment options, including pharmacotherapy for AN, BN, and eating disorders not otherwise specified, as defined by the criteria of the *Diagnostic and Statistical Manual of Mental Disorders, Fourth Edition, Text Revision* of the American Psychiatric Association.[2]

Some new concepts about the etiology of eating disorders are presented, including increasing evidence of a strong genetic component, the role of dieting as a proximal risk factor, and the effects of neuroendocrine abnormalities, such as altered leptin levels. The Sick Control One Stone Fat Food questionnaire (Table 1), a simple screening questionnaire, is suggested as an initial framework for screening. Plotting of weight, height, and body mass index on appropriate growth charts may help to identify deviations from normal and nutritional insufficiency. Other tables cover salient points of history, physical examination findings, diagnosis, differential diagnosis, medical complications, and criteria for hospital admission. This article is very easy to follow and has extensive references. Accordingly, it is an excellent and authoritative source of up-to-date information on this important topic.

C. Lebrun, MD

References

1. American College of Sports Medicine. Position stand: the female athlete triad. *Med Sci Sports Exerc.* 2007;39:1867-1882.
2. American Psychiatric Association. *Diagnostic and Statistical Manual of Mental Disorders, 4th ed. Text Revision (DSM-IV-TR).* Washington, DC: American Psychiatric Association; 2000.

Disordered Eating, Menstrual Disturbances, and Low Bone Mineral Density in Dancers: A Systematic Review

Hincapié CA, Cassidy JD (Toronto Western Hosp, Ontario, Canada; Toronto Western Res Inst, Ontario, Canada; Univ of Toronto, Ontario, Canada)
Arch Phys Med Rehabil 91:1777-1789, 2010

Objective.—To assemble and synthesize the best evidence on the epidemiology, diagnosis, prognosis, treatment, and prevention of disordered eating, menstrual disturbances, and low bone mineral density in dancers.

Data Sources.—Medline, CINAHL, PsycINFO, Embase, and other electronic databases were searched from 1966 to 2010 using key words such as "dance," "dancer," "dancing," "eating disorders," "menstruation disturbances," and "bone density." In addition, the reference lists of relevant studies were examined, specialized journals were hand-searched, and the websites of major dance associations were scanned for relevant information.

Study Selection.—Citations were screened for relevance using a priori criteria, and relevant studies were critically reviewed for scientific merit by the best evidence synthesis method. After 2748 abstracts were screened, 124 articles were reviewed, and 23 (18.5%) of these were accepted as scientifically admissible (representing 19 unique studies).

Data Extraction.—Data from accepted studies were abstracted into evidence tables relating to prevalence and associated factors; incidence and risk factors; diagnosis; and prevention of disordered eating, menstrual disturbances, and/or low bone mineral density in dancers.

Data Synthesis.—The scientifically admissible studies consisted of 13 (68%) cross-sectional studies and 6 (32%) cohort studies. Disordered eating and menstrual disturbances are common in dancers. The lifetime prevalence of any eating disorder was 50% in professional dancers, while the point prevalence ranged between 13.6% and 26.5% in young student dancers. In their first year of intensive dance training, 32% of university-level dancers developed a menstrual disturbance. The incidence of disordered eating and low bone mineral density in dancers is unknown. Several potential risk factors are suggested by the literature, but there is little compelling evidence for any of these. There is preliminary evidence that multifaceted sociocultural prevention strategies may help decrease the incidence of disordered eating.

Conclusions.—The dance medicine literature is heterogeneous. The best available evidence suggests that disordered eating, menstrual disturbances, and low bone mineral density are important health issues for dancers at all skill levels. Future research would benefit from clear and relevant research questions being addressed with appropriate study designs and better reporting of studies in line with current scientific standards.

▶ Disordered eating, menstrual disturbances, and low bone mineral density (BMD) are the interrelated subclinical components of the female athlete triad (Triad). Although the Triad may manifest in any female athlete, it is more relevant to women in activities emphasizing a lean body aesthetic, such as dance.

This meta-analysis revealed a paucity of studies with sufficient scientific merit to accurately estimate the prevalence and incidence of the Triad or disordered eating. There is preliminary evidence that preoccupation with body shape and weight and patterns of restrictive eating are risk factors for disordered eating. With regard to menstrual disorders, the prevalence of late maturation ranged from approximately 40% to 57% in preprofessional ballet dancers, and menstrual disturbance occurred in 37% to 70% of professional ballet dancers during their lifetime. The 4-year incidence of menstrual disturbance was 85% in girls at the preprofessional training level, and 1-year incidence was 32% in university dancers. Hours of training and hormonal status (luteinizing hormone/follicle-stimulating hormone ratio; high dehydroepiandrosterone sulfate level) may be risk factors for the development of menstrual disturbance in dancers. Disordered eating and secondary amenorrhea were more commonly found in preprofessional dancers who dropped out of ballet training than those who continued training. The prevalence of low BMD was approximately 10% to 46% for osteopenia and 9% to 24% for osteoporosis. At the preprofessional and professional levels, the onset or resumption of menses was associated with a significant increase, but not normalization, of BMD. This finding is important because one of the primary concerns in young women is that failure to attain peak bone mass will increase their risk of osteoporosis later in life. Of the 3 Triad components, the only evidence-based screening tool is the 18-item Physiologic Screening Test for disordered eating. At this early stage of Triad research, there is little evidence for effective prevention programs or physiological interrelatedness of the components of the Triad.

C. M. Jankowski, PhD

Folic Acid Supplementation Improves Vascular Function in Amenorrheic Runners

Hoch AZ, Lynch SL, Jurva JW, et al (Med College of Wisconsin, Milwaukee)
Clin J Sport Med 20:205-210, 2010

Objective.—The purpose of this study was to determine if folic acid supplementation improves endothelial vascular function (brachial artery flow-mediated dilation; FMD) in amenorrheic runners.

Design.—Prospective cross-sectional study.

Setting.—Academic medical center in the Midwest.

Participants.—Ten amenorrheic and 10 eumenorrheic women runners from the community volunteered for this study.

Interventions.—Each participant was treated with folic acid (10 mg/d) for 4 weeks.

Main Outcome Measures.—Brachial artery FMD was measured before and after folic acid supplementation with standard techniques.

Results.—The brachial artery FMD response to reactive hyperemia improved after folic acid supplementation in amenorrheic women (3.0% ± 2.3% vs. 7.7% ± 4.5%; $P = 0.02$). In the eumenorrheic control

TABLE 2.—Brachial Artery Studies Before Supplementation

	Eumenorrheic Group, n = 10	Amenorrheic Group, n = 7	P*
Heart rate, beats/min	53.3 ± 10.3	49.1 ± 10.9	0.32
Mean arterial pressure			
Systolic, mmHg	112.2 ± 7.1	103.4 ± 8.2	0.03
Diastolic, mmHg	72.0 ± 6.8	66.6 ± 5.4	0.20
Baseline brachial artery diameter, mm	3.4 ± 0.3	3.5 ± 0.2	0.96
Peak brachial artery diameter, mm	3.4 ± 0.3	3.5 ± 0.3	0.33
Flow-mediated dilation, %	6.7 ± 2.0	3.0 ± 2.3	0.01
Peak change in flow velocity, %	78.2 ± 18.5	74.6 ± 31.9	0.63

Values are mean ± SD.
*P values based on normal approximation to the Wilcoxon rank-sum test.

group, there was no change in brachial artery FMD (6.7% ± 2.0% vs. 5.9% ± 2.6%; $P = 0.52$).

Conclusions.—This study demonstrates that brachial artery FMD, an indicator of vascular endothelial function, improves in amenorrheic female runners after short-term supplementation with folic acid (Table 2).

▶ Some authors attach great significance to endothelial dysfunction as a primary event in the development of atherosclerosis.[1,2] Hoch and associates thus point with concern to the approximate halving of flow-mediated dilatation in female athletes who develop an exercise-related amenorrhea (Table 2). Previous work has shown that the administration of oral contraceptive pills can restore endothelial function in such individuals,[3] but this therapy may in itself increase cardiovascular risk.[4] Large doses of folic acid have a similar normalizing effect,[5] perhaps by encouraging the regeneration of tetrahydro-biopterin (a cofactor for endothelial nitric oxide synthase), lowering homocysteine concentration, or simply serving as an antioxidant. This trial used a massive dose of folic acid (10 mg/d, 25 times the RDA, for a 4-week period) in order to restore dilatation. Before such therapy can be recommended, the safety of such a heavy dose needs to be examined over a longer period of time and in a larger sample of subjects. It may also be pertinent to inquire whether the change in endothelial function is as adverse a sign as Hoch and associates believe when subjects are in good health; such an inference runs counter to the well-accepted reduction of cardiovascular mortality associated with habitual vigorous endurance exercise. Finally, even if it is important to maintain flow dilatation in healthy, active individuals, this could likely be achieved more simply and more physiologically by ensuring that the athlete maintains energy balance when training.

R. J. Shephard, MD (Lond), PhD, DPE

References

1. Walther C, Gielen S, Hambrecht R. The effect of exercise training on endothelial function in cardiovascular disease in humans. *Exerc Sport Sci Rev.* 2004;32: 129-134.

2. Celermajer DS. Endothelial dysfunction: does it matter? Is it reversible? *J Am Coll Cardiol.* 1997;30:325-333.
3. Rickenlund A, Eriksson MJ, Schenck-Gustafsson K, Hirschberg AL. Oral contraceptives improve endothelial function in amenorrheic athletes. *J Clin Endocrinol Metab.* 2005;90:3162-3167.
4. Rossouw JE, Anderson GL, Prentice RL, et al. Risks and benefits of estrogen plus progestin in healthy postmenopausal women: principal results from the Women's Health Initiative randomized controlled trial. *JAMA.* 2002;288:321-333.
5. Hoch AZ, Pajewski NM, Hoffmann RG, et al. Possible relationship of folic acid supplementation and improved flow-mediated dilation in premenopausal, eumenorrheic athletic women. *J Sports Sci Med.* 2009;8:123-129.

Effect of physical training on age-related reduction of GH secretion during exercise in normally cycling women

Coiro V, Volpi R, Gramellini D, et al (Dept of Internal Medicine and Biomed Sciences, Parma, Italy; Dept of Obstetrics and Gynaecology, Italy; et al)
Maturitas 65:392-395, 2010

Objective.—To evaluate whether prolonged physical activity (25 km/week running for 8 years) modifies GH decline.

Design.—The GH response to maximal exercise on bicycle-ergometer was tested in younger (26–30 years) and older (42–46 years) healthy women. Each age group included 2 subgroups of 10 sedentary and 10 runners, which were compared. The workload was increased at 3 min intervals from time 0 until exhaustion. Subjects with a low maximal capacity (as established in a preliminary test) pedalled for 3–4 min against no workload at the beginning of the test, so that exercises lasted about 15 min in all individuals.

Results.—At exhaustion, heart rate and systolic pressure were significantly higher in sedentary than in trained subjects, whereas V_{O_2max}, blood glucose and plasma lactate levels were similar in all groups. Exercise induced similar GH responses in younger sedentary and exercise-trained subjects and in older exercise-trained subjects, with mean peak levels 7.5 times higher than baseline. In contrast, in older sedentary women peak GH level was only 4.4 times higher than baseline and was significantly lower than in the other groups.

Conclusion.—These data suggest that in women prolonged physical training exerts protective effects against age-dependent decline in GH secretion (Fig 1).

▶ A decreased secretion of growth hormone (GH) in older individuals is an important phenomenon, contributing to a progressive loss of muscle and decreases in bone strength with aging. It is well recognized that acute bouts of exercise stimulate the secretion of GH, but the evidence on possible beneficial effects of regular physical activity is conflicting.[1-4] Studies of this question have to date focused on elderly individuals (> 60 years of age). This report is based on a small cross-sectional comparison of physically active and sedentary women in 2 age groups (26-30 and 42-46 years). The active individuals had

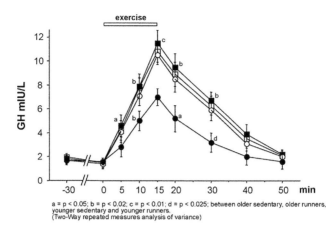

a = p < 0.05; b = p < 0.02; c = p < 0.01; d = p < 0.025; between older sedentary, older runners, younger sedentary and younger runners.
(Two-Way repeated measures analysis of variance)

FIGURE 1.—GH response to exercise in younger sedentary (-■- n.10, 27—29 years), younger runner (-□- n.10, 26—30 years); older sedentary (-●- n.10, 42—46 years), older runner women (-○- n.10, 42—46 years). Each point represents the mean ± SE of 10 observations. (Reprinted from Coiro V, Volpi R, Gramellini D, et al. Effect of physical training on age-related reduction of GH secretion during exercise in normally cycling women. *Maturitas*. 2010;65:392-395, with permission from Elsevier Ireland.)

been running a substantial distance (25 km/wk) for at least 8 years. In the younger individuals, a bout of maximal exercise induced a similar GH release in active and sedentary individuals, but in the older age group, the response of the sedentary subjects was only half as great as that of the runners (Fig 1). The data suggest that regular exercise may help to sustain GH secretion during middle age and provide 1 further reason for encouraging exercise in aging patients. The lesser secretion of GH in the sedentary group does not seem due to a lower level of effort on the cycle ergometer, as all subjects exceeded 75% of maximal oxygen intake, an intensity of exercise when GH secretion is said to be maximal.[5] It remains to be decided how far any reduction of GH response is due to a diminished secretion of GH releasing hormone and how far it is due to increased somatostatin tone.[6,7] The 1 puzzling feature of the present results is that the reported maximal oxygen intake is only a little larger in the active than in the sedentary groups. This is partly because values are reported as an absolute oxygen intake rather than relative to body mass; the more usual way of expressing maximal oxygen intake data (ml/[kg.min]) necessarily favors those who have remained thin because of their habitual physical activity.

R. J. Shephard, MD (Lond), PhD, DPE

References

1. Ambrosio MR, Valentini A, Transforini G, et al. Function of the GH/IGF-1 axis in healthy middle-aged male runners. *Neuroendocrinology*. 1986;63:498-500.
2. Horber FF, Kohler SA, Lippuner K, et al. Effect of regular physical training on age associated alteration of body composition in men. *Eur J Clin Invest*. 1996;26:279-285.
3. Craig BW, Brown R, Everhart J. Effect of progressive resistance training on growth hormone and testosterone levels in young and elderly subjects. *Mech Ageing Dev*. 1989;49:159-169.

4. Rudman D, Mattson DE. Serum insulin-like growth factor 1 in healthy older men in relation to physical activity. *J Am Geriat Soc.* 1994;42:71-76.
5. Luger A, Watschinger B, Deuster P, Svoboda T, Clodi M, Chrousos GP. Plasma growth hormone and prolactin responses to graded levels of acute exercise and to a lactate infusion. *Neuroendocrinology.* 1992;56:112-117.
6. Coiro V, Volpi R, Capretti L, Caffarri G, Davoli C, Chiodera P. Age-dependent decrease in the growth hormone response to growth hormone-releasing hormone in normally cycling women. *Fertil Steril.* 1996;66:230-234.
7. Marcell TJ, Wiswell RA, Hawkins SA, Tarpenning KM. Age-related blunting of growth hormone secretion during exercise may not be solely due to increased somatostatin tone. *Metabolism.* 1999;48:665-670.

Assessment of the Relationship Between Age and the Effect of Risedronate Treatment in Women with Postmenopausal Osteoporosis: A Pooled Analysis of Four Studies

Boonen S, Klemes AB, Zhou X, et al (Leuven Univ, Belgium; Procter & Gamble Pharmaceuticals, Mason, OH; et al)
J Am Geriatr Soc 58:658-663, 2010

Objectives.—To quantify the effect of age on the incidence of osteoporosis-related fractures and of risedronate treatment on fracture risk in different age groups in women with postmenopausal osteoporosis.

Design.—Data from four randomized, double-blind, placebo-controlled, Phase III studies were pooled and analyzed.

Participants.—The analysis population (N = 3,229) consisted of postmenopausal women with osteoporosis as determined on the basis of prevalent vertebral fractures, low bone mineral density (BMD), or both.

Intervention.—Patients had received risedronate 5 mg daily or placebo for 1 to 3 years.

Measurements.—The endpoints of interest were the incidence of osteoporosis-related fractures, clinical fractures, nonvertebral fractures, and morphometric vertebral fractures. The effect of age on fracture risk and treatment benefit was examined using Cox regression models with age and treatment as explanatory variables. The 3-year fracture risk was estimated for patients in each treatment group at a given age.

Results.—Irrespective of treatment, fracture risks were greater in older patients ($P < .001$). On average, for every 1-year increase in age, a patient's risk for osteoporosis-related fracture increased 3.6% (95% confidence interval = 2.3–5.0%). Irrespective of age, risedronate treatment reduced fracture risk 42%. Risedronate-treated patients had fracture risks similar to those of placebo-treated patients 10 to 20 years younger.

Conclusion.—Patients treated with risedronate have a significantly lower fracture risk, similar to that of untreated patients 10 to 20 years younger (Fig 1).

▶ Osteoporotic fracture poses a severe threat to the independence of older women. For example, women who survived a hip fracture lost 20% to 25% of their mobility and related functions. The study by Boonen and colleagues

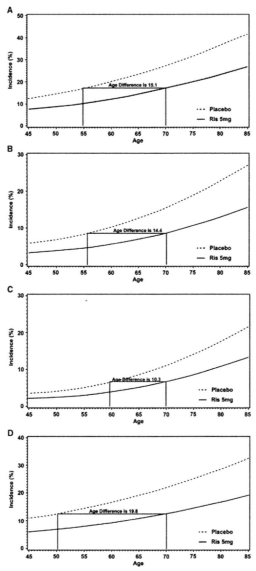

FIGURE 1.—Incidence of (A) osteoporosis-related fractures, (B) clinical fractures, (C) nonvertebral fractures, and (D) morphometric vertebral fractures according to age (placebo [broken line] vs treatment [solid line]). (Reprinted from Boonen S, Klemes AB, Zhou X, et al. Assessment of the relationship between age and the effect of risedronate treatment in women with postmenopausal osteoporosis: a pooled analysis of four studies. *J Am Geriatr Soc.* 2010;58:658-663. Reprinted with permission from 2010, Copyright the Authors. 2010, The American Geriatrics Society, John Wiley and Sons.)

combined fracture data from 4 large clinical trials of the osteoporosis medication risedronate. Importantly, all women enrolled in these studies (> 3000) had a history of osteoporotic fracture, low bone mineral density (BMD), or both. At study entry, the mean age was approximately 68 years, lumbar spine *T*-score was −2.6, and 72% of patients had at least 1 prevalent vertebral fracture. Women were randomized to risedronate (5 mg/d) or placebo and monitored for new fractures for up to 3 years. The main findings of the pooled intention-to-treat data analysis were that the risk of osteoporotic fracture increased with age and that risedronate decreased fracture risk irrespective of age. The risk of a clinical, nonvertebral, or morphometric vertebral osteoporotic fracture increased by 3.6% for every 1-year increase in age. Risedronate treatment decreased fracture risk by 41% to 46% depending on the fracture type (Fig 1). Treatment with risedronate reduced the osteoporotic fracture risk of a 75-year-old woman to that of a woman aged 60 years. On an individual level, the 75-year-old osteoporotic woman who is in otherwise good health would be able to enjoy her independence longer than if she were treated with risedronate. On a population level, the slowing of age-related fracture would unburden the health care system of costs due to hospitalization, rehabilitation, and long-term care. Delaying osteoporotic fracture also provides more time for women to initiate and benefit from other complementary interventions for bone health such as exercise training that targets not only preservation of BMD but also muscle strength and balance.

C. M. Jankowski, PhD

Effect of office-based brief high-impact exercise on bone mineral density in healthy premenopausal women: the Sendai Bone Health Concept Study
Niu K, Ahola R, Guo H, et al (Tohoku Univ Graduate School of Biomed Engineering, Aoba-ku, Sendai, Japan; Univ of Oulu, Finland; et al)
J Bone Miner Metab 28:568-577, 2010

Although there is ample evidence supporting the effectiveness of physical activity in the prevention and treatment of osteoporosis, there are no previous studies to examine the effect of office-based brief high-impact exercise (HIE) on bone mineral density (BMD) in healthy premenopausal women. This study evaluated the effects of office-based HIE on BMD in healthy premenopausal Japanese women. Ninety-one healthy premenopausal women were randomized to receive stretching exercise (SE) or HIE (stretching, along with up to 5×10 vertical and versatile jumps) for 12 months. The BMD of the lumbar spine and proximal femur was measured using dual-energy X-ray absorptiometry. Several cardiovascular risk factors and leg strength also were assessed. An accelerometer-based recorder was used to measure daily impact loading in four 1-week samples. The progression of the HIE program was ensured by the accelerometer. Thirty-three women (71.7%) in the SE group and 34 (75.6%) in the HIE group completed the study. There was a significant difference in the change in the femoral neck BMD between the groups in favor of the HIE group [0.6% (95% CI: −0.4, 1.7) vs. −1.0% (95% CI: −2.2, 0.2)]. Adiponectin, LDL, HDL, and the leg strength of participants in both the groups improved during the intervention. These finding suggested that office-based brief HIE can be recommended for premenopausal women for preventing bone mineral loss (Figs 2 and 3).

▶ The Sendai Bone Health Concept Study is remarkable because it demonstrated that approximately 16 minutes of exercise at the workplace was associated with increased bone mineral density (BMD) and improved cardiovascular disease risk profile in premenopausal Japanese women. Like many women in the workforce, the participants had sedentary desk jobs. The exclusion criteria included the use of steroid hormones, including estrogen. Women were randomly assigned to either high-impact vertical jump exercise (HIE) to impose nonhabitual bone strain or low-impact stretching exercise (LIE). The intervention was conducted at the workplace for 12 months. The sessions were delivered with video instruction and supervised at least 4 times per month by a fitness instructor. The HIE comprised a progressive increase to 50 jumps per session during the first 3 months. After 6 months, the jumping intensity was increased by adding a 10-cm step bench. The LIE comprised stretching exercise. The women wore accelerometers to record the number of vertical acceleration peaks. The frequency of high acceleration peaks was significantly greater in the HIE compared with the LIE in the last 6 months of the study, confirming the greater exposure of bone to high loading forces (Fig 2). The HIE resulted in maintenance of femoral neck BMD after adjusting for changes in body mass index and dietary calcium intake. Within HIE, lumbar spine BMD increased

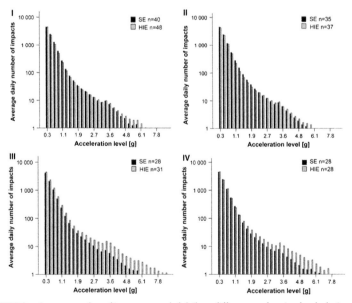

FIGURE 2.—Average number of impacts recorded daily at different acceleration levels during the four 1-week measurement periods (I–IV) in the 12-month study. Stretching exercise (*SE*) and high-impact exercise (*HIE*) groups. (Reprinted from Niu K, Ahola R, Guo H, et al. Effect of office-based brief high-impact exercise on bone mineral density in healthy premenopausal women: the Sendai Bone Health Concept Study. *J Bone Miner Metab*. 2010;28:568-577, with permission from The Japanese Society for Bone and Mineral Research and Springer.)

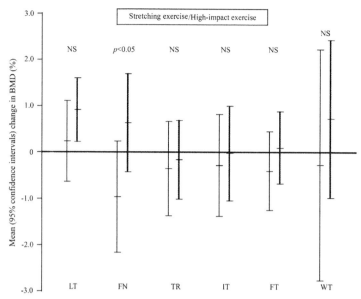

FIGURE 3.—Mean percent changes (95% confidence intervals) in the BMD of the whole lumbar spine and femur over the 12-month study period. *LT* total lumbar spine, *FN* femoral neck, *TR* greater trochanter, *IT* intertrochanteric region, *FT* total femur, and *WT* Ward's triangle. *P* values indicate the difference between the stretching and high-impact exercise groups over the 12-month study period (unpaired *t* test). (Reprinted from Niu K, Ahola R, Guo H, et al. Effect of office-based brief high-impact exercise on bone mineral density in healthy premenopausal women: the Sendai Bone Health Concept Study. *J Bone Miner Metab*. 2010;28:568-577, with permission from The Japanese Society for Bone and Mineral Research and Springer.)

significantly. The changes in BMD at other sites were not significantly different between the impact groups (Fig 3). The changes in femoral BMD can be explained by the compressive and loading forces on that bone region during jump takeoff and landing. There were other health benefits of the intervention independent of vertical impact intensity, such as increased serum adiponectin, increased high-density lipoprotein cholesterol, and decreased low-density lipo-protein cholesterol. The adherence to the intervention was 74% and not different between groups. Dropouts were mainly because of employment changes and transition to menopause. For women who completed the study, the average compliance was 2.4 sessions per week, and there were no adverse events. This study suggests that a very small amount of time (less than a lunch hour) set aside for a targeted bone loading intervention in the workplace has a significant impact on bone health and improved cardiovascular risk profile. Whether the improvements can be sustained after cessation of the intervention is unknown, but this is an important question for osteoporosis prevention in women.

C. M. Jankowski, PhD

Effect of Rhythmic Gymnastics on Volumetric Bone Mineral Density and Bone Geometry in Premenarcheal Female Athletes and Controls

Tournis S, Michopoulou E, Fatouros IG, et al (Univ of Athens, Greece; Democritus Univ of Thrace, Komotini, Greece)
J Clin Endocrinol Metab 95:2755-2762, 2010

Context and Objective.—Weight-bearing exercise during growth exerts positive effects on the skeleton. Our objective was to test the hypothesis that long-term elite rhythmic gymnastics exerts positive effects on volumetric bone mineral density and geometry and to determine whether exercise-induced bone adaptation is associated with increased periosteal bone formation or medullary contraction using tibial peripheral quantitative computed tomography and bone turnover markers.

Design and Setting.—We conducted a cross-sectional study at a tertiary center.

Subjects.—We studied 26 elite premenarcheal female rhythmic gymnasts (RG) and 23 female controls, aged 9—13 yr.

Main Outcome Measures.—We measured bone age, volumetric bone mineral density, bone mineral content (BMC), cortical thickness, cortical and trabecular area, and polar stress strength index (SSIp) by peripheral quantitative computed tomography of the left tibia proximal to the distal metaphysis (trabecular) at 14, 38 (cortical), and 66% (muscle mass) from the distal end and bone turnover markers.

Results.—The two groups were comparable according to height and chronological and bone age. After weight adjustment, cortical BMC, area, and thickness at 38% were significantly higher in RG ($P < 0.005$—0.001). Periosteal circumference, SSIp, and muscle area were higher in RG ($P < 0.01$—0.001). Muscle area was significantly associated with cortical BMC, area, and SSIp, whereas years of training showed positive association with cortical BMC, area, and thickness independent of chronological age.

Conclusions.—RG in premenarcheal girls may induce positive adaptations on the skeleton, especially in cortical bone. Increased duration of exercise is associated with a positive response of bone geometry.

▶ This study adds to the growing body of evidence that muscular stress on bones, particularly during weight-bearing activities, can augment bone health in the childhood age group. This construct is, in fact, one of the most compelling pieces of evidence we have for an exercise-health link in the growing child. It considers the increase in body mass and density in the early years as a means of increasing peak bone mass during the life span and thus helping reduce the risk of osteoporosis and bone fractures in the later years of life. We are just beginning to understand the types of exercise that might be most efficacious in this regard, but clearly inclusion of weight-bearing activities and involvement in sports that put stress on bones can be expected to be high on the list. It would seem, in fact, that a mixture of types of activities—muscle strength, weight bearing, endurance—are important in respect to the future health of children and adolescents.

T. Rowland, MD

Physiologic and behavioral indicators of energy deficiency in female adolescent runners with elevated bone turnover
Barrack MT, Van Loan MD, Rauh MJ, et al (Univ of California Davis, CA; Rocky Mountain Univ of Health Professions, Provo, UT; et al)
Am J Clin Nutr 92:652-659, 2010

Background.—Female adolescent runners have an elevated prevalence of low bone mass for age—an outcome that may be partially due to inadequate energy intake.

Objective.—The objective was to evaluate diet, menstrual history, serum hormone concentrations, and bone mass in female adolescent runners with normal or abnormal bone turnover.

Design.—Thirty-nine cross-country runners (age: 15.7 ± 0.2 y) participated in the study, which included a 7-d dietary assessment with the use of a food record and daily 24-h dietary recalls; serum measures of insulin-like growth factor I, estradiol, leptin, parathyroid hormone, progesterone, triiodothyronine, 25-hydroxycholecalciferol, bone-specific alkaline phosphatase (BAP), and cross-linked C-telopeptides of type I collagen (CTX); an evaluation of height, weight, bone mass, and body composition with the use of dual-energy X-ray absorptiometry; and a questionnaire to assess menses and sports participation. Age- and sex-specific BAP and CTX concentrations of at least the 97th percentile and no greater than the third percentile, respectively, were considered abnormal.

Results.—All abnormal BAP and CTX concentrations fell within the elevated (≥97%) range. Runners with an elevated bone turnover (EBT) ($n = 13$) had a lower body mass, fewer menstrual cycles in the past year, lower estradiol and 25-hydroxycholecalciferol concentrations, and a higher prevalence of body mass index <10% for age, vitamin D insufficiency, amenorrhea, and low bone mass. Girls with EBT consumed less than the recommended amounts of energy and had a higher prevalence of consuming <1300 mg Ca than did those with normal bone turnover.

Conclusions.—Runners with EBT had a profile consistent with energy deficiency. Nutritional support to increase energy, calcium intake, and 25-hydroxycholecalciferol concentrations may improve bone mineral accrual in young runners with EBT. This trial was registered at clinicaltrials.gov as NCT01059968 (Table 6).

▶ In this study of 39 female adolescent runners, one-third ($n = 13$) were classified as having elevated bone turnover (EBT) as determined by sex- and age-specific serum bone-specific alkaline phosphatase (BAP) and cross-linked C-telopeptides of type I collagen (CTX) concentrations. Because bone mineral accrual rate peaks between Tanner stages 2 and 4, with rapid gains until the age of 16 years,

TABLE 6.—Variables that Contributed Significantly to the Prediction of Elevated Bone Turnover

	Odds Ratio (95% CI)
Risk factors	
Secondary amenorrhea	20.83 (2.04, 212.97)
BMI (kg/m^2) <10% for age	7.50 (1.21, 46.50)
Calcium <1300 mg/d	5.5 (1.01, 29.85)
Energy intake <2000 kcal/d	4.2 (0.94, 18.71)
Protective factors	
Began running at older age (y)	0.49 (0.25, 0.99)
Older chronologic age (y)	0.52 (0.27, 0.99)
Higher number of menses in the past year	0.71 (0.57, 0.88)
Higher lean tissue mass (kg)	0.71 (0.56, 0.91)

adolescent girls competing in endurance running may not attain peak bone mass. The EBT runners had significantly lower femoral neck bone mineral content (adjusted for age, height, and weight) compared with the normal bone turnover runners. Sufficient energy status supports normal hormonal regulation of bone formation and resorption. On average, the energy intake of the EBT runners was ≥300 kcal less than age-specific and activity level–specific energy requirements for adolescent girls. EBT runners tended to have a lower dietary calcium intake and a significantly higher prevalence of vitamin D insufficiency (serum 25-hydroxyvitamin D < 30 ng/mL) than normal bone turnover runners. The lower energy intake, low body mass index (BMI) for age, and greater prevalence of amenorrhea (primary and secondary) in the EBT runners are consistent with traits in populations with known chronic energy deficiencies. The EBT runners were significantly younger and began running competitively or training at a younger age than their counterparts with normal bone turnover. The significant predictors of EBT were secondary amenorrhea, BMI < 10% for age, and < 1300 mg/d of dietary calcium intake. Factors protecting against EBT were beginning competitive running at older age, higher gynecologic age, more menses in the past year, and higher lean tissue mass (Table 6). The BAP and CTX concentrations were highly correlated, suggesting increased bone resorption in the EBT runners at a time of peak bone formation rate. These results support the monitoring of bone turnover in adolescent female endurance runners. The limitations of this study include the lack of comparisons to nonathlete controls and nonendurance runners.

C. M. Jankowski, PhD

Prevalence of menopause symptoms and their association with lifestyle among Finnish middle-aged women
Moilanen J, Aalto A-M, Hemminki E, et al (Univ of Tampere, Finland; Natl Inst for Welfare and Health, Helsinki, Finland)
Maturitas 67:368-374, 2010

Background and Aim of the Study.—The aim of this study is to report the prevalence of menopausal symptoms by severity among the Finnish female population and the association of their symptoms with lifestyle (smoking, use of alcohol, physical activity) and body mass index (BMI).

Material and Methods.—Health 2000 is a nationally representative population-based study of Finnish adults. Data were collected by home interview, three self-administered questionnaires and a clinical examination by a physician. This study included women aged 45–64 years ($n = 1427$). All symptoms included menopause-specific symptoms. Both univariate analysis and a factor analysis based on symptom factors were performed by menopausal group. Multiple regression analysis included each symptom factor as a dependent variable and confounding and lifestyle factors (age, education, smoking, alcohol use, physical activity, BMI, use of hormonal replacement therapy (HRT) and chronic disease status).

Results.—Over one-third (38%) of the premenopausal, half of the perimenopausal, and 54% of both postmenopausal and hysterectomized women reported bothersome symptoms. The difference between pre- and perimenopausal women was largest and statistically most significant in the case of back pain and hot flushes. Physically active women reported fewer somatic symptoms than did women with a sedentary lifestyle. Smoking was not related to vasomotor symptoms.

Conclusion.—Bothersome symptoms are common in midlife, regardless of menopausal status. Inverse association between physical activity and menopausal symptoms needs to be confirmed in randomized trials (Table 3).

▶ In many women, menopause is associated with troublesome symptoms.[1-3] This cross-sectional study, using a simple 3-level questionnaire assessment of

---

TABLE 3.—Linear Regression Analyses for Psychological, Somatic/Pain and Vasomotor Symptoms as Dependent Variables. Lifestyle-Specific Standardized Beta Coefficients with 95% Confidence Intervals (CIs) Adjusted for Background Characteristics (Age, Menopausal Status, Education, Chronic Disease, HRT)

Lifestyle	PsychologicalBeta (95% CI)	Somatic/PainBeta (95% CI)	VasomotorBeta (95% CI)
Smoking			
Never (ref.)	—	—	—
Quitter	0.03 (−0.02; 0.08)	0.05 (0.001; 0.10)*	0.04 (−0.004; 0.09)
Smoker	0.01 (−0.05; 0.07)	0.03 (−0.03; 0.09)	0.03 (−0.02; 0.09)
Alcohol portion/week			
<10 (ref.)	—	—	—
10–16	−0.03 (−0.07; 0.01)	0.007 (−0.04; 0.05)	−0.02 (−0.06; 0.02)
>16	−0.02 (−0.06; 0.03)	0.02 (−0.03; 0.07)	0.07 (0.02; 0.11)**
BMI (kg/m²)			
<25 (ref.)	—	—	—
25–29.9	0.08 (0.03; 0.14)**	0.06 (0.003; 0.12)*	0.07 (0.01; 0.12)*
30+	0.12 (0.07; 0.18)***	0.05 (−0.003; 0.11)	0.08 (0.03; 0.13)**
Physical activity			
High (ref.)	—	—	—
Middle	0.03 (−0.03; 0.10)	0.05 (−0.02; 0.11)	0.06 (0.00009; 0.12)
Low	0.14 (0.06; 0.20)***	0.18 (0.10; 0.27)***	0.15 (0.07; 0.22)***

*$p < 0.01$.
**$p < 0.01$.
***$p < 0.001$.

physical activity, confirms earlier reports[3] that symptoms are fewer and hot flushes are of shorter duration in women who remain physically active (Table 3). Although an attempt was made to control for confounding variables, it would be interesting to test benefits using an experimental design. This seems particularly important given the growing appreciation of the risks associated with hormone replacement therapy.

R. J. Shephard, MD (Lond), PhD, DPE

References

1. Nelson HD, Haney E, Humphrey L, et al. Management of menopause-related symptoms. *Evid Rep Technol Assess (Summ)*. 2005:1-6.
2. Woods NF, Mitchell ES. Symptoms during the perimenopause: prevalence, severity, trajectory, and significance in women's lives. *Am J Med*. 2005;118: S14-S24.
3. Col NF, Guthrie JR, Politi M, Dennerstein L. Duration of vasomotor symptoms in middle-aged women: a longitudinal study. *Menopause*. 2009;16:453-457.

Prevalence of menopause symptoms and their association with lifestyle among Finnish middle-aged women

Moilanen J, Aalto A-M, Hemminki E, et al (Univ of Tampere, Finland; Natl Inst for Welfare and Health, Helsinki, Finland; et al)
Maturitas 67:368-374, 2010

Background and Aim of the Study.—The aim of this study is to report the prevalence of menopausal symptoms by severity among the Finnish female population and the association of their symptoms with lifestyle (smoking, use of alcohol, physical activity) and body mass index (BMI).

Material and Methods.—Health 2000 is a nationally representative population-based study of Finnish adults. Data were collected by home interview, three self-administered questionnaires and a clinical examination by a physician. This study included women aged 45–64 years ($n = 1427$). All symptoms included menopause-specific symptoms. Both univariate analysis and a factor analysis based on symptom factors were performed by menopausal group. Multiple regression analysis included each symptom factor as a dependent variable and confounding and lifestyle factors (age, education, smoking, alcohol use, physical activity, BMI, use of hormonal replacement therapy (HRT) and chronic disease status).

Results.—Over one-third (38%) of the premenopausal, half of the perimenopausal, and 54% of both postmenopausal and hysterectomized women reported bothersome symptoms. The difference between pre- and perimenopausal women was largest and statistically most significant in the case of back pain and hot flushes. Physically active women reported fewer somatic symptoms than did women with a sedentary lifestyle. Smoking was not related to vasomotor symptoms.

Conclusion.—Bothersome symptoms are common in midlife, regardless of menopausal status. Inverse association between physical activity and menopausal symptoms needs to be confirmed in randomized trials.

▶ There are a number of risks and side effects associated with hormonal replacement therapy. As a result, lifestyle therapy to alleviate menopausal symptoms has emerged as an important strategy. In this study, women with a sedentary lifestyle reported more psychological symptoms, somatic/pain, and vasomotor symptoms than did women who exercised regularly. Additionally, obese women reported more psychological and vasomotor symptoms than did women of normal weight. Multiple other health benefits are associated with avoidance of obesity and a sedentary lifestyle, and menopause is viewed by the authors as a crucial time to pay attention to personal health. Randomized clinical trials are needed to further address the effect of physical activity on the symptoms experienced by middle-aged women. A few small trials have been conducted, but results are contradictory, and methods have been questionable.[1,2]

D. C. Nieman, DrPH

References

1. Wilbur J, Miller AM, McDevitt J, Wang E, Miller J. Menopausal status, moderate-intensity walking, and symptoms in midlife women. *Res Theory Nurs Pract.* 2005; 19:163-180.
2. Aiello EJ, Yasui Y, Tworoger SS, et al. Effect of a yearlong, moderate-intensity exercise intervention on the occurrence and severity of menopause symptoms in postmenopausal women. *Menopause.* 2004;11:382-388.

Six weeks of structured exercise training and hypocaloric diet increases the probability of ovulation after clomiphene citrate in overweight and obese patients with polycystic ovary syndrome: a randomized controlled trial

Palomba S, Falbo A, Giallauria F, et al (Univ 'Magna Graecia' of Catanzaro, Viale Europa, Italy; Univ 'Federico II' of Naples, Via Pansini, Italy; et al)
Hum Reprod 25:2783-2791, 2010

Background.—Clomiphene citrate (CC) is the first-line therapy for the induction of ovulation in infertile women with polycystic ovary syndrome (PCOS), but ∼20% of patients are unresponsive. The aim of the current study was to test the hypothesis that a 6-week intervention that consisted of structured exercise training (SET) and hypocaloric diet increases the probability of ovulation after CC in overweight and obese CC-resistant PCOS patients.

Methods.—A cohort of 96 overweight and obese CC-resistant PCOS patients was enrolled consecutively in a three-arm randomized, parallel, controlled, assessor-blinded clinical trial. The three interventions were: SET plus hypocaloric diet for 6 weeks (Group A); 2 weeks of observation followed by one cycle of CC therapy (Group B); and SET plus hypocaloric diet for 6 weeks, with one cycle of CC after the first 2 weeks (Group C). The primary end-point was the ovulation rate. Other reproductive data, as well as anthropometric, hormonal and metabolic data, were also collected and considered as secondary end points.

Results.—After 6 weeks of SET plus hypocaloric diet, the ovulation rate was significantly ($P = 0.008$) higher in Group C [12/32 (37.5%)] than in Groups A [4/32 (12.5%)] and B [3/32 (9.4%)] with relative risks of 3.9 [95% confidence interval (CI) 1.1−8.3; $P = 0.035$] and 4.0 (95% CI 1.2−12.8; $P = 0.020$) compared with Groups A and B, respectively. Compared with baseline, in Groups A and C, a significant improvement in clinical and biochemical androgen and insulin sensitivity indexes was observed. In the same two groups, the insulin sensitivity index was significantly ($P < 0.05$) better than that in Group B.

Conclusions.—In overweight and obese CC-resistant PCOS patients, a 6-week intervention of SET and a hypocaloric diet was effective in increasing the probability of ovulation under CC treatment.

The study was registered at Clinicaltrials.gov: NCT0100468.

▶ Clomiphene citrate is a recommended treatment for anovulatory infertility related to polycystic ovary syndrome,[1,2] but unfortunately, a proportion of patients are resistant to this treatment.[3] This blinded and randomized controlled trial lacks a control for those who received clomiphene citrate alone (although it would be difficult to recruit women who are anxious to become pregnant into such a control group). These observations make a fairly convincing case that even a relatively short period (6 weeks) of dietary restriction (4.2 MJ/d energy deficit) and moderate exercise (30 min of cycle ergometry, 3 times a week, at a power output increasing gradually from 60% to 70% of the individual's maximal oxygen intake) is enough to achieve a substantial improvement of ovulation (although this does not necessarily equate with an increased probability of conception and live birth). It is not always easy to persuade obese patients to exercise. Nevertheless, this study demonstrates that exercise and dieting can be a valid alternative to the prescription of additional drug cocktails in patients who are resistant to clomiphene citrate.

R. J. Shephard, MD (Lond), PhD, DPE

References

1. Brown J, Farquhar C, Beck J, Boothroyd C, Hughes E. Clomiphene and anti-oestrogens for ovulation induction in PCOS. *Cochrane Database Syst Rev.* 2009;(4). CD002249.
2. Palomba S, Orio F Jr, Russo T, et al. Is ovulation induction still a therapeutic problem in patients with polycystic ovary syndrome? *J Endocrinol Invest.* 2004; 27:796-805.
3. Kousta E, White DM, Franks S. Modern use of clomiphene citrate in induction of ovulation. *Hum Reprod Update.* 1997;3:359-365.

Age and Gender Interactions in Ultraendurance Performance: Insight from the Triathlon

Lepers R, Maffiuletti NA (Univ of Burgundy, Dijon, France; Schulthess Clinic, Zurich, Switzerland)
Med Sci Sports Exerc 43:134-139, 2011

Purpose.—The purposes of this study were (i) to investigate the effect of age on gender difference in Hawaii Ironman triathlon performance time and (ii) to compare the gender difference among swimming (3.8 km), cycling (180 km), and running (42 km) performances as a function of age.

Methods.—Gender difference in performance times and estimated power output in the three modes of locomotion were analyzed for the top 10 men and women amateur triathletes between the ages of 18 and 64 yr for three consecutive years (2006—2008).

Results.—The gender difference in total performance time was stable until 55 yr and then significantly increased. Mean gender difference in performance time was significantly ($P < 0.01$) smaller for swimming (mean $\pm$ 95% confidence interval = 12.1% $\pm$ 1.9%) compared with cycling (15.4% $\pm$ 0.7%) and running (18.2% $\pm$ 1.3%). In contrast, mean gender difference in cycling estimated power output (38.6% $\pm$ 1.1%) was significantly ($P < 0.01$) greater compared with swimming (27.5% $\pm$ 3.8%) and running (32.6% $\pm$ 0.7%).

Conclusions.—This cross-sectional study provides evidence that gender difference in ultraendurance performance such as an Ironman triathlon was stable until 55 yr and then increased thereafter and differed between the locomotion modes. Further studies examining the changes in training volume and physiological characteristics with advanced age for men and women are required to better understand the age-associated changes in ultraendurance performance.

▶ Elderly athletes are a model of successful aging. Performance in ultraendurance events is limited by the maximal physiological and mental capacity of the athlete. In older athletes, changes in performance are more likely to reflect the effects of primary aging as opposed to reduced physical activity. There is some evidence to suggest a gender gap in aging-related performance changes, with declines in running and swimming performance more pronounced in women than men. Knowledge of gender differences in endurance performance may shed light on sex-specific physiological changes in muscle during active aging. In this study, performance in the Hawaii Ironman triathlon was compared among the top 10 amateur finishers across age and gender groups for 3 years of competition (2006-2008). The youngest and oldest age groups were 18 to 24 and 60 to 64 years, respectively. Age and gender interactions were determined in each of the 3 triathlon disciplines (swimming, cycling, and running) and for total event time. The magnitude of gender difference was the percent difference in time for the average totals of swimming, cycling, running, and total event times between the women and men in each age group. Gender differences in power output were estimated for each discipline using equations that account for differences in air and water resistance. For total event time, a significant gender divergence was found in the oldest age groups (55-59 and 60-64 years) compared with the younger groups and greater in the age group of 60 to 64 years than in the age group of 55 to 59 years (Fig 2 in the original article). Training characteristics such as time and intensity may also account for performance declines in the older age groups, although this supposition has not been rigorously examined. Gender differences in power output were greatest for cycling and least for swimming, independent of age. Gender differences in performance time were greatest for running, intermediate for cycling, and least for swimming. Therefore, gender differences in endurance sport performance are influenced by the mode of activity and age. There were no physiological measures to explain the mechanisms underpinning the observed gender disparities. The results may be confounded by having fewer women than men finishers in the older age groups.

C. M. Jankowski, PhD

Urinary Incontinence Among Group Fitness Instructors Including Yoga and Pilates Teachers

Bø K, Bratland-Sanda S, Sundgot-Borgen J (Norwegian School of Sport Sciences, Oslo, Norway)
Neurourol Urodyn 2011 [Epub ahead of print]

Aims.—Controversies exist on the role of physical activity on urinary incontinence (UI), and search on PubMed revealed no studies on UI in fitness instructors. The aim of this study was to investigate the prevalence of UI among female group fitness instructors, including Pilates and yoga teachers.

Methods.—This was a cross-sectional study of 1,473 instructors representing three of the largest fitness companies recruited from 59 fitness centers in Norway. They filled in an online survey (Questback) about general health, educational background, and number of hours teaching per week. Prevalence of UI was evaluated by the International Consensus on Incontinence Questionnaire, short form (ICIQ-UI SF).

Results.—Three out of 152 men (2%) reported UI. Six hundred eighty-five women, mean age 32.7 years (range 18–68) answered the questionnaire. 26.3% of all the female instructors reported to have UI, with 21.4% reporting leakage ≥once a week, 3.2% 2–3 times/week and 1.7% ≥once per day. 24.4% reported the leakage to be small to moderate and the bother score was 4.6 (SD 2.4) out of 21. 15.3% reported leakage during physical activity and 10.9% when coughing/sneezing. 25.9% of yoga and Pilates instructors reported UI.

Conclusions.—This is the first report on UI among fitness instructors and the results indicate that UI is prevalent among female fitness instructors, including yoga and Pilates teachers. More information about this topic seems to be important in the basic education of fitness instructors.

▶ The prevalence of urinary incontinence (UI) varies between 13% and 60% in the general population. A high prevalence of UI has been reported in elite athletes and dancers presumably because the pelvic floor muscles are exposed to high loading forces. In contrast, epidemiological evidence suggests that physical activity protects against UI. Bo and colleagues completed a cross-sectional online survey of UI in nearly 1500 group fitness instructors. This is a population of healthy fit women who are routinely exposed to high-impact forces. The survey purposely included yoga and Pilates instructors in part because pelvic floor muscle training (PFMT) is incorporated into some yoga and Pilates movements. On average, the instructors had been teaching fitness classes for 8 years, 3 hours a week, and exercised on their own at least once a week. Consistent with the general population, 26% of fitness instructors (all or yoga/Pilates) reported UI, with most reporting stress UI. Female instructors who were older, had been teaching longer, and were not using oral contraceptives had a significantly higher prevalence of UI. These results support neither a protective nor a causal relation between high levels of physical activity and UI. This was a cross-sectional study that relied upon self-reported data, so conclusions must be drawn cautiously. It is not known if PFMT is effective in preventing UI in elite athletes, fitness instructors, or the general population. The authors suggest that the training of fitness instructors include PFMT, which could be facilitated by the accrediting bodies of fitness instructors.

C. M. Jankowski, PhD

Time course and mechanisms of adaptations in cardiorespiratory fitness with endurance training in older and young men
Murias JM, Kowalchuk JM, Paterson DH (The Univ of Western Ontario, London, Canada)
J Appl Physiol 108:621-627, 2010

The time-course and mechanisms of adaptation of cardiorespiratory fitness were examined in 8 older (O) (68 ± 7 yr old) and 8 young (Y) (23 ± 5 yr old) men pretraining and at 3, 6, 9, and 12 wk of training. Training was performed on a cycle ergometer three times per week for 45 min at ~70% of maximal oxygen uptake ($\dot{V}o_{2\,max}$). $\dot{V}o_{2\,max}$ increased within 3 wk with further increases observed posttraining in both O (+31%) and Y (+18%), ($P < 0.05$). Maximal cardiac output ($\dot{Q}_{max}$, open-circuit acetylene) and stroke volume were higher in O and Y after 3 wk with further increases after 9 wk of training ($P < 0.05$). Maximal arterial-venous oxygen difference (a-vO_{2diff}) was higher at *weeks* 3 and 6 and posttraining compared with pretraining in O and Y ($P < 0.05$). In O, ~69% of the increase in $\dot{V}o_{2\,max}$ from pre- to posttraining was explained by an increased $\dot{Q}_{max}$ with the remaining ~31% explained by a widened a-vO_{2diff}. This proportion of $\dot{Q}$ and a-vO_{2diff} contributions to the increase in $\dot{V}o_{2\,max}$ was consistent throughout testing in O. In Y, 56% of the pre- to posttraining increase in $\dot{V}o_{2\,max}$ was attributed to a greater $\dot{Q}_{max}$ and 44% to a widened a-vO_{2diff}. Early adaptations (first 3 wk) mainly relied on a widened maximal a-vO_{2diff} (~66%) whereas further increases in $\dot{V}o_{2\,max}$ were exclusively explained by a greater $\dot{Q}_{max}$.

In conclusion, with short-term training O and Y significantly increased their $\dot{V}o_{2\,max}$; however, the proportion of $\dot{V}o_{2\,max}$ increase explained by $\dot{Q}_{max}$ and maximal a-vO_{2diff} throughout training showed a different pattern by age group (Table 2).

▶ The speed of adaptation to cardiorespiratory training is an important consideration when deciding whether it is more difficult to induce training in the elderly than in those who are younger. Comparisons are usually made after a fixed time, and if the process is slower in an older person, the ultimate extent of response may be underestimated. It is less certain how far the present study can answer this question. The subject samples ($n = 8$ younger and 8 older) are very small, and neither may be representative of their age group (both young and old groups were said to be healthy, active nonsmokers, but not to have been involved in specific endurance training for at least 12 months). The intensity of training was set at 70% of what seems a carefully determined maximal oxygen intake test for each individual. Both groups were examined after identical periods of training, although the collection of data at 3, 6, 9, and 12 weeks possibly gives some possibility to detect differences in the speed of response; contrary to the authors' comments, the data suggest a trend to slower increase of oxygen transport in the 65-year-olds (Table 2). Perhaps the most controversial part of the article is the attempt to differentiate changes in maximal cardiac

TABLE 2.—Maximal Exercise Responses for PO, $\dot{V}o_{2\,max}$, HR, $\dot{Q}$, SV, and a-vO_{2diff} in O and Y From Pretraining Through Posttraining

	Pretraining	Week 3	Week 6	Week 9	Posttraining
PO_{peak}, W					
O[e]	188 (44)	201 (40)[a]	208 (44)[a,b]	215 (49)[a,b]	219 (49)[a,b,c,d]
Y	314 (41)	346 (47)[a]	359 (45)[a,b]	365 (57)[a,b]	377 (50)[a,b,c,d]
$\dot{V}o_{2\,max}$, l/min					
O[e]	2.29 (0.49)	2.48 (0.42)[a]	2.65 (0.58)[a]	2.77 (0.53)[a]	2.95 (0.48)[a,b,c,d]
Y	3.82 (0.47)	4.27 (0.52)[a]	4.22 (0.44)[a]	4.28 (0.49)[a]	4.47 (0.34)[a,b,c,d]
$\dot{V}o_{2\,max}$, ml·kg^{-1}·min^{-1}					
O[e]	28.3 (7.1)	30.7 (6.0)[a]	32.8 (7.6)[a]	34.5 (8.0)[a]	36.6 (6.5)[a,b,c,d]
Y	48.0 (6.1)	53.8 (7.6)[a]	52.5 (6.4)[a]	53.1 (6.5)[a]	55.4 (5.5)[a,b,c,d]
HR_{max}, beats/min					
O[e]	144 (22)	139 (23)[a]	141 (21)	142 (19)	145 (17)[b,d]
Y	189 (7)	185 (5)[a]	185 (5)	185 (6)	187 (7)[b,d]
$\dot{Q}_{max}$, l/min					
O[e]	16.8 (3.0)	18.0 (3.8)[a]	18.7 (4.2)[a]	19.8 (3.5)[a,b,c]	20.3 (3.7)[a,b,c]
Y	25.9 (2.8)	26.7 (2.2)[a]	27.3 (2.1)[a]	28.6 (1.6)[a,b,c]	28.4 (1.8)[a,b,c]
SV_{max}, ml/beat					
O	122.1 (21.7)	130.4 (19.4)[a]	133.2 (22.0)[a]	140.6 (21.5)[a,b,c]	140.2 (21.3)[a,b]
Y	137.3 (17.2)	144.7 (12.6)[a]	148.2 (15.2)[a]	154.6 (10.6)[a,b,c]	152.3 (12.6)[a,b]
Maximal a-vO_{2diff}, ml O_2/100 ml blood					
O	13.5 (2.2)	14.0 (2.2)[a]	14.2 (1.7)[a]	14.0 (1.9)	14.7 (2.1)[a]
Y	14.7 (0.9)	15.8 (1.2)[a]	15.4 (1.3)[a]	14.8 (1.4)	15.7 (0.9)[a]

Values are means (SD). PO_{peak}, peak power output; $\dot{V}o_{2\,max}$, maximal O_2 uptake; HR_{max}, maximal heart rate; $\dot{Q}_{max}$, maximal cardiac output; SV_{max}, maximal stroke volume; maximal a-vO_{2diff}, maximal arterial-venous O_2 difference.
[a]Significantly different from pretraining values ($P < 0.05$).
[b]Significantly different from *week 3* ($P < 0.05$).
[c]Significantly different from *week 6*.
[d]Significantly different from *week 9*.
[e]Significantly different from Y ($P < 0.05$).

output and maximal arteriovenous oxygen differences between the young and the old; a much larger sample would be needed to make this distinction with confidence. One of the important lessons from this report is that given a sufficiently rigorous training program, the elderly can enhance maximal oxygen intake by 31%, at least as large a percentage as seen in younger individuals.

R. J. Shephard, MD (Lond), PhD, DPE

Objective Light-Intensity Physical Activity Associations With Rated Health in Older Adults

Buman MP, Hekler EB, Haskell WL, et al (Stanford Univ School of Medicine, CA; et al)
Am J Epidemiol 172:1155-1165, 2010

The extent to which light-intensity physical activity contributes to health in older adults is not well known. The authors examined associations between physical activity across the intensity spectrum (sedentary to vigorous) and health and well-being variables in older adults. Two 7-day assessments of accelerometry from 2005 to 2007 were collected 6 months apart in the observational Senior Neighborhood Quality of Life Study of adults aged > 65 years in Baltimore, Maryland, and Seattle, Washington. Self-reported health and psychosocial variables (e.g., lower-extremity function, body weight, rated stress) were also collected. Physical activity based on existing accelerometer thresholds for moderate/vigorous, high-light, low-light, and sedentary categories were examined as correlates of physical health and psychosocial well-being in mixed-effects regression models. Participants ($N = 862$) were 75.4 (standard deviation, 6.8) years of age, 56% female, 71% white, and 58% overweight/obese. After adjustment for study covariates and time spent in moderate/vigorous physical activity and sedentary behavior, low-light and high-light physical activity were positively related to physical health (all $P < 0.0001$) and well-being (all $P < 0.001$). Additionally, replacing 30 minutes/day of sedentary time with equal amounts of low-light or high-light physical activity was associated with better physical health (all $P < 0.0001$). Objectively measured light-intensity physical activity is associated with physical health and well-being variables in older adults.

▶ There is strong evidence for the health benefits of moderate/vigorous physical activity (MVPA) and the disease-promoting effects of sedentary behavior.[1] Less is known about the effect of light-intensity activity (eg, easy walking) on health, an important issue for the elderly who find it difficult to initiate and maintain MVPA. In this study of older adults, time spent in physical activities at both the low-light physical activity (LLPA) and high-light physical activity (HLPA) levels of light intensity activity were positively associated with physical health and well-being. Replacing 30 minutes/day of sedentary time with an equal amount of LLPA, HLPA, or MVPA was associated with a higher physical health score. The physical health benefits of HLPA were in the same range as those for MVPA, and HLPA appeared to confer greater psychosocial well-being. Lighter intensity activities are more feasible and appealing to older adults than MVPA, and this study supports their substitution for sedentary time to promote health.

D. C. Nieman, DrPH

Reference

1. Patel AV, Bernstein L, Deka A, et al. Leisure time spent sitting in relation to total mortality in a prospective cohort of US adults. *Am J Epidemiol.* 2010;172:419-429.

Physical Activity at Midlife in Relation to Successful Survival in Women at Age 70 Years or Older
Sun Q, Townsend MK, Okereke OI, et al (Harvard School of Public Health, Boston, MA; Brigham and Women's Hosp and Harvard Med School, Boston, MA; et al)
Arch Intern Med 170:194-201, 2010

Background.—Physical activity is associated with reduced risks of chronic diseases and premature death. Whether physical activity is also associated with improved overall health among those who survive to older ages is unclear.

Methods.—A total of 13 535 Nurses' Health Study participants who were free of major chronic diseases at baseline in 1986 and had survived to age 70 years or older as of the 1995-2001 period made up the study population. We defined successful survival as no history of 10 major chronic diseases or coronary artery bypass graft surgery and no cognitive impairment, physical impairment, or mental health limitations.

Results.—After multivariate adjustment for covariates, higher physical activity levels at midlife, as measured by metabolic-equivalent tasks, were significantly associated with better odds of successful survival. Significant increases in successful survival were observed beginning at the third quintile of activity: odds ratios (ORs) (95% confidence intervals [CIs]) in the lowest to highest quintiles were 1 [Reference], 0.98 (0.80-1.20), 1.37 (1.13-1.65), 1.34 (1.11-1.61), and 1.99 (1.66-2.38) (P<.001 for trend). Increasing energy expenditure from walking was associated with a similar elevation in odds of successful survival: the ORs (95% CIs) of successful survival across quintiles of walking were 1 [Reference], 0.99 (0.80-1.21), 1.19 (0.97-1.45), 1.50 (1.24-1.82), and 1.47 (1.22-1.79) (P<.001 for trend).

Conclusion.—These data provide evidence that higher levels of midlife physical activity are associated with exceptional health status among women who survive to older ages and corroborate the potential role of physical activity in improving overall health (Table 2).

▶ The benefits of physical activity are often assessed in terms of a reduction in all-cause or disease-specific mortality (eg, in the classical studies of Paffenbarger et al[1,2]). The use of death certificates to identify the cause of death

TABLE 2.—Odds of Successful Survival Among Women 70 Years or Older in the Nurses' Health Study[22] by Physical Activity Level at Midlife

Characteristic	Total Physical Activity Quintile[a]					P Value for Trend[b]
	1 (Lowest)	2	3	4	5 (Highest)	
Activity level, METs (h/wk), median (range)	0.9 (0.2-2.3)	3.6 (2.4-5.1)	7.9 (5.2-11.4)	16.2 (11.5-22.8)	37.1 (≥22.9)	NA
Usual/successful survivors, No./No.	2603/213	2349/195	2466/307	2382/303	2279/438	NA
Age-adjusted model	1 [Reference]	1.01 (0.83-1.24)	1.53 (1.28-1.84)	1.57 (1.31-1.89)	2.39 (2.01-2.85)	<.001
Multivariate model 1[c]	1 [Reference]	0.98 (0.80-1.20)	1.37 (1.13-1.65)	1.34 (1.11-1.61)	1.99 (1.66-2.38)	<.001
Multivariate model 2[d]	1 [Reference]	0.96 (0.78-1.18)	1.30 (1.08-1.57)	1.25 (1.03-1.51)	1.76 (1.47-2.12)	<.001
Walking Quintile[a]						
Activity level, METs (h/wk), median (range)	0 (0-0.5)	2.0 (0.6-2.5)	3.0 (2.7-4.5)	7.5 (5.0-11.2)	20.0 (≥12.5)	NA
Usual/successful survivors, No./No.	2231/195	2536/230	2553/295	2423/379	2336/357	NA
Age-adjusted model	1 [Reference]	1.04 (0.86-1.28)	1.32 (1.09-1.60)	1.82 (1.52-2.18)	1.80 (1.50-2.17)	<.001
Multivariate model 1[c]	1 [Reference]	0.99 (0.80-1.21)	1.19 (0.97-1.45)	1.50 (1.24-1.82)	1.47 (1.22-1.79)	<.001
Multivariate model 2[d]	1 [Reference]	0.99 (0.80-1.22)	1.15 (0.94-1.40)	1.42 (1.17-1.72)	1.37 (1.10-1.67)	<.001

Abbreviations: BMI, body mass index (calculated as weight in kilograms divided by height in meters squared); CI, confidence interval; METs, metabolic-equivalent tasks (measured in hours per week; each MET-hour is the caloric need per kilogram of body weight per hour of activity divided by the caloric need per kilogram of weight per hour at rest); NA, not applicable.

Editor's Note: Please refer to original journal article for full references.

[a]Unless otherwise noted, data are reported as odds ratios (95% confidence intervals).

[b]Estimates of P value for linear trend are based on the medians of each physical activity category.

[c]Multivariate model was adjusted for age at baseline (in years); education (registered nurse, bachelor's degree, master's degree, or doctorate); if married, husband's education (less than high school, some high school, high school graduate, college graduate, or graduate school); marital status (unmarried, married, widow, separated, or divorced); smoking status (never, past, current 1-14 cigarettes/d or 15-24 cigarettes/d or ≥25 cigarettes/d); family history of heart disease, diabetes, or cancer (yes or no); postmenopausal hormone use (never, past, or current use); dietary polyunsaturated to saturated fat ratio (in quintiles); intakes of trans fat, alcohol, and cereal fiber (all in quintiles); and intakes of fruits and vegetables and red meat (in tertiles). For walking METs, vigorous physical activity METs were further adjusted.

[d]Further adjusted for BMI category (<18.5, 18.5-22.9, 23.0-24.9, or ≥25.0), history of hypertension (yes or no), and history of hypercholesterolemia (yes or no).

seemingly gives validity to the relationships thus established. However, as medical advances permit survival to an ever greater age, a problem arises from the fact that a specific, internationally accepted, immediate cause of death must always be reported, although in fact many old people are really dying of old age. The main health benefits of physical activity are seen in the prevention of a fatal heart attack at the age of 50 rather than the avoidance of a fatal abnormality of cardiac rhythm at the age of 95. From the practical viewpoint, the important question is whether midlife physical activity will enhance quality of life and the prospects of disease- and disability-free survival,[3-5] and in this regard, the evidence is more equivocal, particularly if multivariate analysis adjusts for some of the likely mediators of the benefits of physical activity.[6] Sun and associates examine this question further, using data from the Nurses Health Study, a prospective evaluation of 13 535 initially disease-free registered nurses from the Eastern United States who entered the investigation when aged 30 to 55 years and have now been followed for 10 or more years. Physical activity in metabolic-equivalent task (MET)-hours per week was assessed by a detailed questionnaire. Self-reports of successful, disease-free, and healthy aging to 70 years (found in only about 10% of the sample) were strongly associated with habitual physical activity after adjustment for confounding factors (Table 2); benefit was seen in the third to fifth quintiles (those practicing an average of more than 7.9 MET-hours of activity per week) but not in the second quintile (those averaging 3.6 MET-hours per week). The implication is that benefit is first seen with somewhere between 1.2 and 2.6 hours of moderate activity (>3 METs) per week, in line with many currently recommended minimum amounts of physical activity. Benefit was also more likely to be observed in those who walked rapidly. Interestingly, the optimal body mass index (BMI) for successful aging was lower than in some previous mortality-based reports (18.5-22.9 kg/m^2), although physical activity did benefit the prognosis of those with a higher BMI.

R. J. Shephard, MD (Lond), PhD, DPE

References

1. Paffenbarger RS Jr, Hyde RT, Wing AL, Lee IM, Jung DL, Kampert JB. The association of changes in physical activity level and other lifestyle characteristics with mortality among men. *N Engl J Med*. 1993;328:538-545.
2. Paffenbarger RT, Hyde RT, Wing AL, et al. Some inter-relationships of physical activity, physiological fitness, health and longevity. In: Bouchard C, Shephard RJ, Stephens T, eds. *Physical Activity, Fitness and Health*. Champaign, IL: Human Kinetics; 1994:119-133.
3. Newman AB, Arnold AM, Naydeck BL, et al. Cardiovascular Health Study Research Group. "Successful aging": effect of subclinical cardiovascular disease. *Arch Intern Med*. 2003;163:2315-2322.
4. Vaillant GE, Mukamal K. Successful aging. *Am J Psychiatry*. 2001;158:839-847.
5. He XZ, Baker DW. Body mass index, physical activity, and the risk of decline in overall health and physical functioning in late middle age. *Am J Public Health*. 2004;94:1567-1573.
6. Willcox BJ, He Q, Chen R, et al. Midlife risk factors and healthy survival in men. *JAMA*. 2006;296:2343-2350.

Exercise Effects on Risk Factors and Health Care Costs in the Elderly. Final Results of the Senior Fitness and Prevention Study (SEFIP)

Kemmler W, von Stengel S, Mayer S, et al (Friedrich-Alexander Universität Erlangen-Nürnberg, Germany)
Dtsch Z Sportmed 61:264-269, 2010

Physical exercise positively affects many risk factors and diseases of the elderly and may thus reduce health costs. The aim of this study was to determine whether a single exercise program positively affects health care costs and important risk factors of community-living elderly females. 246 females (69.1 ± 4.0 yrs) living independently in the area of Erlangen-Nürnberg (Germany) were randomly assigned either to a multi-purpose exercise program with special emphasis on exercise intensity (EG, n=123) or to a low intensity, low frequency program that primarily focused on well-being (CG, n=123). Beside total health care costs (HCC), fracture, coronary-heart-disease (CHD) and sarcopenia risk-factors were assessed. Significant exercise effects were observed for BMD of the lumbar spine (EG: $1.8 \pm 2.7\%$ vs. CG: $0.3 \pm 3.1\%$, p<0.001) femoral neck (EG: $1.0 \pm 3.3\%$ vs. CG: $-1.1 \pm 3.3\%$, p<0.001) and fall rate/18 months (EG: 1.00 ± 1.3 vs. CG: 1.66 ± 1.8, p $= 0.002$). Appendicular skeletal muscle mass also significantly differed between both groups (EG: 0.02 ± 0.76 vs. CG: -0.28 ± 0.91 kg, p<0.007). Despite different changes (EG: -12% vs. CG: $\pm 0\%$) no significant differences (p=0.07) between both groups were observed for Metabolic Symbol prevalence. Cost benefit analysis did not show significant differences between the groups (EG: 2255 ± 2596 € vs. CG: 2780 ± 3318 €/18 months, p=.20). Our exercise program positively affects central risk factors of the elderly; however, improvements were not directly reflected in HCC. Future studies should address this issue with more adequate cohorts or/and higher statistical power.

▶ Many investigators today unfortunately ignore articles that are written in foreign languages, often because they lack the necessary linguistic skills to read material in languages other than English. It is true that some investigators submit their first-rank material to North American journals, but interesting articles sometimes appear in journals from other nations, and there is much to commend the practice of the University of London, which at least in my student days required the ability to read, translate, and understand scientific articles in at least 2 foreign languages before a student was awarded a bachelor's degree in physiology. The study of Kemmler and associates explores by a controlled prospective trial a question of considerable practical importance, the impact of an exercise programme on health care costs in elderly women (a substantial group of 246 independently living females with an average initial age of 69 years). Those assigned to the training group undertook a 60-minute activity programme twice a week for 18 months; their classes included 20 minutes of aerobic activity at 70% of peak effort and an isometric training routine, whereas the control group merely participated in four 10 week blocks of wellness programming over the same period. The actual health care costs of the 2 groups were ascertained from Bavarian Health Funding and a health fund operated by the Siemens Company. The authors concluded that the exercisers did not incur smaller health care costs, but their data show a trend to a substantial difference (2255 vs 2780€, a difference of about $715, Fig 1 in the original article). Although not statistically significant ($P = .20$), the trend is in keeping with previous studies from our laboratory,[1-4] and the study merits repeating on a larger sample of subjects, preferably with a more demanding exercise programme.

R. J. Shephard, MD (Lond), PhD, DPE

References

1. Shephard RJ, Corey P, Renzland P, Cox M. The influence of an employee fitness and lifestyle modification program upon medical care costs. *Can J Public Health*. 1982;73:259-263.
2. Shephard RJ, Corey P, Renzland P, Cox M. The impact of changes in fitness and lifestyle upon health care utilization. *Can J Public Health*. 1983;74:51-54.
3. Katzmarzyk PT, Gledhill N, Shephard RJ. The economic burden of physical inactivity in Canada. *CMAJ*. 2000;163:1435-1440.
4. Aoyagi Y, Shephard RJ. A model to estimate the potential for a physical activity-induced reduction in health care costs for the elderly, based on pedometer/accelerometer data from the Nakanojo Study. *Sports Med*. In press.

Does physical activity reduce seniors' need for healthcare?: a study of 24 281 Canadians
Woolcott JC, PACC Research Team (Univ of British Columbia, Vancouver, Canada; et al)
Br J Sports Med 44:902-904, 2010

Objectives.—Physical inactivity has been associated with significant increases in disease morbidity and mortality. This study assessed the association between physical activity and (1) health resource use and (2) health resource use costs.

Design and Participants.—The responses from 24 281 respondents >65 years to the Canadian Community Health Survey Cycle 1.1 were used to find activity levels and determine health resource use and costs. Logistic regression models were used to assess risks of hospitalisation.

Results.—Physical inactivity was associated with statistically significant increases to hospitalisations, lengths of stay and healthcare visits (p<0.01). Average healthcare costs (based on the 2007 value of the Canadian dollar) for the physically inactive were $C1214.15 higher than the healthcare costs of the physically active ($C2005.27 vs $C791.12, p<0.01).

Conclusion.—Among those >65 years, physical activity is strongly associated with reduced health resource use and costs (Table 3).

▶ Most older adults are physically inactive, a perplexing public health problem that exists despite strong evidence for the beneficial effects of physical activity

TABLE 3.—Total Health Resource Use Cost by Activity Level

Weekly Physical Activity Level, kcal/wk (kj/wk)	Mean (95% CI), $C
0–499 (0–2089)	2069.82 (1890.65 to 2301.30)
500–999 (2090–4186)	1155.45 (1079.54 to 1622.43)
1000–1499 (4187–6276)	982.65 (940.89 to 1101.60)
1500–1999 (6277–8369)	769.79 (720.12 to 883.75)
>2000 (>8370)	843.12 (613.05 to 877.48)

on quality of life and prevention of disease.[1] In this large group of elderly Canadians, the risk of hospitalization for inactive individuals was almost twice as great, with longer lengths of stay, when compared with that of those who were physically active (1000 kcal/wk or more). Furthermore, the health resource use costs of inactive versus active seniors were more than 2.5 times greater. As summarized in Table 3, when stratifying costs by physical activity, health resource use costs decreased with increase in levels of activity. The authors urged that physical activity promotion be given more attention among the elderly to decrease health resource use and their related costs.

D. C. Nieman, DrPH

Reference

1. Motl RW, McAuley E. Physical activity, disability, and quality of life in older adults. *Phys Med Rehabil Clin N Am.* 2010;21:299-308.

Does physical activity reduce seniors' need for healthcare?: a study of 24 281 Canadians

Woolcott JC, PACC Research Team (Univ of British Columbia, Vancouver, Canada; et al)
Br J Sports Med 44:902-904, 2010

Objectives.—Physical inactivity has been associated with significant increases in disease morbidity and mortality. This study assessed the association between physical activity and (1) health resource use and (2) health resource use costs.

Design and Participants.—The responses from 24 281 respondents >65 years to the Canadian Community Health Survey Cycle 1.1 were used to find activity levels and determine health resource use and costs. Logistic regression models were used to assess risks of hospitalisation.

Results.—Physical inactivity was associated with statistically significant increases to hospitalisations, lengths of stay and healthcare visits (p<0.01). Average healthcare costs (based on the 2007 value of the Canadian dollar) for the physically inactive were $C1214.15 higher than the healthcare costs of the physically active ($C2005.27 vs $C791.12, p<0.01).

TABLE 3.—Total Health Resource Use Cost By Activity Level

Weekly Physical Activity Level, kcal/wk (kj/wk)	Mean (95% CI), $C
0–499 (0–2089)	2069.82 (1890.65 to 2301.30)
500–999 (2090–4186)	1155.45 (1079.54 to 1622.43)
1000–1499 (4187–6276)	982.65 (940.89 to 1101.60)
1500–1999 (6277–8369)	769.79 (720.12 to 883.75)
>2000 (>8370)	843.12 (613.05 to 877.48)

Conclusion.—Among those >65 years, physical activity is strongly associated with reduced health resource use and costs (Table 3).

▶ The article by Woolcott and associates makes an interesting cross-sectional estimate of health and medical care expenses among a representative sample of Canadian seniors older than 65 years, based on the length and duration of their leisure activities, as reported in a telephone survey. The overall sample was large (24 281 respondents), but more than 75% reported no leisure activity. As might be expected, the most important source of medical expense was hospital admission, at almost $600 per day. Those who were inactive had both a greater relative risk of hospital admission (1.84) and a longer average length of stay (3.18 vs 0.82 days) relative to those who were active. Subjects were classified in terms of their estimated weekly leisure energy expenditures, and there was surprisingly little difference in costs between those grossing 2.1 to 4.2 MJ per week and those spending more than 8.4 MJ per week (Table 3). This may be because benefits of being active tend to plateau, but it may also reflect the limitations of the few questions that were asked about weekly activities. (These are unlikely to have done more than make a crude comparison of behaviors between individuals.) One important item omitted from overall costing is the likelihood of an early loss of independence among seniors who are inactive.[1] Because the study is cross-sectional in design, it is possible that ill health caused physical inactivity rather than the converse. Furthermore, even if the relationship is indeed causal, there is no guarantee that greater physical activity would improve the health of those who are presently inactive or that any individual health care savings would reduce overall national medical expenditures.

R. J. Shephard, MD (Lond), PhD, DPE

Reference

1. Shephard RJ, Montelpare W. Geriatric benefits of exercise as an adult. *J Gerontol.* 1988;43:M86-M90.

Former Athletes' Health-Related Lifestyle Behaviours and Self-Rated Health in Late Adulthood

Bäckmand H, Kujala U, Sarna S, et al (Natl Inst for Health and Welfare (THL), Helsinki, Finland; Univ of Jyväskylä, Finland; Univ of Helsinki, Finland)
Int J Sports Med 31:751-758, 2010

The aim of this study was to examine the associations between self-rated health (SRH), physical activity and other lifestyle habits among former athletes and referents in late adulthood. Male athletes (N = 514) who represented Finland from 1920 through 1965 and referents (N = 368) who were classified healthy at the age of 20 years participated in this population-based cohort study. The present analysis was based on a questionnaire study in 2001. SRH was assessed by a single question. Univariate binary and multivariate logistic regression analyses were used to examine the associations of health-related behaviours with SRH. The majority of former athletes (64%) rated their health better than referents (48%). A higher percentage of the athletes (54%) compared to the referents (44%) belonged to the most physically active groups (MET quintiles IV-V). A high percentage of the athletes (77%) and referents (79%) were occasional or moderate alcohol users. The proportion of never smokers among athletes was 59% and among referents 37%. Among current smokers there were no differences in nicotine dependence between athletes and referents (p = 0.07). In the univariate analysis the odds of reporting good SRH was 2 times higher for athletes (OR 2.01, 95% CI 1.53-2.64, p < 0.001) than for referents. In multivariate logistic regression analysis, former participation in team and power athletic groups had significantly higher SRH than the referents even after adjusting for age, level of physical activity, alcohol and smoking habit, and occupation. People who participated in very active physical exercise in their youth, as indexed by participation in competitive sports by elite athletes, continue a physically active lifestyle, and maintained healthier lifestyle. They had significantly higher SRH than the referents in their senior years, which was not totally explained by their physically active and healthier lifestyles (Table 4).

▶ Sarna and colleagues have made a number of valuable long-term follow-up studies of Finnish athletes.[1] Some studies from the United States, such as those conducted by Henry Montoye and colleagues,[2] have suggested that once their formal athletic careers are ended, university athletic letter winners become more obese and have a poorer lifestyle than their noncompetitive peers. However, Sarna and Kaprio[1] found that top competitors retained an advantage of lifespan relative to their nonathletic counterparts. This case-control study focuses on lifestyle and self-reported health of initially healthy athletic and nonathletic cohorts, followed into their 70s and 80s. Given the longer lifespan of the athletic cohort and knowing the relationship between self-reported health and lifespan,[3] it is not surprising that more of the athletes than the controls had a good perception of their health (Table 4). This cannot be explained entirely by such lifestyle factors as a better diet and a smaller proportion of smokers in the athletic group; it seems that continuing physical activity and

TABLE 4.—Multivariate Logistic Regression Analysis of Odds Ratio (OR) and 95 % Confidence Intervals (CI) for Self-Rated Health#. The Outcome is Good Self-Rated Health in 2001

Dependent Variables		Number of Subject, (%)	Odds Ratio (with 95 % Confidence Intervals)	p-Value*	Cumulative R^2
good self-rated health					
age	≤ 64 years	259, (36.3)	2.44 (1.42−4.20)	0.001	0.034
	65−74 years	344, (48.2)	2.38 (1.43−3.97)	0.001	
	(age, ≥ 75 years ref.)	111, (15.5)	1.00		
sports	endurance sports	74, (10.4)	1.75 (0.93−3.30)	0.081	0.090
	power sports	174, (24.4)	1.69 (1.08−2.63)	0.021	
	team sports	177, (24.8)	1.63 (1.04−2.58)	0.034	
	(sports, referents ref.)	289, (40.4)	1.00		
lifestyle					
physical	MET quintile 2^	136, (19.0)	2.15 (1.26−3.67)	0.005	0.209
activity	MET quintile 3^	86, (12.2)	5.27 (2.71−10.23)	< 0.001	
	MET quintile 4^	258, (36.1)	3.28 (2.02−5.32)	< 0.001	
	MET quintile 5^	101, (14.1)	5.28 (2.74−10.17)	< 0.001	
	(MET quintile 1^ ref.)	133, (18.6)	1.00		
alcohol	abstainers	84, (11.8)	1.25 (0.60−2.60)	0.552	
consumption	occasional users	350, (49.0)	1.74 (0.96−3.14)	0.066	
	moderate users	207, (29.0)	2.12 (1.14−3.92)	0.017	
	(alcohol, heavy users ref.)	73, (10.2)	1.00		
smoking	never smoked	351, (49.2)	1.70 (1.01−2.86)	0.047	
	ex-smoker	265, (37.1)	1.33 (0.79−2.23)	0.290	
	(smoke, current smoker ref.)	98, (13.7)	1.00		
anthropometric data					
body mass	BMI ≤ 24.99	256, (35.9)	1.63 (0.95−2.80)	0.077	0.215
index	BMI 25.00−29.99	353, (49.4)	1.37 (0.84−2.26)	0.208	
	(BMI ≥ 30.00 ref.)	105, (14.7)	1.00		
marital status					
	married	593, (83.1)	0.90 (0.58−1.42)	0.663	0.215
	(marital status, unmarried ref.)	121, (16.9)	1.00		
socioeconomic status					
	executives	138, (19.3)	1.50 (0.91−2.47)	0.115	0.237
	skilled workers	240, (33.6)	0.66 (0.44−0.98)	0.038	
	unskilled workers	14, (2.0)	0.34 (0.10−1.11)	0.073	
	agricultural workers	52, (7.3)	0.79 (0.39−1.57)	0.496	
	(socioeconomics status, clerical workers ref.)	270, (37.8)	1.00		

*Wald's test.
^Metabolic equivalent (MET) index was calculated by assigning a multiple of resting metabolic rate to each activity and calculating the product of intensity x duration x frequency.
#In multivariate logistic regression analysis, the explanatory factors were introduced in 6 separate blocks of variables (1) age, 2) sporting group / the former athletes vs. referents, 3) lifestyle; MET quintiles, use of alcohol and tobacco, 4) BMI, 5) marital, and 6) socioeconomic status), all forced in the model.

possibly other less easily determined factors, such as a higher social status and differences of personality and genotype, contribute to their better-perceived health. In old age, former power and team athletes were less active than endurance competitors, but at least as assessed by questionnaires, they still had a significantly greater average level of physical activity than their nonathletic peers.

R. J. Shephard, MD (Lond), PhD, DPE

References

1. Sarna S, Kaprio J. Life expectancy of former elite athletes. *Sports Med.* 1994;17: 149-151.
2. Montoye HJ, Van Huss WD, Olson HW, Person WO, Hudec AJ. *The longevity and morbidity of college athletes.* Lansing, MI: Michigan State University; 1957.
3. Idler EL, Benyamyi Y. Self-rated health and mortality: a review of twenty-seven community studies. *J Health Soc Behav.* 1997;38:21-37.

Objectively measured physical capability levels and mortality: systematic review and meta-analysis
Cooper R, Mortality Review Group on behalf of the FALCon and HALCyon study teams (Univ College London, UK)
BMJ 341:c4467, 2010

Objective.—To do a quantitative systematic review, including published and unpublished data, examining the associations between individual objective measures of physical capability (grip strength, walking speed, chair rising, and standing balance times) and mortality in community dwelling populations.

Design.—Systematic review and meta-analysis.

Data sources.—Relevant studies published by May 2009 identified through literature searches using Embase (from 1980) and Medline (from 1950) and manual searching of reference lists; unpublished results were obtained from study investigators.

Study Selection.—Eligible observational studies were those done in community dwelling people of any age that examined the association of at least one of the specified measures of physical capability (grip strength, walking speed, chair rises, or standing balance) with mortality.

Data Synthesis.—Effect estimates obtained were pooled by using random effects meta-analysis models with heterogeneity between studies investigated.

Results.—Although heterogeneity was detected, consistent evidence was found of associations between all four measures of physical capability and mortality; those people who performed less well in these tests were found to be at higher risk of all cause mortality. For example, the summary hazard ratio for mortality comparing the weakest with the strongest quarter of grip strength (14 studies, 53 476 participants) was 1.67 (95% confidence interval 1.45 to 1.93) after adjustment for age, sex, and body size (I^2=84.0%, 95% confidence interval 74% to 90%; P from Q statistic <0.001). The summary hazard ratio for mortality comparing the slowest with the fastest quarter of walking speed (five studies, 14 692 participants) was 2.87 (2.22 to 3.72) (I^2=25.2%, 0% to 70%; P=0.25) after similar adjustments. Whereas studies of the associations of walking speed, chair rising, and standing balance with mortality have only been done in older populations (average age over 70 years), the association of grip strength

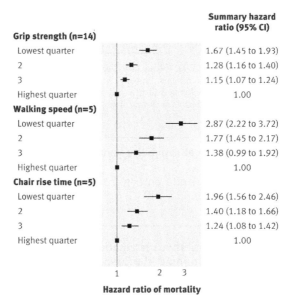

FIGURE 5.—Summary hazard ratios of mortality from meta-analyses comparing each quarter of grip strength, walking speed, and chair rise time with highest quarter, including results adjusted for age, sex (where appropriate), and body size (n=number of data points included in meta-analysis). (Reprinted from Cooper R, Mortality Review Group on behalf of the FALCon and HALCyon study teams. Objectively measured physical capability levels and mortality: systematic review and meta-analysis. *BMJ*. 2010;341:c4467, reproduced with permission from the BMJ Publishing Group Ltd.)

with mortality was also found in younger populations (five studies had an average age under 60 years).

Conclusions.—Objective measures of physical capability are predictors of all cause mortality in older community dwelling populations. Such measures may therefore provide useful tools for identifying older people at higher risk of death (Fig 5).

▶ This meta-analysis draws together up to 14 studies examining relationships between physical capability and mortality, with a total of up to 53 476 participants. Where appropriate, unpublished studies were also included in the analysis to minimize the risk of a positive publication bias. As might be expected from individual, smaller studies, such indices of physical ability as grip strength, walking speed, speed of rising from a chair, and standing balance were all positively correlated with survival after adjustment for the individual's age, size, and body build (Fig 5). The problem with the demonstration of such associations is to know whether poor initial health compromised test performance or whether poor physical performance scores were indeed true harbingers of subsequent mortality. With the exception of grip strength, the data analyzed were collected almost exclusively in old or very old people. The studies of grip strength in some cases had a follow-up period of 20 years or more, and here it is difficult to believe that poor survival could be explained in terms of poor initial ill health.

The analysis may have been compromised to some extent by important unmeasured covariates; for instance, socioeconomic status is an important determinant of survival in many countries. There seems a need for further studies of this type, with data collection beginning at a much earlier age and a preliminary period of several years of observation being allowed to eliminate from the analysis those with incipient disease.

R. J. Shephard, MD (Lond), PhD, DPE

Exercise Capacity and Mortality in Older Men: A 20-Year Follow-up Study
Kokkinos P, Myers J, Faselis C, et al (Veterans Affairs Med Ctr, Washington, DC; Veterans Affairs Palo Alto Health Care System, CA; et al)
Circulation 122:790-797, 2010

Background.—Epidemiological findings, based largely on middle-aged populations, support an inverse and independent association between exercise capacity and mortality risk. The information available in older individuals is limited.

Methods and Results.—Between 1986 and 2008, we assessed the association between exercise capacity and all-cause mortality in 5314 male veterans aged 65 to 92 years (mean ± SD, 71.4 ± 5.0 years) who completed an exercise test at the Veterans Affairs Medical Centers in Washington, DC, and Palo Alto, Calif. We established fitness categories based on peak metabolic equivalents (METs) achieved. During a median 8.1 years of follow-up (range, 0.1 to 25.3), there were 2137 deaths. Baseline exercise capacity was 6.3 ± 2.4 METs among survivors and 5.3 ± 2.0 METs in those who died ($P<0.001$) and emerged as a strong predictor of mortality. For each 1-MET increase in exercise capacity, the adjusted hazard for death was 12% lower (hazard ratio=0.88; confidence interval, 0.86 to 0.90). Compared with the least fit individuals (≤4 METs), the mortality risk was 38% lower for those who achieved 5.1 to 6.0 METs (hazard ratio=0.62; confidence interval, 0.54 to 0.71) and progressively declined to 61% (hazard ratio=0.39; confidence interval, 0.32 to 0.49) for those who achieved >9 METs, regardless of age. Unfit individuals who improved their fitness status with serial testing had a 35% lower mortality risk (hazard ratio=0.65; confidence interval, 0.46 to 0.93) compared with those who remained unfit.

Conclusions.—Exercise capacity is an independent predictor of all-cause mortality in older men. The relationship is inverse and graded, with most survival benefits achieved in those with an exercise capacity >5 METs. Survival improved significantly when unfit individuals became fit (Table 3).

▶ It is widely accepted that in middle-aged adults, fitness level is a good predictor of prognosis, particularly the risk of all-cause mortality.[1-3] However, it is a little less clear whether vigorous physical activity extends longevity in the final 2 decades of life, and at least 1 report has suggested that at this

TABLE 3.—Mortality Risk Hazard Ratios for Exercise Capacity of Entire Cohort and the 2 Age Categories

Variables	No. of Deaths	Hazard Ratio	95% CI	P
All participants (n=5314)	2137			
Exercise capacity (for each 1-MET increment), unadjusted model		0.87	0.84−0.88	<0.001
Exercise capacity (for each 1-MET increment) adjusted for age, BMI, resting BP, race, cardiovascular risk factors,* cardiovascular medications,† and CVD‡		0.88	0.86−0.90	<0.001
Group aged 65−70 y (n=2560)	953			
Exercise capacity (for each 1-MET increment), unadjusted model		0.87	0.85−0.90	<0.001
Exercise capacity (for each 1-MET increment) adjusted for age, BMI, resting BP, race, cardiovascular risk factors, cardiovascular medications, and CVD		0.88	0.85−0.90	<0.001
Group aged >70 y (n=2754)	1184			
Exercise capacity (for each 1-MET increment), unadjusted model		0.86	0.83−89	<0.001
Exercise capacity (for each 1-MET increment) adjusted for age, BMI, resting BP, race, cardiovascular risk factors, cardiovascular medications, and CVD		0.88	0.85−0.91	<0.001

*Cardiovascular risk factors include hypertension, diabetes mellitus, dyslipidemia, and smoking.
†Cardiovascular medications include β-blockers, calcium channel blockers, angiotensin-converting enzyme inhibitors, diuretics, nitrates, vasodilators, aspirin, and statins.
‡CVD includes documented coronary artery disease, cardiac surgery for coronary artery disease, myocardial infarction, stroke, heart failure, and peripheral vascular disease.

stage in life, there may be a small negative effect.[4] This 8-year prospective study of US male veterans aged 65 to 92 years suggested some advantage to more active members of the group, although the advantage (a 12% decrease in the risk of dying per 1 metabolic equivalent [MET] advantage in a treadmill ramp test) remained substantial (Table 3), particularly in individuals with initial values >5 METs (equivalent to a peak oxygen transport of 17.5 mL/ [kg min]). It could be argued that much of the observed mortality was because of pre-existing disease, which also reduced the patient's initial exercise tolerance (ie, a reverse causality). However, the authors' findings were not substantially modified when they excluded those who died in the first 2 years of observation, those with a body mass index less than 20 kg/m^2, and those unable to reach 85% of their theoretical maximal heart rate at the initial testing. Moreover, benefit was seen in those who were unfit initially but subsequently improved their fitness status. These observations strengthen the view that exercise should be encouraged, irrespective of a patient's age. However, the authors neglect the even more important contributions of regular physical activity to successful aging, the maintenance of quality of life and independence.[5]

R. J. Shephard, MD (Lond), PhD, DPE

References

1. Kokkinos P, Myers J, Kokkinos JP, et al. Exercise capacity and mortality in black and white men. *Circulation.* 2008;117:614-622.
2. Blair SN, Kampert JB, Kohl HW III, et al. Influences of cardiorespiratory fitness and other precursors on cardiovascular disease and all-cause mortality in men and women. *JAMA.* 1996;276:205-210.
3. Myers J, Prakash M, Froelicher V, Do D, Partington S, Atwood JE. Exercise capacity and mortality among men referred for exercise testing. *N Engl J Med.* 2002;346:793-801.
4. Linsted KD, Tonstad K, Kuzma JW. Self-reports of physical activity and patterns of mortality in Seventh-Day Adventist men. *J Clin Epidemiol.* 1991;44:355-364.
5. Shephard RJ. *Aging, Physical Activity and Health.* Champaign, IL: Human Kinetics; 1997.

Exercise Capacity and Mortality in Older Men: A 20-Year Follow-Up Study
Kokkinos P, Myers J, Faselis C, et al (Veterans Affairs Med Ctr, Washington, DC; Veterans Affairs Palo Alto Health Care System, CA; et al)
Circulation 122:790-797, 2010

Background.—Epidemiological findings, based largely on middle-aged populations, support an inverse and independent association between exercise capacity and mortality risk. The information available in older individuals is limited.

Methods and Results.—Between 1986 and 2008, we assessed the association between exercise capacity and all-cause mortality in 5314 male veterans aged 65 to 92 years (mean ± SD, 71.4 ± 5.0 years) who completed an exercise test at the Veterans Affairs Medical Centers in Washington, DC, and Palo Alto, Calif. We established fitness categories based on peak metabolic equivalents (METs) achieved. During a median 8.1 years of follow-up (range, 0.1 to 25.3), there were 2137 deaths. Baseline exercise capacity was 6.3 ± 2.4 METs among survivors and 5.3 ± 2.0 METs in those who died ($P<0.001$) and emerged as a strong predictor of mortality. For each 1-MET increase in exercise capacity, the adjusted hazard for death was 12% lower (hazard ratio=0.88; confidence interval, 0.86 to 0.90). Compared with the least fit individuals (≤4 METs), the mortality risk was 38% lower for those who achieved 5.1 to 6.0 METs (hazard ratio=0.62; confidence interval, 0.54 to 0.71) and progressively declined to 61% (hazard ratio=0.39; confidence interval, 0.32 to 0.49) for those who achieved >9METs, regardless of age. Unfit individuals who improved their fitness status with serial testing had a 35% lower mortality risk (hazard ratio=0.65; confidence interval, 0.46 to 0.93) compared with those who remained unfit.

Conclusions.—Exercise capacity is an independent predictor of all-cause mortality in older men. The relationship is inverse and graded, with most survival benefits achieved in those with an exercise capacity >5 METs. Survival improved significantly when unfit individuals became fit.

▶ Exercise capacity has been associated with decreased all-cause and cardiovascular disease (CVD) mortality in middle-aged adults, primarily males, but Kokkinos and colleagues provide compelling evidence that the exercise-mortality association persists into old age and that becoming fit in old age reduces mortality risk. They compiled 20 years of exercise test results from more than 5000 male veterans of the armed forces, aged 65 to 92 years. The men were referred for exercise tolerance testing as a part of routine medical care or suspected exercise-induced ischemia. For this study, cases were excluded by history of diagnosed cardiac or vascular disease. Peak exercise capacity was determined by total test time using treadmill protocols at 2 Department of Veterans Affairs locations. Peak metabolic equivalent tasks (METs) were estimated from peak test time using published equations. In an improvement from previous studies, the large size of the cohort allowed for peak METs to be categorized into 1-MET increment (from ≤4 METs to ≥9 METs) and for comparisons to be made by age groups (65-70 years and >70 years). The risk of all-cause mortality was about 13% lower for each 1-MET increment in exercise capacity, which remained stable after adjustment for confounders such as the presence of CVD, cardiovascular medications, and risk factors. There was a break point in the hazard ratios for mortality across fitness categories such that mortality was progressively lower when exercise capacity was above 5.0 METs (Fig 1 in the original article). When comparing the least fit (≤4 METs; lowest 20th percentile rank of the sample) with the other fitness categories, mortality risk decreased from 32% to 63% in the 65- to 70-year age group and 45% to 60% in the older group. Reverse causality was investigated by repeating the analyses after exclusion of men who may have been in poor health at the time of the test (ie, died within 2 years of the follow-up; did not achieve 85% of age-predicted maximum heart rate). The association between exercise capacity and mortality risk was unchanged in the face of these analyses. Perhaps the most unique results came from a subset analysis of change in fitness in 867 men who had 2 treadmill tests at least 6 months apart. Men were classified as unfit (≤5 METs) or fit (>5 METs) using the baseline test and then reclassified using the follow-up test. Two key points emerged. Men who were initially unfit and became fit had a 35% lower mortality risk compared with men who were unfit at both test periods. Individuals who were fit and became unfit had a lower mortality risk than men who were unfit at both evaluations. Thus, becoming more fit in later life has benefits, and being fit helps to keep mortality risk lower if fitness slides. The least favorable outcome was to be unfit and stay unfit later in life. The authors propose that a fitness level greater than 5 METs can be achieved through 20 to 40 minutes of moderate daily exercise. Although this is sound advice, an intervention study would be needed to confirm the efficacy of this approach. The 2 main limitations of this very important study were that only men were included in the analyses and there were no measures of physical activity.

C. M. Jankowski, PhD

Exercise Capacity and Mortality in Older Men: A 20-Year Follow-up Study
Kokkinos P, Myers J, Faselis C, et al (Veterans Affairs Med Ctr, Washington, DC; Veterans Affairs Palo Alto Health Care System, CA; et al)
Circulation 122:790-797, 2010

Background.—Epidemiological findings, based largely on middle-aged populations, support an inverse and independent association between exercise capacity and mortality risk. The information available in older individuals is limited.

Methods and Results.—Between 1986 and 2008, we assessed the association between exercise capacity and all-cause mortality in 5314 male veterans aged 65 to 92 years (mean ± SD, 71.4 ± 5.0 years) who completed an exercise test at the Veterans Affairs Medical Centers in Washington, DC, and Palo Alto, Calif. We established fitness categories based on peak metabolic equivalents (METs) achieved. During a median 8.1 years of follow-up (range, 0.1 to 25.3), there were 2137 deaths. Baseline exercise capacity was 6.3 ± 2.4 METs among survivors and 5.3 ± 2.0 METs in those who died ($P<0.001$) and emerged as a strong predictor of mortality. For each 1-MET increase in exercise capacity, the adjusted hazard for death was 12% lower (hazard ratio=0.88; confidence interval, 0.86 to 0.90). Compared with the least fit individuals ($\leq$4 METs), the mortality risk was 38% lower for those who achieved 5.1 to 6.0 METs (hazard ratio=0.62; confidence interval, 0.54 to 0.71) and progressively declined to 61% (hazard ratio=0.39; confidence interval, 0.32 to 0.49) for those who achieved >9 METs, regardless of age. Unfit individuals who improved their fitness status with serial testing had a 35% lower mortality risk (hazard ratio=0.65; confidence interval, 0.46 to 0.93) compared with those who remained unfit.

Conclusions.—Exercise capacity is an independent predictor of all-cause mortality in older men. The relationship is inverse and graded, with most survival benefits achieved in those with an exercise capacity >5 METs. Survival improved significantly when unfit individuals became fit.

▶ Few studies have examined the health and disease prevention benefits of physical fitness in older populations. These data support a strong inverse graded association between exercise capacity (especially 5 metabolic equivalents [METS] and higher) and mortality risk in subjects 65 years of age and older. The 5-MET level of fitness is achievable by most older individuals through 20 to 40 minutes of moderate daily exercise, such as brisk walking.

The US population is aging, and the association between physical fitness capacity and mortality in older individuals reported in this study is of particular public health significance. The authors emphasize that "these results support the concept that exercise capacity should be given as much attention by clinicians as other major risk factors. Thus, physicians and other healthcare professionals should encourage older individuals to initiate and maintain a physically active lifestyle consisting of moderate-intensity activities (brisk walking or similar activities) at any age. Such programs are likely to improve exercise capacity and lower the risk of mortality in older individuals."

D. C. Nieman, DrPH

Trail Making Test Predicts Physical Impairment and Mortality in Older Persons

Vazzana R, Bandinelli S, Lauretani F, et al (Univ "G. D' Annunzio," Chieti, Italy; Azienda Sanitaria di Firenze, Florence, Italy; Tuscany Health Regional Agency, Florence, Italy; et al)

J Am Geriatr Soc 58:719-723, 2010

Objectives.—To examine whether performance in the Trail Making Test (TMT) predicts mobility impairment and mortality in older persons.

Design.—Prospective cohort study.

Setting.—Community-dwelling older persons enrolled in the Invecchiare in Chianti (InCHIANTI) Study.

Participants.—Five hundred eighty-three participants aged 65 and older and free of major cognitive impairment (Mini-Mental State Examination score >21) with baseline data on TMT performance. Of these, 427 performed the Short Physical Performance Battery (SPPB) for the assessment of lower extremity function at baseline and after 6 years. Of the initial 583 participants, 106 died during a 9-year follow-up.

Measurements.—The TMT Parts A and B (TMT-A and TMT-B) and SPPB were administered at baseline and 6-year follow-up. Impaired mobility was defined as an SPPB score less than 10. Vital status was ascertained over a 9-year follow-up.

Results.—InCHIANTI participants in the fourth quartile of the time to complete TMT-B minus time to complete TMT-A (TMT (B-A)) were significantly more likely to develop an SPPB score less than 10 during the 6-year follow-up than those in the first quartile (relative risk (RR) = 2.4, 95% confidence interval (CI) = 1.4−3.9, $P = .001$). After adjusting for potential confounders, these findings were substantially unchanged (RR = 2.2, 95% CI = 1.4−3.6, $P = .001$). Worse performance on the TMT was associated with significantly greater decline in SPPB score over the 6-year follow-up, after adjusting for age, sex, and baseline SPPB scores ($\beta = -0.01$, standard error = 0.003, $P = .004$). During the 9-year follow-up, 18.2% of the participants died. After adjustment for age and sex, the proportion of participants who died was higher in participants in the worst than the best performance quartile of TMT (B-A) scores (hazard ratio (HR) = 1.7, 95% CI = 1.0−2.9, $P = .048$). Results were similar in a parsimonious adjusted model (HR = 1.8, 95% CI = 1.0−3.2, $P = .04$).

Conclusion.—Performance on the TMT is a strong, independent predictor of mobility impairment, accelerated decline in lower extremity function, and death in older adults living in the community. The TMT could be a useful addition to geriatric assessment.

▶ The study by Vazanna and colleagues is the first longitudinal study of the relation of executive cognitive function with physical function and mortality in older adults. Poor cognitive function is associated with shorter life expectancy. Executive function, 1 domain of cognitive function, involves the ability to plan, initiate, sequence, monitor, and stop complex behaviors. In a previous cross-sectional analysis, impaired executive function was significantly associated with slower walking speed.[1] There are numerous tests of executive function, but these investigators selected the Trail A and Trail B tests. Trail A requires connecting numbered circles in ascending order (1-2-3, etc). Trail B requires connecting circles that alternate in number and letter sequences (1-A-2-B-3-C and so on). The difference in time to complete Trails A and B increases as executive function declines. Men and women aged 65 years and older enrolled in the Invecchiare in Chianti Study, completed Trails A and B at study entry, and performed the Short Physical Performance Battery (SPPB) test of mobility at baseline and 6 years of follow-up. The SPPB test includes 4 tasks of lower extremity performance that require psychomotor integration and visual-motor speed. All-cause mortality was determined at 9 years of follow-up. At baseline, the participants were generally in good health with some mobility impairment, given the mean SPPB score of 11 (range 0-12; higher scores indicate better mobility). Participants with overt cognitive impairment at baseline were excluded. After 3 years of follow-up, women and men with the poorest performance on the Trail A and B tests were more likely to have developed mobility impairment (SPPB < 10) and had a more rapid decline in mobility than peers with better executive function. After 9 years of follow-up, persons with the poorest executive function at baseline were 1.7 times more likely to have died than their peers. It is not clear what mechanisms explain the association of executive function and mobility or survival. The authors suggest including an executive function screening in routine geriatric assessment so that risk of mobility impairments can be revealed and monitored.

C. M. Jankowski, PhD

Reference

1. Ble A, Volpato S, Zuliani G, et al. Executive function correlate with walking speed in older persons: the InCHIANTI study. *J Am Geriatr Soc*. 2005;53:410-415.

Trail-Walking Exercise and Fall Risk Factors in Community-Dwelling Older Adults: Preliminary Results of a Randomized Controlled Trial
Yamada M, Tanaka B, Nagai K, et al (Kyoto Univ, Japan)
J Am Geriatr Soc 58:1946-1951, 2010

Objectives.—To evaluate the effects of a trail-walking exercise (TWE) program on the rate of falls in community-dwelling older adults.
Design.—Pilot randomized controlled trial (RCT).

Setting.—This trial was conducted in Japan and involved community-dwelling older adults as participants.

Participants.—Sixty participants randomized into a TWE group (n = 30) and a walking (W) group (n = 30).

Intervention.—Exercise class combined with multicomponent trail walking program, versus exercise class combined with simple indoor walking program.

Measurement.—Measurement was based on the difference in fall rates between the TWE and W groups.

Results.—Six months after the intervention, the incidence rate ratio (IRR) of falls for the TWE group compared with the W group was 0.20 (95% confidence interval (CI) = 0.04–0.91); 12 months after the intervention, the IRR of falls for the TWE group compared with the W group was 0.45 (95% CI = 0.16–1.77).

Conclusion.—The results of this pilot RCT suggest that the TWE program was more effective in improving locomotion and cognitive performance under trail-walking task conditions than walking. In addition, participants who took part in the TWE demonstrated a decrease in the incidence rate of falls 6 months after trial completion. Further confirmation is needed, but this preliminary result may promote a new understanding of accidental falls in older adults.

▶ Trail walking is a very popular form of exercise for senior citizens in British Columbia. Depending on the individual's fitness, walks vary from 5 km covered over an hour to all-day treks over the hills. The beautiful scenery and companionship on the walks, coupled with refreshment at the end of the hike add greatly to the motivation. Good organizers choose the route carefully with an eye on the weather, the shade of woodland on a hot summer day, but avoid the dangers of woodland if there are high winds. They also watch for reports of bears, cougars, and other wildlife and ensure that there is an experienced walker at the rear to help anyone who is lagging behind or encountering other difficulties. Regular exercise is well recognized as decreasing the risk of falls,[1] but the randomized controlled trial of Yamada and associates suggests that when combined with other exercises, a 16-week trail-walking program may increase protection relative to walking over a regular course in a gymnasium. Further study of this question seems needed, as the Japanese trail walking consisted simply of moving around irregularly placed flags, apparently on a smooth ground surface. I suspect that real trail walking, particularly in a glacial area with many boulders buried in the ground, would confer much greater benefit than the laboratory simulation of a hike; certainly, it demands a continuous use of balancing skills throughout the walk.

R. J. Shephard, MD (Lond), PhD, DPE

Reference

1. Robertson MC, Campbell AJ, Gardner MM, Devlin N. Preventing injuries in older people by preventing falls: a meta-analysis of individual-level data. *J Am Geriatr Soc.* 2002;50:905-911.

The Energetic Pathway to Mobility Loss: An Emerging New Framework for Longitudinal Studies on Aging
Schrack JA, Simonsick EM, Ferrucci L (The Johns Hopkins Univ, Baltimore, MD; Natl Insts of Health, Baltimore, MD)
J Am Geriatr Soc 58:S329-S336, 2010

The capacity to walk independently is a central component of independent living. Numerous large and well-designed longitudinal studies have shown that gait speed, a reliable marker of mobility, tends to decline with age and as a consequence of chronic disease. This decline in performance is of utmost importance because slow walking speed is a strong, independent predictor of disability, healthcare utilization, nursing home admission, and mortality. Based on these robust findings, it has been postulated that age-associated decline in walking speed is a reliable barometer of the effect of biological aging on health and functional status. Despite the extraordinary prognostic information that walking speed provides, which is often superior to traditional medical information, there is a limited understanding of the mechanisms that underlie age- and disease-related gait speed decline. Identifying the mechanisms that underlie the prognostic value of walking speed should be a central theme in the design of the next generation of longitudinal studies of aging, with appropriate measures introduced and analytical approaches incorporated.

This study hypothesized that a scarcity of available energy induces the decline in customary walking speed with aging and disease. Based on work in the Baltimore Longitudinal Study of Aging, examples of measures, operationalized dimensions, and analytical models that may be implemented to address this are provided. The main premise is simple: the biochemical processes that maintain life, secure homeostatic equilibrium, and prevent the collapse of health require energy. If energy becomes deficient, adaptive behaviors develop to conserve energy (Figs 1 and 2).

▶ The hypothesis of the energetic pathway to mobility loss is that there is a direct connection between mortality and metabolic rate and this connection underlies the degree of decline in mobility in older adults. Across species, organisms that remain mobile later in life tend to survive longer, and even simple movements critical for life decline with age. These observations imply that age-related mobility decline is because of core physiological changes with aging rather than cultural expectations. Energy scarcity is found when homeostatic regulation is on the verge of collapse. Poor mobility develops when a critical threshold of energy scarcity has been passed. Although gait decline with age is a strong predictor of adverse outcomes, the reasons for the slowing of gait are unknown. In the Baltimore Longitudinal Study of Aging (BLSA), a higher resting metabolic rate was associated with greater mortality, suggesting that the energy requirement to maintain resting homeostasis had increased.[1] Because Vo_2max decreases with age, an increase in resting metabolism leaves less energy in reserve for activities such as walking, and the energy of the individual becomes compressed (Fig 1). During energetic compression, basic

Maximal Energy (VO$_{2max}$)

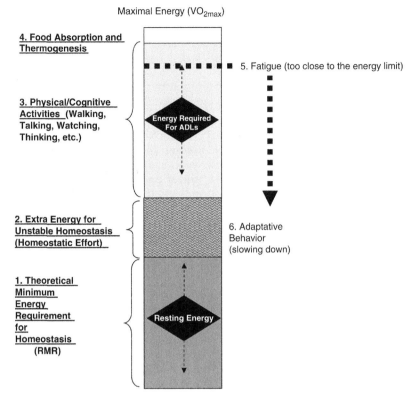

4. Food Absorption and Thermogenesis

5. Fatigue (too close to the energy limit)

3. Physical/Cognitive Activities (Walking, Talking, Watching, Thinking, etc.)

Energy Required For ADLs

2. Extra Energy for Unstable Homeostasis (Homeostatic Effort)

6. Adaptative Behavior (slowing down)

1. Theoretical Minimum Energy Requirement for Homeostasis (RMR)

Resting Energy

FIGURE 1.—An extended model of aging energetics. The box represents the total amount of energy available to an individual over 24 hours. An individual's maximal oxygen consumption (VO$_2$ max), or the maximum amount of energy an individual can expend during physical activity determines the height of the box. Total energy availability can be divided into sections that reflect energy utilization. Section 1 represents the theoretical minimal energy required to maintain life, or resting metabolic rate (RMR). Section 2 depicts extra energy required for unstable homeostasis. In older individuals, this may reflect the energy needed to combat multiple comorbidities as the body attempts to heal itself or the extra energy needed to perform physical tasks because of poorer biomechanical efficiency. Section 3 represents the energy used for daily activities, ranging from activities of daily living to volitional exercise. Section 4 represents the energy needed to break down food and maintain body temperature. In older adults, declines in VO$_2$ max compress the size of the box, resulting in less energy availability overall. Furthermore, more energy is required to maintain homeostasis and perform daily tasks because of poorer metabolic and biomechanical efficiency, which results in less energy available for "essential" tasks related to independent living and greater feelings of fatigue (Section 5). These feelings represent a signal to the brain that energy resources are limited and that there is a need to slow down (Section 6). (Reprinted with permission from 2010 Schrack JA, Simonsick EM, Ferrucci L. The energetic pathway to mobility loss: an emerging new framework for longitudinal studies on aging. *J Am Geriatr Soc.* 2010;58:S329-S336 Copyright the Authors. 2010, The American Geriatrics Society, John Wiley and Sons.)

movement tasks in older adults become challenging, anaerobic, and fatiguing. To test the energetic compression model, energy expenditure at rest, during submaximal walking, and at peak walking pace during the 400-m long-distance corridor walk test was measured in 350 BLSA participants (mean age, 70 years). Total energy was divided into essential energy (submaximal + rest), potential energy (peak − submaximal), and available energy (peak − resting).

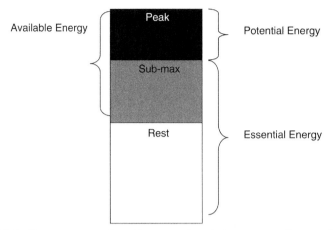

FIGURE 2.—Energy constructs. Essential energy (submaximal energy expenditure + resting energy expenditure). Potential energy (peak energy expenditure − submaximal energy expenditure). Available energy (peak energy expenditure − resting energy expenditure). (Reprinted with permission from 2010 Schrack JA, Simonsick EM, Ferrucci L. The energetic pathway to mobility loss: an emerging new framework for longitudinal studies on aging. *J Am Geriatr Soc.* 2010;58:S329-S336 Copyright the Authors. 2010, The American Geriatrics Society, John Wiley and Sons.)

Essential energy increased with age, suggesting a greater energy demand for submaximal activity (Fig 2). Potential energy and available energy decreased with age, suggesting declined energy and reserve capacity. A significant contributor to the regression of age on the energy constructs was the ratio of fat to lean mass. People with higher levels of fat mass had lower reserve capacity and lower overall energy for physical activity. The authors acknowledge that energy availability is a complex phenomenon. However, if the energetic hypothesis is correct, interventions for disability prevention should be maximally effective in late middle to old age, just before gait speed begins to slow down.

C. M. Jankowski, PhD

Reference

1. Ruggerio C, Metter EJ, Melenovsky V, et al. High basal metabolic rate is a risk factor for mortality: the Baltimore Longitudinal Study of Aging. *J Gerontol A Biol Sci Med Sci.* 2008;63:698-706.

What is the Relationship Between Fear of Falling and Gait in Well-Functioning Older Persons Aged 65 to 70 Years?
Rochat S, Büla CJ, Martin E, et al (Univ of Lausanne Hosp Ctr, Switzerland; et al)
Arch Phys Med Rehabil 91:879-884, 2010

Objective.—To investigate the association between fear of falling and gait performance in well-functioning older persons.

Design.—Survey.

Setting.—Community.

Participants.—Subjects (N = 860, aged 65–70y) were a subsample of participants enrolled in a cohort study who underwent gait measurements.

Interventions.—Not applicable.

Main Outcome Measures.—Fear of falling and its severity were assessed by 2 questions about fear and related activity restriction. Gait performance, including gait variability, was measured using body-fixed sensors.

Results.—Overall, 29.6% (210/860) of the participants reported fear of falling, with 5.2% (45/860) reporting activity restriction. Fear of falling was associated with reduced gait performance, including increased gait variability. A gradient in gait performance was observed from participants without fear to those reporting fear without activity restriction and those reporting both fear and activity restriction. For instance, stride velocity decreased from $1.15 \pm .15$ to $1.11 \pm .17$ to $1.00 \pm .19$ m/s ($P<.001$) in participants without fear, with fear but no activity restriction and with fear and activity restriction, respectively. In multivariate analysis, fear of falling with activity restriction remained associated with reduced gait performance, independent of sex, comorbidity, functional status, falls history, and depressive symptoms.

Conclusions.—In these well-functioning older people, those reporting fear of falling with activity restriction had reduced gait performance and increased gait variability, independent of health and functional status. These relationships suggest that early interventions targeting fear of falling might potentially help to prevent its adverse consequences on mobility and function in similar populations (Fig 1).

▶ In older adults, fear of falling has been associated with mobility impairment and activity restriction. Fear of falling can be a barrier to encouraging an older patient to become more physically active. Although reduced gait speed, one aspect of gait performance, has been associated with fear of falling, Rochat and colleagues suggest that the relation between gait performance and fear of falling may be reciprocal. They measured gait performance and fear of falling in relatively healthy adults who did not have specific gait impairments. The selection of young-old (aged 64-70 years) for this study was unique in the fear of falling literature, given that most studies focused on participants who were frail and/or fallers. Approximately 29% of participants reported fear of falling, a rate comparable to that of the older US population. The participants were classified as having no fear of falling, fear without activity restriction, and fear with restricted activity based on self-report. Gait performance was measured using 4 body-fixed sensors to determine stride velocity, stride length, total double support (percent of the gait cycle with both feet on the ground), and step cadence and the variability of these measures. Across the 3 categories of fear and activity restriction, there was a gradual and significant deterioration and variability in stride velocity (slower and with more pace changes), stride length, double support, and step cadence in those with no fear compared with the fear- and activity-restricted group (Fig 1). These differences prevailed

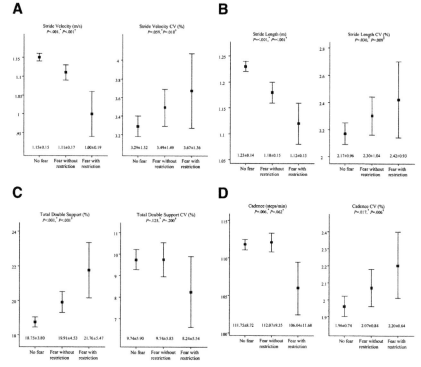

FIGURE 1.—Comparison of gait performance among subjects reporting no fear of falling, fear without activity restriction, and fear with activity restriction (mean and 95% CIs). (A) Stride velocity and stride velocity CV. (B) Stride length and stride length CV. (C) Total double support and total double support CV. (D) Cadence and cadence CV. NOTE. Values are mean ± SD. Squares represent mean values; bars represent 95% CIs. CV: coefficient of variation, where CV = (SD/mean) × 100. *Kruskal-Wallis test for continuous variables. †Nonparametrical Cuzick test for trend. (Reprinted from Archives of Physical Medicine and Rehabilitation, Rochat S, Büla CJ, Martin E, et al. What is the relationship between fear of falling and gait in well-functioning older persons aged 65 to 70 years? *Arch Phys Med Rehabil.* 2010;91:879-884. Copyright 2010, with permission from the American Congress of Rehabilitation Medicine and the American Academy of Physical Medicine and Rehabilitation.)

after adjustment for covariates including age, falls within the last 12 months, depressive symptoms, and comorbidities. When further adjusted for muscle strength (grip strength and 5 chair stand time), fear of falling with activity restriction remained significantly associated with decreased stride velocity. The authors suggested that activity restriction in older adults is a prognostic indicator of the severity of fear of falling, although the prognostic value remains untested. When fear of falling is not accompanied by activity restriction, reduced gait performance is likely mediated by confounders such as comorbidities or functional impairment. The temporal relation of gait abnormalities and fear of falling could not be addressed in this cross-sectional study.

C. M. Jankowski, PhD

Chronic Musculoskeletal Pain and the Occurrence of Falls in an Older Population

Leveille SG, Jones RN, Kiely DK, et al (Beth Israel Deaconess Med Ctr, Boston, MA; Inst for Aging Res, Boston, MA; et al)

JAMA 302:2214-2221, 2009

Context.—Chronic pain is a major contributor to disability in older adults; however, the potential role of chronic pain as a risk factor for falls is poorly understood.

Objective.—To determine whether chronic musculoskeletal pain is associated with an increased occurrence of falls in a cohort of community-living older adults.

Design, Setting, and Participants.—The Maintenance of Balance, Independent Living, Intellect, and Zest in the Elderly (MOBILIZE) Boston Study is a population-based longitudinal study of falls involving 749 adults aged 70 years and older. Participants were enrolled from September 2005 through January 2008.

Main Outcome Measure.—Participants recorded falls on monthly calendar postcards mailed to the study center during an 18-month period.

Results.—There were 1029 falls reported during the follow-up. A report of 2 or more locations of musculoskeletal pain at baseline was associated with greater occurrence of falls. The age-adjusted rates of falls per person-year were 1.18 (95% confidence interval [CI], 1.13-1.23) for the 300 participants with 2 or more sites of joint pain, 0.90 (95% CI, 0.87-0.92) for the 181 participants with single-site pain, and 0.78 (95% CI, 0.74-0.81) for the 267 participants with no joint pain. Similarly, more severe or disabling pain at baseline was associated with higher fall rates ($P < .05$). The association persisted after adjusting for multiple confounders and fall risk factors. The greatest risk for falls was observed in persons who had 2 or more pain sites (adjusted rate ratio [RR], 1.53; 95% CI, 1.17-1.99), and those in the highest tertiles of pain severity (adjusted RR, 1.53; 95% CI, 1.12-2.08) and pain interference with activities (adjusted RR, 1.53; 95% CI, 1.15-2.05), compared with their peers with no pain or those in the lowest tertiles of pain scores.

Conclusions.—Chronic pain measured according to number of locations, severity, or pain interference with daily activities was associated with greater risk of falls in older adults.

▶ Falls among seniors cause significant personal suffering and add substantially to health costs. Sport and exercise medicine has a role to play as exercise programs have reduced falls by around 35% (Cochrane). This study adds a new risk factor for consideration—chronic pain. The authors suggest that the common complaint of the aches and pains of old age is related to a greater hazard than previously thought. Thus, chronic pain may be an important risk factor for falls and possibly fall-related injuries among seniors. This research identifies chronic pain as an important risk factor for falls in older adults. I was surprised that the authors were able to ignore depression in the model.

Depression is an independent risk factor for falls and is associated with chronic pain.

The authors provide 3 possible mechanisms that need to be addressed in future research: (1) local joint pathology, such as is seen in arthritis; (2) neuro-muscular effects of pain; and (3) central mechanisms in which pain interferes with cognition or executive function.

K. Khan, MD

Efficacy of a Short Multidisciplinary Falls Prevention Program for Elderly Persons With Osteoporosis and a Fall History: A Randomized Controlled Trial

Smulders E, Weerdesteyn V, Groen BE, et al (Sint Maartenskliniek, Nijmegen, The Netherlands; et al)
Arch Phys Med Rehabil 91:1705-1711, 2010

Objective.—To evaluate the efficacy of the Nijmegen Falls Prevention Program (NFPP) for persons with osteoporosis and a fall history in a random-ized controlled trial. Persons with osteoporosis are at risk for fall-related fractures because of decreased bone strength. A decrease in the number of falls therefore is expected to be particularly beneficial for these persons.

Design.—Randomized controlled trial.

Setting.—Hospital.

Participants.—Persons with osteoporosis and a fall history (N = 96; mean ± SD age, 71.0 ± 4.7 y; 90 women).

Intervention.—After baseline assessment, participants were randomly assigned to the exercise (n = 50; participated in the NFPP for persons with osteoporosis [5.5 wk]) or control group (n = 46; usual care).

Main Outcome Measures.—Primary outcome measure was fall rate, measured by using monthly fall calendars for 1 year. Secondary outcomes were balance confidence (Activity-specific Balance Confidence Scale), quality of life (QOL; Quality of Life Questionnaire of the European Foun-dation for Osteoporosis), and activity level (LASA Physical Activity Ques-tionnaire, pedometer), assessed posttreatment subsequent to the program and after 1 year of follow-up.

Results.—The fall rate in the exercise group was 39% lower than for the control group (.72 vs 1.18 falls/person-year; risk ratio, .61; 95% confi-dence interval, .40–.94). Balance confidence in the exercise group increased by 13.9% ($P = .001$). No group differences were observed in QOL and activity levels.

Conclusion.—The NFPP for persons with osteoporosis was effective in decreasing the number of falls and improving balance confidence. There-fore, it is a valuable new tool to improve mobility and independence of persons with osteoporosis.

▶ This is the first randomized controlled trial to demonstrate the efficacy of a short-term falls prevention intervention in older adults who have osteoporosis and a history of falls. The intervention was the Nijmegen Falls Prevention Program (NFPP).[1] The NFPP comprises 6 elements: education, an obstacle course, walking exercises, weight-bearing exercises, correction of gait abnormalities, and training in fall techniques. The fall techniques were adjusted to reduce peak impact forces to ensure the safety of persons with osteoporosis. The elements were rotated throughout 11 sessions in 5.5 weeks and provided by physical and occupational therapists. To be eligible, participants had a femoral neck or lumbar spine T score of ≤ -2.5 and at least 1 fall in the previous year. Additional inclusion criteria were the ability to walk 15 minutes without a walking device and no history of severe comorbidities associated with increased fall risk (eg, severe pulmonary disease, neurological disorders). The primary outcome, fall rate (average number of falls per person a year), was determined from fall calendars kept by participants from the start of the intervention through 1 year of follow-up and compared with a control group. In the intent-to-treat analysis, fall rate was 39% lower in the exercise group compared with control group. There were also fewer falls with major injuries (fractures, concussion, wounds requiring suturing) in the exercise group than control group (1 vs 5, respectively). Balance confidence was significantly greater in the exercise group than control group at the 1-year follow-up. This is an important finding because balance confidence was low prior to the intervention (~ 55 on a 0-100 scale) and improved about 14% in the exercise group. Physical activity, as determined by questionnaire and pedometer step counts, did not change significantly in response to the intervention. There has been concern on the part of clinicians that increasing the awareness of fall risk may cause some older adults to reduce their movements out of fear of falling. However, this study refutes that concern. There were no adverse events reported, which can be attributed to the careful planning and supervision of the intervention. The modified NFPP is a new tool for prevention of falls in persons with osteoporosis and a fall history. It can be implemented over a short period of time, thereby enhancing adherence and, potentially, insurability and affordability.

C. M. Jankowski, PhD

Reference

1. Weerdesteyn V, Rijken H, Geurts AC, Smits-Engelsman BC, Mulder T, Duysens J. A five-week exercise program can reduce falls and improve obstacle avoidance in the elderly. *Gerontology.* 2006;52:131-141.

Physical Activity Over the Life Course and Its Association with Cognitive Performance and Impairment in Old Age

Middleton LE, Barnes DE, Lui L-Y, et al (Sunnybrook Health Sciences Ctr, Toronto, Ontario, Canada; Univ of California at San Francisco; California Pacific Med Ctr, San Francisco)

J Am Geriatr Soc 58:1322-1326, 2010

Objective.—To determine how physical activity at various ages over the life course is associated with cognitive impairment in late life.

Design.—Cross-sectional study.

Setting.—Four U.S. sites.

Participants.—Nine thousand three hundred forty-four women aged 65 and older (mean 71.6) who self-reported teenage, age 30, age 50, and late-life physical activity.

Measurements.—Logistic regression was used to determine the association between physical activity status at each age and likelihood of cognitive impairment (modified Mini-Mental State Examination (mMMSE) score >1.5 standard deviations below the mean, mMMSE score≤22). Models were adjusted for age, education, marital status, diabetes mellitus, hypertension, depressive symptoms, smoking, and body mass index.

Results.—Women who reported being physically active had a lower prevalence of cognitive impairment in late life than women who were inactive at each time (teenage: 8.5% vs 16.7%, adjusted odds ratio (AOR) = 0.65, 95% confidence interval (CI) = 0.53−0.80; age 30: 8.9% vs 12.0%, AOR = 0.80, 95% CI = 0.67−0.96); age 50: 8.5% vs 13.1%, AOR = 0.71, 95% CI = 0.59−0.85; old age: 8.2% vs 15.9%, AOR = 0.74, 95% CI = 0.61−0.91). When the four times were analyzed together, teenage physical activity was most strongly associated with lower odds of late-life cognitive impairment (OR = 0.73, 95% CI = 0.58−0.92). However, women who were physically inactive as teenagers and became active in later life had lower risk than those who remained inactive.

Conclusions.—Women who reported being physically active at any point over the life course, especially as teenagers, had a lower likelihood

TABLE 2.—Association Between Physical Activity Status Across the Life Course and Odds of Late-Life Cognitive Impairment (>1.5 Standard Deviations Below the Mean Modified Mini-Mental State Examination Score (≤22)) in Older Women

Physical Activity Status	Prevalence, %	Odds Ratio (95% Confidence Interval) Unadjusted	Adjusted*
Teenage			
Inactive	16.7	1.0 (Reference)	1.0 (Reference)
Active	8.5	0.46 (0.39−0.54)	0.65 (0.53−0.80)
Age 30			
Inactive	12.0	1.0 (Reference)	1.0 (Reference)
Active	8.9	0.71 (0.61−0.82)	0.80 (0.67−0.96)
Age 50			
Inactive	13.1	1.0 (Reference)	1.0 (Reference)
Active	8.5	0.62 (0.54−0.71)	0.71 (0.59−0.85)
Late life			
Inactive	15.9	1.0 (Reference)	1.0 (Reference)
Active	8.2	0.47 (0.41−0.55)	0.74 (0.61−0.91)

Teenage: age, education, marital status, diabetes mellitus, depressive symptoms, smoking, body mass index (BMI).
Age 30: education, diabetes mellitus, depressive symptoms, smoking, BMI.
Age 50: age, education, marital status, diabetes mellitus, depressive symptoms, smoking, BMI.
Late Life: age, education, marital status, diabetes mellitus, hypertension, depressive symptoms, BMI.
*Adjusted models include significant confounders from descriptive analyses:

of cognitive impairment in late life. Interventions should promote physical activity early in life and throughout the life course (Table 2).

▶ Senile dementia is a growing problem in our aging population, with corresponding interest in reports that regular physical activity earlier in life can minimize this risk.[1-3] However, randomized controls of physical activity have had less consistent effects on elderly populations.[4] This study suffers from the uncertainties of an epidemiological approach, but it has the merit that an attempt has been made to assess the habitual physical activity in a large sample of women at 3 points in their lifespan, using the Paffenbarger questionnaire. At all 3 points, but particularly in youth, the risk is substantially lower for those who report physical activity (Table 2). Nevertheless, it is a little surprising that there is no dose-response curve, and subjects are thus classed simply as active or inactive. Those who are active as teenagers gain no additional benefit from remaining active in later life. Moreover, the apparent benefit of physical activity is substantially attenuated when the model is adjusted for other risk factors, such as smoking and obesity. The possibility thus remains that all of the supposed exercise effect might disappear if a full allowance could be made for interfering variables; further work is needed before we can claim confidently that regular exercise will avert senile dementia.

R. J. Shephard, MD (Lond), PhD, DPE

References

1. Laurin D, Verreault R, Lindsay J, MacPherson K, Rockwood K. Physical activity and risk of cognitive impairment and dementia in elderly persons. *Arch Neurol.* 2001;58:498-504.
2. Rovio S, Kareholt I, Helkala EL, et al. Leisure-time physical activity at midlife and the risk of dementia and Alzheimer's disease. *Lancet Neurol.* 2005;4:705-711.
3. Schuit AJ, Feskens EJ, Launer LJ, Kromhout D. Physical activity and cognitive decline, the role of the apolipoprotein e4 allele. *Med Sci Sports Exerc.* 2001;33: 772-777.
4. Angevaren M, Aufdemkampe G, Verhaar HJ, Aleman A, Vanhees L. Physical activity and enhanced fitness to improve cognitive function in older people without known cognitive impairment. *Cochrane Database Syst Rev.* 2008;(3): CD005381.

Physical activity predicts gray matter volume in late adulthood: The Cardiovascular Health Study

Erickson KI, Raji CA, Lopez OL, et al (Univ of Pittsburgh, PA; et al)
Neurology 75:1415-1422, 2010

Objectives.—Physical activity (PA) has been hypothesized to spare gray matter volume in late adulthood, but longitudinal data testing an association has been lacking. Here we tested whether PA would be associated with greater gray matter volume after a 9-year follow-up, a threshold could be identified for the amount of walking necessary to spare gray matter volume, and greater gray matter volume associated with PA would be associated with a reduced risk for cognitive impairment 13 years after the PA evaluation.

Methods.—In 299 adults (mean age 78 years) from the Cardiovascular Health Cognition Study, we examined the association between gray matter volume, PA, and cognitive impairment. Physical activity was quantified as the number of blocks walked over 1 week. High-resolution brain scans were acquired 9 years after the PA assessment on cognitively normal adults. White matter hyperintensities, ventricular grade, and other health variables at baseline were used as covariates. Clinical adjudication for cognitive impairment occurred 13 years after baseline.

Results.—Walking amounts ranged from 0 to 300 blocks (mean 56.3; SD 69.7). Greater PA predicted greater volumes of frontal, occipital, entorhinal, and hippocampal regions 9 years later. Walking 72 blocks was necessary to detect increased gray matter volume but walking more than 72 blocks did not spare additional volume. Greater gray matter volume with PA reduced the risk for cognitive impairment 2-fold.

Conclusion.—Greater amounts of walking are associated with greater gray matter volume, which is in turn associated with a reduced risk of cognitive impairment.

▶ Gray matter (GM) volume shrinks in late adulthood, often preceding and leading to cognitive impairment.[1] Physical activity may protect against the deterioration of brain tissue, but this hypothesis has not been tested in longitudinal studies. This study found that walking distance assessed at baseline predicted greater volume of GM tissue 9 years later, even after adjustment for multiple confounders. GM volume in the highest quartile of walking differed from the other 3 quartiles, and this effect was consistent in the frontal cortex, the temporal lobes, and the hippocampal formation (Fig 3 in the original article). Rodent research indicates that aerobic activity induces cellular cascades that increase GM volume, enhances learning, and promotes the proliferation and survival of new neurons in the hippocampus.[2]

D. C. Nieman, DrPH

References

1. Raz N, Lindenberger U, Rodrigue KM, et al. Regional brain changes in aging healthy adults: general trends, individual differences and modifiers. *Cereb Cortex.* 2005;15:1676-1689.
2. van Praag H, Kempermann G, Gage FH. Running increases cell proliferation and neurogenesis in the adult mouse dentate gyrus. *Nat Neurosci.* 1999;2:266-270.

Resistance exercise for muscular strength in older adults: A meta-analysis
Peterson MD, Rhea MR, Sen A, et al (Univ of Michigan, Ann Arbor; AT Still Univ/Arizona School of Health Sciences, Mesa, AZ)
Ageing Res Rev 9:226-237, 2010

Purpose.—The effectiveness of resistance exercise for strength improvement among aging persons is inconsistent across investigations, and there is a lack of research synthesis for multiple strength outcomes.

Methods.—The systematic review followed the Preferred Reporting Items for Systematic Reviews and Meta-Analyses (PRISMA) recommendations. A meta-analysis was conducted to determine the effect of resistance exercise (RE) for multiple strength outcomes in aging adults. Randomized-controlled trials and randomized or non-randomized studies among adults ≥50 years, were included. Data were pooled using random-effect models. Outcomes for 4 common strength tests were analyzed for main effects. Heterogeneity between studies was assessed using the Cochran Q and I^2 statistics, and publication bias was evaluated through physical inspection of funnel plots as well as formal rank-correlation statistics. A linear mixed model regression was incorporated to examine differences between outcomes, as well as potential study-level predictor variables.

Results.—Forty-seven studies were included, representing 1079 participants. A positive effect for each of the strength outcomes was determined however there was heterogeneity between studies. Regression revealed that higher intensity training was associated with greater improvement. Strength increases ranged from 9.8 to 31.6 kg, and percent changes were 29 ± 2, 24 ± 2, 33 ± 3, and 25 ± 2, respectively for leg press, chest press, knee extension, and lat pull.

Conclusions.—RE is effective for improving strength among older adults, particularly with higher intensity training. Findings therefore suggest that RE may be considered a viable strategy to prevent generalized muscular weakness associated with aging (Figs 2-5).

▶ Peterson and colleagues compiled 47 studies that included resistance exercise training interventions performed by older adults to determine average muscle strength gains. The need for this meta-analysis stems from the lack of data supporting a dose-response relationship for exercise and strength in aging because most resistance exercise studies have not compared different training regimes over a broad range of age and health status. In the meta-analysis, participants ranged in age from 50 to 92 years (mean ± standard deviation was 67 ± 4 years) and included women and men. The length of training was 6 to

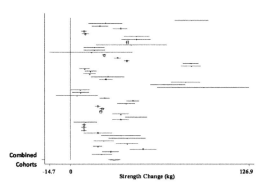

FIGURE 2.—Forest plot of effect sizes and 95% confidence intervals for all 51 cohorts (32 studies) representing leg press, based on the random-effects meta-analysis results. (Reprinted from Peterson MD, Rhea MR, Sen A, et al. Resistance exercise for muscular strength in older adults: a meta-analysis. *Ageing Res Rev.* 2010;9:226-237, with permission from Elsevier Ireland Ltd.)

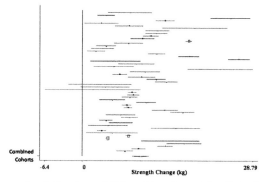

FIGURE 3.—Forest plot of effect sizes and 95% confidence intervals for all 55 cohorts (36 studies) representing chest press, based on the random-effects meta-analysis results. (Reprinted from Peterson MD, Rhea MR, Sen A, et al. Resistance exercise for muscular strength in older adults: a meta-analysis. *Ageing Res Rev.* 2010;9:226-237, with permission from Elsevier Ireland Ltd.)

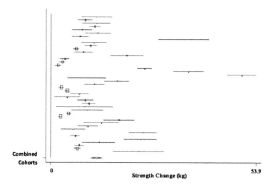

FIGURE 4.—Forest plot of effect sizes and 95% confidence intervals for all 43 cohorts (28 studies) representing knee extension, based on the random-effects meta-analysis results. (Reprinted from Peterson MD, Rhea MR, Sen A, et al. Resistance exercise for muscular strength in older adults: a meta-analysis. *Ageing Res Rev.* 2010;9:226-237, with permission from Elsevier Ireland Ltd.)

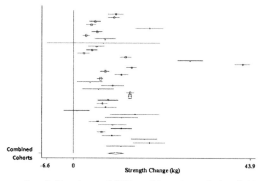

FIGURE 5.—Forest plot of effect sizes and 95% confidence intervals for all 38 cohorts (19 studies) representing lat pull, based on the random-effects meta-analysis results. (Reprinted from Peterson MD, Rhea MR, Sen A, et al. Resistance exercise for muscular strength in older adults: a meta-analysis. *Ageing Res Rev.* 2010;9:226-237, with permission from Elsevier Ireland Ltd.)

52 weeks, frequency of 1 to 3 times per week, and intensity from 40% to 85% of one-repetition maximum (1RM). Compliance was very good given that 85% to 100% of exercise sessions were attended. The total body response to training was determined by including strength changes in upper (chest press and lat pull-down) and lower body (leg press and knee extension) exercises. The training effect was a 24% to 33% improvement in strength compared with pretraining values, indicating a significant total body response in older adults (Figs 2-5). The largest improvement in strength occurred with knee extension, although this may be partly attributed to publication bias. That is, published increases in knee extension may be overestimated because studies with negative results were not published. Publication bias was not evident for the other 3 exercises. The only significant predictor of strength gain was the training intensity, which was categorized into 4 subgroups (low, < 60% 1RM; low/moderate, 60%-69% 1RM; moderate/high, 70%-79% 1RM; and high intensity, ≥80% 1RM). There was a 5.3% greater increase in strength for each increment of training intensity. Importantly, strength gains were not predicted by gender, age, length of training, or average training volume. Although this meta-analysis supports significant improvements in total body strength among older adults in response to resistance exercise training, there is a clear need for studies designed a priori to determine the dose-response effects of resistance training and whether variable training regimes (ie, periodization) may provide additional strength benefits.

C. M. Jankowski, PhD

Can aerobic training improve muscle strength and power in older men?
Lovell DI, Cuneo R, Gass GC (School of Health and Sport Sciences, University of the Sunshine Coast, Queensland, Australia)
J Aging Phys Act 18:14-26, 2010

This study examined the effect of aerobic training on leg strength, power, and muscle mass in previously sedentary, healthy older men (70–80 yr). Training consisted of 30–45 min of cycle ergometry at 50–70% maximal oxygen consumption (VO2max), 3 times weekly for 16 wk, then 4 wk detraining, or assignment to a nontraining control group (n = 12 both groups). Training increased leg strength, leg power, upper leg muscle mass, and VO2max above pretraining values (21%, 12%, 4%, and 15%, respectively; p < .05). However, all gains were lost after detraining, except for some gain in VO2max. This suggests that cycle ergometry is sufficient stimulus to improve neuromuscular function in older men, but gains are quickly lost with detraining. For the older population cycle ergometry provides the means to not only increase aerobic fitness but also increase leg strength and power and upper leg muscle mass. However, during periods of inactivity neuromuscular gains are quickly lost.

▶ Muscle strengthening exercises might seem the logical approach to the prevention of sarcopenia, but given the popularity of walking among the elderly, the question arises whether regular engagement in such activity can contribute to the prevention of muscle wasting. Our cross-sectional study of both men and women aged 65 to 85 years showed an association between whole body dual X-ray absorptiometry (DXA) scores and year-long walking activity as assessed by an accurate pedometer/accelerometer.[1] The association was substantial, with inactive members of the group having 2 to 5 times the risk of sarcopenia relative to those taking at least 23 minutes per day of walking activity at an intensity > 3 metabolic equivalents; however, the favorable association of DXA score was more obvious for the legs than for the arms. The obvious limitations of our observations were (1) that preservation of muscle mass may have allowed the seniors concerned to walk vigorously for longer periods, and (2) walking may have served as a marker of individuals with an overall commitment to physical activity. The study of Lovell and associates is experimental and thus serves to confirm the causality of the relationships that we observed between aerobic exercise and the development of muscle mass. Lovell and colleagues again used DXA, supplemented by measures of muscle strength, but they tested only men and looked only at changes in thigh muscle volume. This is particularly unfortunate, as overall body mass decreased during the 16 weeks of cycle ergometer training. Moreover, cycle ergometry offers a rather specific stimulation of the quadriceps, and there may well have been no change or even a decrease in arm muscle mass in response to the cycle training. The lesson from both studies seems that if the muscle of an elderly adult is to be developed by an aerobic activity such as walking, it is important to add some stimulation for the muscles of the arms and back, whether by use of walking poles or the carrying of groceries.

R. J. Shephard, MD (Lond), PhD, DPE

Reference

1. Park H, Park S, Shephard RJ, Aoyagi Y. Yearlong physical activity and sarcopenia in older adults: the Nakanojo study. *Eur J Appl Physiol.* 2010;109:953-961.

Adverse Events Reported in Progressive Resistance Strength Training Trials in Older Adults: 2 Sides of a Coin

Liu C-J, Latham N (Indiana Univ at Indianapolis; Boston Univ, MA)
Arch Phys Med Rehabil 91:1471-1473, 2010

Objectives.—To summarize adverse events reported in randomized controlled trials that applied progressive resistance strength training in older adults and to examine factors that might be associated with these events.

Design.—After systematic searches of databases, 2 reviewers independently screened and extracted adverse event—related information from identified trials.

Setting.—Not applicable.

Participants.—Older adults 60 years of age and above (N = 6700).

Intervention.—Muscle strength training exercise that increases load gradually.

Main Outcome Measures.—Adverse events and reasons for dropout. Adverse events include any undesirable outcomes that may be directly related or unrelated to the intervention.

Results.—Among 121 trials identified, 53 trials provided no comments about adverse events, 25 trials reported no adverse events occurred, and 43 trials reported some types of adverse events. Most adverse events reported were musculoskeletal problems such as muscle strain or joint pain. Adverse events were reported more often in trials that recruited participants with certain health conditions, functional limitations, or sedentary lifestyle; in trials that applied high intensity; and in trials that were published after the 2001 Consolidated Standards of Reporting Trials statement had been published. Reasons reported for dropout in 58 trials might be related to adverse events. The most frequent reasons for dropout were illness or medical problems.

Conclusions.—Adverse events may be underreported because there is no consensus on the definition. Reporting adverse events associated with progressive resistance strength training in older adults is informative for practitioners to translate clinical research to clinical practice by knowing both the benefits and risks. Future trials should clearly define adverse events and report them in the published article.

▶ Clinicians are challenged to translate the results of exercise randomized controlled trials (RCTs) to individual recommendations for patients. Unlike many other types of RCTs, there is little guidance for the reporting and classification of adverse events (AEs) in exercise trials. In addition to a lack of reporting guidelines, many, if not most, exercise RCTs are not required by the sponsoring agency to have a data and safety monitoring board (DSMB). A DSMB and investigators establish a reporting system and definitions of AEs in the active exercise and control groups. Most AEs will not be life threatening, but the overall profile of AEs relative to controls provides a risk-to-benefit assessment of the resistance training intervention. In their review of 121 RCTs of resistance exercise training, Liu and Latham found that only about half (68 RCTs) included an account of AEs, and 25 of these trials stated that there were no AEs. AEs were reported more often in RCTs that included subpopulations with chronic comorbidities (eg, osteoarthritis) or with high-intensity (vs low- or moderate-intensity) exercise. It is reasonable to assume that investigators of these studies had decided a priori to track and classify AEs within their high-risk populations or more aggressive interventions. However, it is equally important to know what the risks and benefits of resistance exercise are for relatively healthy older adults who see their primary care physician for annual examinations, seek exercise advice, or are advised to become more physically active. Compared with cardiovascular exercise, resistance exercise can be more difficult to describe during an office visit. Even minor injuries or discomforts can disrupt the frequency and progression of training and thereby thwart the establishment of a resistance exercise habit. Advice from clinicians regarding the expected temporary discomforts of resistance exercise—specific recommendations for patients with comorbidities—would likely contribute to exercise adherence. Reporting of AEs in progressive resistance exercise RCTs has improved since the publication of the Consolidated Standard of Reporting Trials recommendations in 2001. However, this is an aspect of exercise research that requires maturation, particularly in regards to intervention studies of older adults.

C. M. Jankowski, PhD

A prospective study of the associations between 25-hydroxy-vitamin D, sarcopenia progression and physical activity in older adults
Scott D, Blizzard L, Fell J, et al (Univ of Tasmania, Hobart, Australia; Univ of Tasmania, Launceston, Australia)
Clin Endocrinol 73:581-587, 2010

Objective.—Low 25-hydroxyvitamin D (25OHD) levels may be associated with both sarcopenia (the age-related decline in muscle mass and function) and low physical activity (PA). Our objective was to describe prospective associations between 25OHD, muscle parameters, and PA in community-dwelling older adults.

Design.—Prospective, population-based study with a mean follow-up of $2·6 ± 0·4$ years.

Patients.—Six hundred and eighty-six community-dwelling older adults (49% women; mean ± SD 62 ± 7 years old).

Measurements.—Appendicular lean mass percentage (%ALM) and body fat assessed by Dual-energy X-ray Absorptiometry, leg strength by dynamometer, leg muscle quality (LMQ), PA assessed by pedometer, self-reported sun exposure by questionnaire, and serum 25OHD measured by radioimmunoassay.

Results.—Participants with 25OHD ≤50 nM had lower mean %ALM, leg strength, LMQ and PA (all $P < 0·05$). As a continuous function, baseline 25OHD was a positive independent predictor of change in leg strength ($β = 5·74$ kg, 95% CI 0·65, 10·82) and LMQ ($β = 0·49$ kg/kg, 95% CI 0·17, 0·82). Also, change in 25OHD was positively predicted by baseline %ALM ($β = 2·03$ pM/p.a., 95% CI 0·44, 3·62) leg strength ($β = 0·30$ pM/p.a., 95% CI 0·06, 0·53), LMQ ($β = 4·48$ pM/p.a., 95% CI 0·36, 8·61) and PA ($β = 2·63$ pM/p.a., 95% CI 0·35, 4·92) after adjustment for sun exposure and body fat.

Conclusions.—25OHD may be important for the maintenance of muscle function, and higher skeletal muscle mass and function as well as general PA levels may also be beneficial for 25OHD status, in community-dwelling older adults.

▶ Scott and colleagues raise the intriguing prospect that physical activity and skeletal muscle may increase serum vitamin D and thereby protect older adults from sarcopenia. In the Tasmanian Older Adult Cohort Study, the development and progression of osteoarthritis and osteoporosis in women and men aged

50 to 70 years was evaluated over an average of 2.6 years. The investigators posed 2 questions: does vitamin D predict change in muscle mass, strength, and quality (strength/mass) and, conversely, do muscle quantity, quality, and physical activity predict improvements in vitamin D? Approximately 700 participants were included in the analyses. Physical activity was measured by pedometers, maximum isometric leg strength by dynamometry, and appendicular lean tissue mass by dual-energy X-ray absorptiometry. The participants were classified as having low 25-hydroxyvitamin D (25OHD) ($\leq$50 nM) or normal 25OHD ($>$50 nM) at study entry. The regression analyses were adjusted for potentially confounding factors, including age, sex, baseline physical activity, self-reported sun exposure, and vitamin D supplementation. Blood samples were obtained in summer/autumn and winter/spring to account for seasonal variation in sun exposure. Serum 25OHD at baseline was a significant predictor of improvements in leg strength and leg muscle quality but not appendicular lean mass. Conversely, having greater appendicular lean mass, strength, leg muscle quality, and greater physical activity at study entry independently predicted higher serum 25OHD. The mechanisms underlying these associations are not well known but could include influences on vitamin D absorption, synthesis, or metabolism. For example, 25OHD may activate vitamin D receptors in skeletal muscle, which are linked to protein synthesis and/or may impart anti-inflammatory actions on muscle. These suppositions suggest that vitamin D affects the anabolic and catabolic sides of the muscle balance equation. Skeletal muscle may serve as a storage receptacle for vitamin D raising the question of whether sufficient storage can be manipulated at an earlier age or more physically active stage of life for protection from functional decline later in life.

C. M. Jankowski, PhD

A prospective study of the associations between 25-hydroxy-vitamin D, sarcopenia progression and physical activity in older adults

Scott D, Blizzard L, Fell J, et al (Univ of Tasmania, Hobart, Australia; Univ of Tasmania, Launceston, Australia)
Clin Endocrinol 73:581-587, 2010

Objective.—Low 25-hydroxyvitamin D (25OHD) levels may be associated with both sarcopenia (the age-related decline in muscle mass and function) and low physical activity (PA). Our objective was to describe prospective associations between 25OHD, muscle parameters, and PA in community-dwelling older adults.

Design.—Prospective, population-based study with a mean follow-up of $2 \cdot 6 \pm 0 \cdot 4$ years.

Patients.—Six hundred and eighty-six community-dwelling older adults (49% women; mean $\pm$ SD 62 $\pm$ 7 years old).

Measurements.—Appendicular lean mass percentage (%ALM) and body fat assessed by Dual-energy X-ray Absorptiometry, leg strength by dynamometer, leg muscle quality (LMQ), PA assessed by pedometer, self-reported sun exposure by questionnaire, and serum 25OHD measured by radioimmunoassay.

Results.—Participants with 25OHD ≤50 nM had lower mean %ALM, leg strength, LMQ and PA (all $P < 0.05$). As a continuous function, baseline 25OHD was a positive independent predictor of change in leg strength ($\beta = 5.74$ kg, 95% CI 0.65, 10.82) and LMQ ($\beta = 0.49$ kg/kg, 95% CI 0.17, 0.82). Also, change in 25OHD was positively predicted by baseline %ALM ($\beta = 2.03$ pM/p.a., 95% CI 0.44, 3.62) leg strength ($\beta = 0.30$ pM/p.a., 95% CI 0.06, 0.53), LMQ ($\beta = 4.48$ pM/p.a., 95% CI 0.36, 8.61) and PA ($\beta = 2.63$ pM/p.a., 95% CI 0.35, 4.92) after adjustment for sun exposure and body fat.

Conclusions.—25OHD may be important for the maintenance of muscle function, and higher skeletal muscle mass and function as well as general PA levels may also be beneficial for 25OHD status, in community-dwelling older adults (Table 1).

▶ Any possible clues to the control of sarcopenia are welcome. The association between low vitamin D intake and muscle weakness (Table 1) as seen in this longitudinal study is thus interesting, as is the relationship between baseline vitamin D and changes in muscle strength over a 2- to 3-year period of observation. The authors of this article suggest that the storage of vitamin D in muscle may be a relevant factor,[1,2] and muscle is certainly rich in vitamin D receptors[3]; they also suggest that activation of vitamin D receptors may stimulate the formation of muscle protein[4] and that vitamin D may reduce the local inflammatory processes that are associated with sarcopenia.[5] Nevertheless, there are a number of possible sources for spurious correlations that need to be carefully weighed and excluded. An active senior is likely to spend more

TABLE 1.—Descriptive Characteristics (Mean ± SD) of TASOAC Participants at Baseline, Classified by 25OHD Status

	25OHD <50 nM (N = 297)	25OHD >50 nM (N = 389)	*P*-Value for Difference in Mean
Mean 25OHD (nM)	37·1 ± 8·4	67·8 ± 13·4	**<0·001**
Age (years)	62·2 ± 7·6	61·5 ± 6·7	0·212
Female (%)	53·9	45·8	**0·035***
Height (cm)	166·9 ± 8·6	168·3 ± 9·0	**0·040**
Weight (kg)	78·1 ± 14·6	76·6 ± 13·6	0·164
BMI (kg/m²)	28·1 ± 5·0	27·0 ± 3·8	**0·001**
Body fat (%)	34·5 ± 8·0	32·2 ± 7·5	**<0·001**
Appendicular lean mass (%)	59·3 ± 9·9	62·2 ± 9·6	**<0·001**
Ambulatory activity (steps/day)	8470·3 ± 3347·5	9401·7 ± 3612·9	**<0·001**
Leg strength (kg)	91·5 ± 47·8	100·8 ± 50·1	**0·014**
Leg muscle quality (kg/kg)	5·5 ± 2·3	5·9 ± 2·3	**0·026**
Current smoker (%)	10·1	10·5	0·852*
Vitamin D supplementation (%)	7·7	6·4	0·503*
Summer sun exposure (1–5)	2·7 ± 1·4	3·2 ± 1·4	**<0·001**
Winter sun exposure (1–5)	2·5 ± 1·2	3·0 ± 1·4	**<0·001**

BMI, body mass index.
All bolded values are significant at a level $P < 0.05$.
*Chi-square tests; all others independent *t*-tests.

time outdoors, and the additional exposure to sunlight may increase synthesis of vitamin D.[6] The active person will also have a greater total daily energy expenditure and thus a greater ingestion of foods that will likely include a variety of vitamins. Finally, active individuals may be health conscious and thus likely to ingest vitamin supplements. Sunlight exposure was estimated by questionnaire rather than by objective polysulphone badges. It was found to be somewhat lower in those subjects with low vitamin D levels, although statistical allowance was made for this difference in multivariate analysis. There are other minor criticisms of technique. Physical activity was assessed based on a 7-day pedometer step count (without reference to season or possible reactive effects from wearing the instrument); furthermore, there was a change in the type of instrument used from baseline to final data collection. Finally, the follow-up period was rather short for a realistic evaluation of any changes in individual liability to sarcopenia.

R. J. Shephard, MD (Lond), PhD, DPE

References

1. Clements MR, Fraser DR. Vitamin D supply to the rat fetus and neonate. *J Clin Invest.* 1988;81:1768-1773.
2. Heaney RP, Horst RL, Cullen DM, Armas LA. Vitamin D3 distribution and status in the body. *J Am Coll Nutr.* 2009;28:252-256.
3. Bischoff-Ferrari HA, Borchers M, Gudat F, Dürmüller U, Stähelin HB, Dick W. Vitamin D receptor expression in human muscle tissue decreases with age. *J Bone Min Res.* 2004;19:265-269.
4. Boland R. Role of vitamin D in skeletal muscle function. *Endocr Rev.* 1986;7: 434-448.
5. Schleithoff SS, Zittermann A, Tenderich G, Berthold HK, Stehle P, Koerfer R. Vitamin D supplementation improves cytokine profiles in patients with congestive heart failure: a double-blind, randomized, placebo-controlled trial. *Am J Clin Nutr.* 2006;83:754-759.
6. Holick MF. Vitamin D deficiency. *N Engl J Med.* 2007;357:266-281.

A prospective study of the associations between 25-hydroxy-vitamin D, sarcopenia progression and physical activity in older adults
Scott D, Blizzard L, Fell J, et al (Univ of Tasmania, Hobart, Australia; Univ of Tasmania, Launceston, Australia)
Clin Endocrinol 73:581-587, 2010

Objective.—Low 25-hydroxyvitamin D (25OHD) levels may be associated with both sarcopenia (the age-related decline in muscle mass and function) and low physical activity (PA). Our objective was to describe prospective associations between 25OHD, muscle parameters, and PA in community-dwelling older adults.

Design.—Prospective, population-based study with a mean follow-up of 2·6 ± 0·4 years.

Patients.—Six hundred and eighty-six community-dwelling older adults (49% women; mean ± SD 62 ± 7 years old).

Measurements.—Appendicular lean mass percentage (%ALM) and body fat assessed by Dual-energy X-ray Absorptiometry, leg strength by dynamometer, leg muscle quality (LMQ), PA assessed by pedometer, self-reported sun exposure by questionnaire, and serum 25OHD measured by radioimmunoassay.

Results.—Participants with 25OHD ≤ 50 nM had lower mean %ALM, leg strength, LMQ and PA (all $P < 0.05$). As a continuous function, baseline 25OHD was a positive independent predictor of change in leg strength ($\beta = 5 \cdot 74$ kg, 95% CI $0 \cdot 65$, $10 \cdot 82$) and LMQ ($\beta = 0 \cdot 49$ kg/kg, 95% CI $0 \cdot 17$, $0 \cdot 82$). Also, change in 25OHD was positively predicted by baseline %ALM ($\beta = 2 \cdot 03$ pM/p.a., 95% CI $0 \cdot 44$, $3 \cdot 62$) leg strength ($\beta = 0 \cdot 30$ pM/p.a., 95% CI 0.06, $0 \cdot 53$), LMQ ($\beta = 4 \cdot 48$ pM/p.a., 95% CI $0 \cdot 36$, $8 \cdot 61$) and PA ($\beta = 2 \cdot 63$ pM/p.a., 95% CI $0 \cdot 35$, $4 \cdot 92$) after adjustment for sun exposure and body fat.

Conclusions.—25OHD may be important for the maintenance of muscle function, and higher skeletal muscle mass and function as well as general PA levels may also be beneficial for 25OHD status, in community-dwelling older adults.

▶ This prospective study of community-dwelling older adults demonstrated that higher 25-hydroxyvitamin D (25OHD) has a modest linkage with greater muscle mass and strength. Skeletal muscle parameters and physical activity predicted higher 25OHD levels, supporting an influence on the absorption, synthesis, or metabolism of vitamin D. Potential mechanisms by which 25OHD may benefit muscle function in older adults include the activation of the skeletal muscle vitamin D receptor (VDR) leading to protein synthesis and muscle cell growth.[1] Skeletal muscle VDR expression decreases with age, and this may partially explain age-related sarcopenia. Also, vitamin D supplementation is associated with decreases in inflammatory cytokines, another sarcopenia-related pathway. Limited evidence suggests that physical activity and skeletal muscle hypertrophy may be a source of vitamin D separate from exposure to sunlight.[2,3] Outdoor physical activity improves 25OHD status in older adults, but even indoor muscle-building programs improve 25OHD levels.[2] In general, age-related sarcopenia and disability can be partially countered by multiple interventions, including resistance training, physical activity, and improvements in 25OHD levels.

D. C. Nieman, DrPH

References

1. Bischoff-Ferrari HA, Borchers M, Gudat F, Dürmüller U, Stähelin HB, Dick W. Vitamin D receptor expression in human muscle tissue decreases with age. *J Bone Miner Res.* 2004;19:265-269.
2. Annweiler C, Schott AM, Berrut G, Fantino B, Beauchet O. Vitamin D related changes in physical performance: a systematic review. *J Nutr Health Aging.* 2009;13:893-898.
3. Visser M, Deeg DJ, Lips P. Low vitamin D and high parathyroid hormone levels as determinants of loss of muscle strength and muscle mass (sarcopenia): the Longitudinal Aging Study Amsterdam. *J Clin Endocrinol Metab.* 2003;88:5766-5772.

Article Index

Chapter 1: Epidemiology, Prevention of Injuries, Lesions of Head and Neck

Chapter 2: Other Musculoskeletal Injuries

Chapter 3: Biomechanics, Muscle Strength and Training

Chapter 4: Physical Activity, Cardiorespiratory Physiology and Immune Function

Chapter 5: Metabolism and Obesity, Nutrition and Doping

Chapter 6: Cardiorespiratory Disorders

Chapter 7: Other Medical Problems

Chapter 8: Environmental Factors

Chapter 9: Special Considerations: Children, Women, the Elderly, and Special Populations

Author Index

Printed and bound by CPI Group (UK) Ltd, Croydon, CR0 4YY

08/05/2025

01864678-0014